Gatekeeping in the Mental Health Professions

edited by
Alicia M. Homrich
Kathryn L. Henderson

American Counseling Association

6101 Stevenson Avenue, Suite 600 | Alexandria, VA 22304 | www.counseling.org

Gatekeeping in the Mental Health Professions

American Counseling Association
6101 Stevenson Avenue, Suite 600 | Alexandria, VA 22304

Associate Publisher | Carolyn C. Baker

Senior Production Manager | Bonny E. Gaston

Digital and Print Development Editor | Nancy Driver

Copy Editor | Beth Ciha

Cover and text design by Bonny E. Gaston

Library of Congress Cataloging-in-Publication Data

Names: Homrich, Alicia M., editor. | Henderson, Kathryn L., editor. | American Counseling Association, issuing body.
Title: Gatekeeping in the mental health professions / Alicia M. Homrich, Kathryn L. Henderson, editors.
Description: Alexandria, VA : American Counseling Association, [2018] | Includes bibliographical references and index.
Identifiers: LCCN 2018007027 | ISBN 9781556203282 (pbk. : alk. paper)
Subjects: | MESH: Counseling—education | Mentoring—methods | Mental Health Services—standards | Clinical Competence—standards | United States
Classification: LCC RC466 | NLM WM 18 | DDC 362.2/04256—dc23 LC record available at https://lccn.loc.gov/2018007027

To mentors, who we often want to be when we become professionals, and the careers they model of integrity and compassion, who do the hard work with the students who need it the most.

—KLH

• • •

To clinical faculty and supervisors, the frontline gatekeepers for our respective professions, for your courage and commitment to developing future ethical, effective clinical professionals and redirecting those who are unable to attain expected standards. Thank you for protecting the quality of the mental health community and those who seek our expertise to pursue their fullest potential.

—AMH

Table of Contents

Preface

The term *gatekeeper* is a metaphor for those who monitor or oversee the progress of others while simultaneously controlling admission or access to an entity. In the context of career preparation programs, the gatekeeper is an experienced member of a profession who oversees the academic and clinical development of individuals preparing to enter the field while upholding professional standards for the welfare of future clients. Allowing qualified individuals to successfully progress through training and pass through "gates," such as graduation and licensure, implies that those individuals have met minimal clinical training standards.

Gatekeeping is the inherent responsibility of educators and supervisors in the mental health professions. Jurisdictional regulatory and licensing boards, accrediting bodies, and professional associations mandate gatekeeping in laws, rules, standards, and ethics codes. The health professions are increasingly being held accountable for developing standards and enacting practices that fulfill quality assurance expectations that protect the public and safeguard clients. The effects of *gateslipping* can be life threatening and/or result in long-term psychological injury. Passing unqualified students for graduation or endorsing incapable supervisees for licensure endangers the welfare of others. Ignoring gatekeeping mandates risks harming a trainee or other colleagues who may be affected by his or her actions, compromises the integrity of the clinical professions, and diminishes the trustworthiness and reputation of mental health training programs and related agencies. Gatekeeping is also a very challenging professional responsibility. The literatures in each of the allied professions—counseling, social work, psychology, and marriage and family therapy—reflect the challenges of the gatekeeper's role.

The goal of this book is to support faculty and supervisors to engage effectively in the tasks and challenges of the gatekeeping process. The book has been written with the intention of bringing together the developing body of professional performance standards for trainees from multiple behavioral health fields. It is accompanied by suggested standards for best practices across the myriad gatekeeping tasks and processes. This book aims to be a guidebook for clinical faculty and supervisors that supports the development of gatekeeping practices and policies found in the current literature. This volume can also be useful in training new supervisors and doctoral students preparing to assume the role of gatekeeper. The philosophical foundations supporting gatekeeping are examined, along with suggestions for best practices and tools and templates that can be used with trainees.

A trainee's fitness in the domains of academic and clinical ability can be readily established through the use of evaluative measures that assess commonly held standards for performance. However, evaluating trainee competency in the domains of interpersonal behavior, intrapersonal functioning, and professional conduct to determine readiness to practice is much more subjective. This critical domain of trainee development—the heart of the gatekeeping focus—is less clearly defined and lacks common agreement within and across the mental health professions; thus, it is typically the area of greatest concern for clinical educators and supervisors.

Chapters in this book discuss the following topics addressing gatekeeping in terms of the professional conduct and personal behavior of students and supervisees.

Chapter 1 provides an introduction to gatekeeping by reviewing the foundational principles that guide gatekeeping practices. It begins the discussion of ethical principles and legal concepts pertinent to gatekeeping that are woven throughout the book as they pertain to various practices or stages of the process.

Chapter 2 defines the lexicon that is specifically relevant to the practice of gatekeeping, offering a compilation and background review of key terminology. Professional terminology is introduced that should be avoided, along with the background or history of the word usage and current recommended language for practice. General legal perspectives, such as due process and liability, are applied to the practice of gatekeeping, in addition to vocabulary and definitions found in other guiding documents in the clinical professions.

The challenge of addressing problematic trainees, a concern of every faculty member and supervisor, is the focus of Chapter 3. The author of this chapter proposes the development of policies, systems, and strategies for assisting students and supervisees who are exhibiting problematic behavior in their developmental process as clinical professionals.

Recognizing that training is a developmental process and that all trainees have unique personal identities, Chapter 4 encourages gatekeepers to be sensitive to and respectful of the broader contextual factors that may overlay trainee functioning. This chapter represents one of the inherent tensions in gatekeeping: upholding professional standards and the duty to protect future clients while simultaneously being sensitive to trainees' developmental processes and caring for their individual experiences and differences.

Chapter 5 offers descriptions of the roles and responsibilities faculty and supervisors have in gatekeeping activities as defined by professional standards. This chapter considers the various mandates for training practitioners, including licensure laws, accreditation standards, and codes of ethics from the mental health professions.

An important aspect of efficacious gatekeeping is garnering active support and participation from multiple constituencies. Chapter 6 describes the multiple institutional influences that interact to support or hinder the gatekeeping process. This chapter identifies potential stakeholders and suggests methods of collaboration essential to successful gatekeeping.

How does a clinical program or agency site inform students and supervisees about expectations for personal behavior and professional conduct? Chapter 7 identifies procedures for clearly advising prospective trainees about graduate program or agency expectations, standards, and gatekeeping policies at various points of contact, starting with admissions.

Chapter 8 reviews the literature from the mental health professions about trainee problems of professional competency. Empirical research on the personal behavior and professional conduct of trainees is reviewed in order to assist programs in constructing their own set of expectations and standards for trainee performance.

Once programs identify expectations or standards for trainee behavior, they must undertake the process of evaluating the meeting of those behavioral standards. Chapter 9 suggests methods for assessing and evaluating trainee conduct and behavior and offers a review of formal measures currently available in the field.

Chapter 10 describes best practices for intervening when trainees demonstrate problems with professional competency. In some situations, trainees may struggle with change, may be incapable of meeting required standards of behavior and conduct, or may be unwilling to comply with standards. A range of possible strategies and interventions is offered in this chapter, including formal remediation plans and accompanying remedial interventions.

Throughout the gatekeeping process, documentation is critical for legal and ethical reasons. Chapter 11 suggests best practice procedures in documenting, such as verifying that published procedures were followed, documenting subsequent actions taken, and verifying trainee actions and reactions. Examples of documentation formats are illustrated in this chapter.

Avoiding the need to engage in gatekeeping processes, the situation preferred by most professors and supervisors, can lie in prevention efforts. Chapter 12 offers strategies for preempting the development of problematic behavior in trainees and for curtailing problems through education, relationship building, and other early intervention approaches, including the admissions process.

The appendices offer a detailed review of ethics codes from several professions that directly address gatekeeping functions. Sample documentation and forms that may be adapted for use in practice are also included for readers of this book. These include sample correspondence and examples of evaluation and prevention strategies.

In sum, this book aims to be a practical resource to assist educators and supervisors in the practice of gatekeeping and to give doctoral students and future supervisors a foundational understanding of the gatekeeping process. As a fundamental responsibility of faculty and supervisors, gatekeeping represents an ethical imperative to address the struggles and challenges trainees may experience in their development, which could lead to harming clients. The ethical mandate speaks not only to protecting the clinical professions and the public from harm but also to providing trainees with transparent feedback regarding their competence and their likelihood of success as professional clinicians. During their time of struggle and challenge, effective feedback and remedial support from gatekeepers can offer trainees an opportunity, should they choose to accept it, to achieve success and develop into competent, ethical, and professionally effective clinicians.

About the Editors

Alicia M. Homrich, PhD, is a professor in the Graduate Studies in Counseling program (accredited by the Council for Accreditation of Counseling and Related Educational Programs) at Rollins College in Winter Park, Florida. She is a licensed psychologist and licensed marriage and family therapist in the State of Florida, a national certified counselor, and a qualified supervisor. Dr. Homrich has been researching, publishing, and presenting on the topic of gatekeeping for more than 15 years. Her goals for publishing this book are to encourage faculty and supervisors to support optimal clinical trainee development by engaging in gatekeeping processes during pre- and postgraduate training, to safeguard clients, and to uphold the practice standards of the clinical professions.

• • •

Kathryn L. Henderson, PhD, is an assistant professor in the Department of Counseling and Applied Behavioral Studies at the University of Saint Joseph (accredited by the Council for Accreditation of Counseling and Related Educational Programs) in West Hartford, Connecticut. Dr. Henderson is a licensed professional counselor in Texas and a national certified counselor. Dr. Henderson has researched, published, and presented on student remediation and gatekeeping for more than 8 years. She is an advocate of early intervention and transparency in the gatekeeping process and views counselor self-care and wellness as cornerstones of ethical practice.

About the Contributors

Kyle D. Baldwin, EdD, is the clinical practice and assessment coordinator and a clinical professor of counseling in the Graduate Studies in Counseling program (accredited by the Council for Accreditation of Counseling and Related Educational Programs) at Rollins College in Winter Park, Florida. She is a licensed mental health counselor, national certified counselor, master addictions counselor, certified clinical mental health counselor, clinical sexologist, and qualified supervisor. Dr. Baldwin's research interests include counselor wellness and counselor education and supervision.

Theresa A. Coogan, PhD, is a counselor educator and educational consultant in Raleigh, North Carolina. She is a licensed/certified school counselor in Massachusetts and New York, a national certified school counselor, and national certified counselor. Dr. Coogan has worked as a counselor educator and program director for school counselor training for 10 years. She recently started an educational consulting business serving kindergarten–Grade 12 and higher education clients providing professional and curriculum development as well as program evaluation, gatekeeping, and accreditation compliance.

Leigh D. DeLorenzi, PhD, is an assistant professor in the Graduate Studies in Counseling program (accredited by the Council for Accreditation of Counseling and Related Educational Programs) at Rollins College in Winter Park, Florida, and a licensed mental health counselor in the State of Florida. Dr. DeLorenzi began researching and writing on the professional, interpersonal, and intrapersonal conduct behaviors of helping professionals in 2013. She has developed and implemented gatekeeping-focused assessment systems for graduate programs to streamline and simplify the gatekeeping process from preadmission to graduation.

Roxane L. Dufrene, PhD, is an associate professor in the Counselor Education Program at the University of New Orleans (accredited by the Council for Accreditation of Counseling and Related Educational Programs) in Louisiana. She is a licensed professional counselor and licensed marriage and family therapist in the State of Louisiana as well as a national certified counselor. Dr. Dufrene has been researching and presenting on the topic of remediation for more than 10 years.

Page L. Thanasiu, PhD, is an assistant professor of counselor education at Stetson University (accredited by the Council for Accreditation of Counseling and Related Educational Programs) in DeLand, Florida. She is a licensed mental health counselor and qualified supervisor in the State of Florida. At the national level, she is credentialed as a registered play therapist supervisor and a national certified counselor. Dr. Thanasiu has been supporting master's-level students through remediation and gatekeeping processes for the past 10 years and truly appreciates the opportunity to join trainees on their developmental journey.

Acknowledgments

A special thanks to Dr. Burt Bertram, who has been a longtime advocate and supporter for this project. Without his encouragement and professional mentorship, this book would not have been written.

We would also like to acknowledge the work of Michelle Sullivan, a graduate assistant at Rollins College, who offered invaluable support as an early copy editor and research assistant. A huge thank-you for your help with this project!

Chapter 1

Introduction to Gatekeeping

Alicia M. Homrich

The term *gatekeeping* is thought to have first originated in the arena of communications wherein an editor or editorial board determined which information or news stories would be pursued and which would be shelved (Kerl & Eichler, 2005). Gatekeeping was a point of control that advanced or deterred progression through the publication process. This activity is akin to the credentialing process, through which an individual prepares for and applies for entry into a profession, documenting satisfactory achievement of the requisite training in knowledge and skills and the professional qualities necessary to be recognized as a full practitioner. In all cases, approval of an individual to enter a profession is sanctioned by appointed senior practitioners with professional experience and the credentials to make such a determination. Within the context of the allied mental health professions, multiple scholars have defined the term *gatekeeping* as the ongoing responsibility of faculty members and clinical supervisors to monitor trainee progress and appropriateness to enter professional practice.

The Purposes of Gatekeeping

The two primary purposes of gatekeeping are to protect the integrity of the clinical professions and to prevent harm to clientele receiving services from incompetent clinicians (Brear, Dorrian, & Luscri, 2008). A secondary goal of gatekeeping is to consider the best interests of others, be it the trainee, the training community, the clinical or educational setting, or the population at large (Brear & Dorrian, 2010). Bodner (2012) noted that an additional responsibility of gatekeeping is to uphold professional standards, including the principles of beneficence, nonmaleficence, fidelity, personal dignity, and justice, as described in most ethics codes of the clinical professions.

The charge to the professions' gatekeepers is to enforce gatekeeping policies and procedures in order to reduce the incidence of advancing poorly or marginally suited trainees through graduate training and onto licensure in a clinical profession without intervention. This phenomenon was defined by Gaubatz and Vera (2002) as *gateslipping*. They found that clinical training programs that implemented formalized gatekeeping practices "reduce the number of deficient students who slip through programs' gates (i.e., graduate without remedial attention)" (p. 296). Thoughtful gatekeeping practices protect the public and the clinical professions from inept practitioners.

The Role of the Gatekeeper

Gatekeepers are the persons responsible for ethically monitoring trainees' progression through gatekeeping checkpoints prior to endorsing them for independent professional practice. In the clinical professions, educators and supervisors serve in this role both before and after trainees receive a degree. Gatekeeping is one responsibility expected of supervisors and/or faculty members who have oversight of trainees. Gatekeeping is an aspect of the assessment and evaluation processes incumbent on every supervisor and professor who has a role in preparing future clinicians. Gizara and Forrest (2004) described gatekeepers as quality control agents for the clinical training experience because they determine the readiness and fit of candidates for their particular profession. Gatekeepers institute evaluative procedures, deliver feedback aimed at improvement, provide trainees with the opportunity to respond to and address concerns, and take responsibility for deciding whether and when to permit trainees to continue to the next phase of the training process or to stop their progression for the purpose of remediating behaviors of concern (Gaubatz & Vera, 2002; Ziomek-Daigle & Christensen, 2010). Gatekeepers act to "ensure that those who graduate are capable of interacting with clients, colleagues, and the community in an ethical and competent manner" (J. Miller & Koerin, 2002, p. 1) and "control the access of impaired, unethical or incompetent counselors to clients, thereby protecting clients who are likely to be at a highly vulnerable stage of their lives" (Bhat, 2005, p. 399). The trainee's ability and/or willingness to achieve the requisite competencies of a given clinical profession predicts his or her progression through the various gatekeeping checkpoints across the training process (see Figure 1.1).

Most educators and supervisors in clinical programs are energized by the prospect of training individuals to become competent, ethically

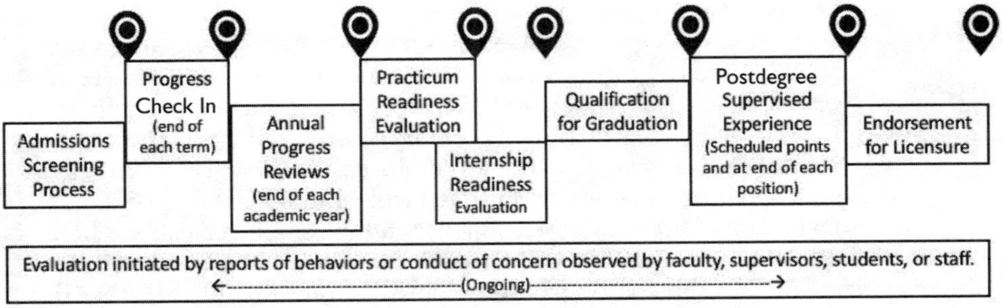

Figure 1.1 • Gatekeeping Checkpoints

Use these points for evaluating personal behavior and professional conduct to determine continuation of clinical training.

practicing professionals. This enthusiasm and commitment applies to training programs across the behavioral health fields, including the professions of mental health counseling; marriage and family therapy; psychology; social work; and specialized practice fields such as school counseling, school psychology, rehabilitation counseling, or neuropsychology. Whether professors in academic programs, faculty supervising students in practicum or internship courses, field site clinicians engaged in supervisory experiences with graduate students, or supervisors of postdegree trainees obtaining experience in fulfillment of licensure requirements, clinical trainers have one thing in common: the opportunity to influence the development of clinical knowledge, skills, and professionalism in novice members of the profession. In legal terms, this role is known as the respondeat superior (see On the Legal Side 1.1): the professional responsible for the actions of trainees (Wheeler & Bertram, 2015).

Inherent in the position of respondeat superior are multiple professional obligations. According to Saccuzzo (1997), these duties include monitoring the training and supervisory processes to:

1. protect the welfare of current and future clients (patients) from harm by ensuring that they receive effective treatment, that their rights are protected, and that they are treated with dignity and respect;
2. protect the welfare of the student or supervisee;
3. protect the well-being of other trainees or colleagues who may be affected by the individual student or supervisee;
4. protect the integrity of the clinical professions by graduating and endorsing for licensure only those practitioners who demonstrate the competencies necessary to be effective practitioners; and
5. protect the trustworthiness and reputation of the program, institution, or agency (although not a direct duty of respondeat superiors, this secondary influence is often the concern of administrators and other affiliates of the institution, such as alumni).

On the Legal Side 1.1

A Latin term, *respondeat superior* means "let the master answer or respond." This legal doctrine holds that a person such as an employer or a supervisor is legally responsible for the wrongful acts of those over which he or she has charge, such as an employee or supervisee. Essentially, when the respondeat superior premise is invoked in a legal proceeding, a plaintiff will look to hold both the employer and the employee liable. There is no national standard for respondeat superiors. Because states create their own standards for the doctrine, different jurisdictions use different tests to prove the responsibility of the respondeat superior (Cornell Law School Legal Information Institute, 2017). Clinical supervisors of predegree and prelicensed counselors can be identified as respondeat superiors, which means that they can be held legally responsible for the actions of their supervisees (Saccuzzo, 1997; Wheeler & Bertram, 2015).

These responsibilities also converge to inform the direction of activities and procedures known as gatekeeping.

The Process of Gatekeeping

Clinical trainees are expected to progress through a series of gates or checkpoints, as illustrated in Figure 1.1, that are carefully placed across the training experience to substantiate attainment or demonstration of competencies in three domains: acquired knowledge, execution of clinical skill, and demonstration of personal behaviors or professional conduct appropriate for a practicing clinician. Fundamental to this process are the procedures of monitoring and evaluating trainee development to ascertain whether expected levels of performance have been achieved to support continued advancement toward graduation, licensure, and eventual independent professional practice (Brear et al., 2008; Council for Accreditation of Counseling and Related Educational Programs [CACREP], 2015). The process of gatekeeping also incorporates engagement in activities that support trainee development or remedy stalled progress. Gatekeeping may also involve stopping a trainee from graduating or gaining licensure in his or her chosen profession (Koerin & Miller, 1995) because of an inability or lack of willingness to meet standards or professional expectations. Multiple processes are involved in gatekeeping and are the topics featured in this book.

The Mandate for Gatekeeping

All clinical professions reference the obligation of preventing inept practitioners from entering into the profession primarily to protect clients from harm. This mandate is identified by multiple governing bodies within each professional group and extends to all members of the profession. In the realm of preprofessional preparation, the gatekeeping obligation is typically fulfilled by clinical faculty and supervisors serving as respondeat superiors accountable for overseeing the training process and trainees. The responsibilities of gatekeeping include monitoring, evaluating, and determining which trainees can appropriately enter the given profession while remediating or stopping those who cannot. Where and how this mandate is explained or defined across the clinical professions varies.

Professional Associations' Codes of Ethics

General expectations for gatekeeping are addressed in the ethics codes of the four primary clinical professions: the American Counseling Association (ACA), American Psychological Association (APA), National Association of Social Workers (NASW), and American Association for Marriage and Family Therapy (AAMFT).

Above all, professional ethics uphold the standards of beneficence and nonmaleficence: striving to do no harm and protect the rights and welfare of those with whom counselors and therapists interact, especially clients. Standards in professional ethics also identify some criteria for professional demeanor and behavior for members of their respective organizations beyond the competencies of having the knowledge and skills to practice effectively. Most ethical standards delineate or infer that students and supervisees will adhere to the same ideals as professional members. Chapter 7 provides examples of these expectations.

The general tenets of ethics codes stipulate the role of the gatekeeper for members who are educators or supervisors; however, the amount of detail varies considerably across the four major mental health professions. For example, the APA *Ethical Principles of Psychologists and Code of Conduct* (APA, 2017c) states in Standard 7.04(2) that psychologists do not disclose personal information about trainees except when

> the information is necessary to evaluate or obtain assistance for students whose personal problems could reasonably be judged to be preventing them from performing their training- or professionally related activities in a competent manner or posing a threat to the students or others.

Other APA standards address timely assessment and feedback processes; however, they do not specifically address the role or responsibility of respondeat superiors in training positions to protect clients or the profession from inappropriate trainees via the gatekeeping process. Bodner (2012) extrapolated the ethical principles that she believed apply to gatekeeping practices in psychology.

The *NASW Code of Ethics* (NASW, 2017) details the obligation of social workers to address their own impairment or the impaired, incompetent, or unethical conduct of colleagues—as do all clinical professions' ethics codes; however, the ethical standards are very vague in reference to trainees and include only that "social workers who function as educators or field instructors for students should evaluate students' performance in a manner that is fair and respectful" (Standard 3.02[b]). Descriptions of "fair and respectful" are undefined and left to the assumptions of the members.

The 2015 revision of AAMFT's *Code of Ethics* (AAMFT, 2015) reveals standards that are similarly ambiguous when describing the role and expectations of gatekeepers. Standard 4.4 reads: "Oversight of Supervisee Competence. Marriage and family therapists do not permit students or supervisees to perform or to hold themselves out as competent to perform professional services beyond their training, level of experience, and competence." This standard is generally known as the scope of practice clause and is included in every ethics code as a principle that applies to all practicing professionals. Standard 4.5 reads: "Oversight of Supervisee Professionalism. Marriage and family therapists take reasonable measures to ensure that services provided by supervisees are professional." This standard does not offer an explanation or definition of behaviors that qualify as "professional," which could be interpreted broadly in a gatekeeping proceeding.

The *ACA Code of Ethics* (ACA, 2014a) offers the most comprehensive ethical guidelines for supervisors and educators engaged in training by describing key components of the gatekeeping process, including monitoring, evaluating, protecting clients, and determining continuation in the profession. This code is unique in specifying that trainees are obligated to follow the *ACA Code of Ethics* and includes an entire section of standards that support gatekeepers by defining expectations for professional behavior:

> **Section F: Supervision, Training, and Teaching**
>
> **F.1. Counselor Supervision and Client Welfare**
>
> **F.1.a. Client Welfare** A primary obligation of counseling supervisors is to monitor the services provided by supervisees. Counseling supervisors monitor client welfare and supervisee performance and professional development. To fulfill these obligations, supervisors meet regularly with supervisees to review the supervisees' work and help them become prepared to serve a range of diverse clients. Supervisees have a responsibility to understand and follow the *ACA Code of Ethics.*
>
> **F.4. Supervisor Responsibilities**
>
> **F.4.a. Informed Consent for Supervision** Supervisors are responsible for incorporating into their supervision the principles of informed consent and participation. Supervisors inform supervisees of the policies and procedures to which supervisors are to adhere and the mechanisms for due process appeal of individual supervisor actions. The issues unique to the use of distance supervision are to be included in the documentation as necessary.
>
> **F.5. Student and Supervisee Responsibilities**
>
> **F.5.a. Ethical Responsibilities** Students and supervisees have a responsibility to understand and follow the *ACA Code of Ethics.* Students and supervisees have the same obligation to clients as those required of professional counselors.

F.6. Counseling Supervision Evaluation, Remediation, and Endorsement

F.6.a. Evaluation Supervisors document and provide supervisees with ongoing feedback regarding their performance and schedule periodic formal evaluative sessions throughout the supervisory relationship.

F.6.b. Gatekeeping and Remediation Through initial and ongoing evaluation, supervisors are aware of supervisee limitations that might impede performance. Supervisors assist supervisees in securing remedial assistance when needed. They recommend dismissal from training programs, applied counseling settings, and state or voluntary professional credentialing processes when those supervisees are unable to demonstrate that they can provide competent professional services to a range of diverse clients. Supervisors seek consultation and document their decisions to dismiss or refer supervisees for assistance. They ensure that supervisees are aware of options available to them to address such decisions.

F.8. Student Welfare

F.8.d. Addressing Personal Concerns Counselor educators may require students to address any personal concerns that have the potential to affect professional competency.

F.9. Evaluation and Remediation

F.9.a. Evaluation of Students Counselor educators clearly state to students, prior to and throughout the training program, the levels of competency expected, appraisal methods, and timing of evaluations for both didactic and clinical competencies. Counselor educators provide students with ongoing feedback regarding their performance throughout the training program.

F.9.b. Limitations Counselor educators, through ongoing evaluation, are aware of and address the inability of some students to achieve counseling competencies. Counselor educators do the following:

1. assist students in securing remedial assistance when needed,
2. seek professional consultation and document their decision to dismiss or refer students for assistance, and
3. ensure that students have recourse in a timely manner to address decisions requiring them to seek assistance or to dismiss them and provide students with due process according to institutional policies and procedures. (pp. 12–15)

The *ACA Code of Ethics* is much more specific and helpful in providing guidance to faculty and supervisors than most codes across the clinical professions, as illustrated above. Appendix A provides excerpts from ethics codes that guide gatekeeping processes in additional professional specialties: the *ASCA Ethical Standards for School Counselors* (American School Counselor Association, 2016), the *AMHCA Code of Ethics* (American Mental Health Counselors Association [AMHCA], 2015), and the *Code of Professional Ethics for Rehabilitation Counselors* (Commission on Rehabilitation Counselor Certification, 2017).

A general limitation of ethics codes with regard to gatekeeping is their lack of specificity, which is typically considered to be acceptable because ethics codes are intended to be aspirational standards applicable to multiple contexts. Although considered foundational descriptions for ideal professional functioning, codes of ethics are only enforceable among members of the particular professional association who have agreed to abide by the code as a condition of membership. Nevertheless, codes of ethics are considered to reflect standards for best practice and have at times been relied on in court cases and licensure board hearings to define expectations for practicing clinicians, even if the individuals appearing in those proceedings are not members of their professional group. Also, some state licensure laws reference the ethics code of a given profession as the legal standard for practice. APA, for example, proposed a model state licensure act in 2010 that included adoption of its ethics code as the standard for conduct for psychologists (APA, 2011). Similarly, of the 52 jurisdictions that license mental health counselors, 19 have adopted the *ACA Code of Ethics* as the standard for ethical practice and professional conduct (ACA, 2014b), and other states have adopted the *AMHCA Code of Ethics* (AMHCA, 2015) as the benchmark criteria for licensees' practice.

As demonstrated by the differences among the ethics codes of the mental health professions, there is significant disparity, which contributes to the confusion of identifying expected actions of the gatekeeper. Only the counseling profession addresses this role in detail in its ethics code, which provides guidelines for easy reference. The directives for other professional groups are inconsistent and not necessarily identified elsewhere in the standards of those particular professions.

Accrediting Bodies for Training Programs

Professional accrediting bodies such as the Commission on Accreditation for Marriage and Family Therapy Education, CACREP, APA's Commission on Accreditation, and the Council on Social Work Education (CSWE) accreditation program also define specific academic standards for clinical training programs. The role of accrediting bodies is important in clinical education because the process of accreditation

> assures the educational community and the general public that an institution or a program has clearly defined and appropriate objectives and maintains conditions under which their achievement can reasonably be expected. . . . through the development of principles and guidelines for assessing educational effectiveness. (APA, 2017a, para. 1)

Although not all training programs are professionally accredited, the highest standards for training are influential in defining the ideals of academic gatekeeping as well as licensing. In the domain of gatekeeping, there is variation across these major accrediting bodies in terms of defining and specifying processes required of accredited programs to ensure the protection of clients and the profession. Along with codes of ethics, program accreditation standards for the professions of counseling and psychology offer the most specificity and guidance for the gatekeeping mandate in clinical training programs.

In counselor education, CACREP (2015) establishes the standards for training for accredited counseling programs. Of the four accrediting bodies named previously, CACREP's standards are the only ones that designate and define the gatekeeping process as a function of clinical training:

> Gatekeeping [is] the ethical responsibility of counselor educators and supervisors to monitor and evaluate an individual's knowledge, skills, and professional dispositions required by competent professional counselors and to remediate or prevent those that are lacking in professional competence from becoming counselors. (p. 45)

The CACREP standards for accreditation also offer a related definition for this particular area of student functioning: "Professional dispositions [are] the commitments, characteristics, values, beliefs, interpersonal functioning, and behaviors that influence the counselor's professional growth and interactions with clients and colleagues" (p. 47). This definition is less explicit than that of gatekeeping but offers the importance of personal and professional functioning as a critical factor in student development worthy of evaluation, feedback, remediation, and, if found to be problematic and unchangeable, dismissal from the training program.

The APA Commission on Accreditation (2015) mentions policies and procedures that provide for student performance evaluation, feedback, advisement, retention, and termination decisions and for due process and grievance procedures for students. The APA Commission on Accreditation also designates that newly admitted students receive written policies and procedures regarding program and institution requirements and expectations regarding students' performance and continuance in the program and procedures for terminating students. Another foundational gatekeeping practice is also addressed by this accrediting body:

> Feedback and Remediation. Students receive, at least annually and as the need is observed for it, written feedback on the extent to which they are meeting the program's requirements and performance expectations. Such feedback should include:
>
> a. timely, written notification of any problems that have been noted and the opportunity to discuss them;
> b. guidance regarding steps to remediate any problems (if remediable);
> c. substantive, written feedback on the extent to which corrective actions have or have not been successful in addressing the issues of concern. (Standard III.C.3.)

Psychology trainees are also expected to conduct professional activities with respect and sensitivity for human and cultural diversity; maintain professional conduct, including self-reflection and responsiveness to feedback and supervision; and fulfill expectations for the communication and interpersonal skills of students and interns. These are some of the characteristics of trainees that align with the interpersonal, intrapersonal, and professional standards considered in gatekeeping efforts. To support faculty and supervisors in their training role, APA (2012) has published a website of resources that includes *A Practical Guidebook for the Competency Benchmarks.* This document and the accompanying website offer a toolkit of resources and guidance for evaluating trainees, communicating feedback, and remediating professionalism and related competencies.

NASW's CSWE, the program accreditation body for training in social work, includes as its first competency the expectation for trainees to demonstrate ethical and professional behavior. Although limited in definition, the accreditation standards (CSWE Commission on Accreditation, 2015) also identify the requirement for students (a) to demonstrate their abilities to use self-awareness, self-reflection, and self-regulation to manage personal values and maintain professionalism in practice situations; and (b) to demonstrate professional demeanor in their behavior, appearance, and communication. The CSWE standards also prescribe a process for student development that includes evaluating students' professional performance, informing students of policies and criteria for evaluation, and terminating students from training programs for problems with professional performance. Designated faculty and field personnel are expected to oversee organized procedures for the ongoing assessment of student outcomes according to this accrediting body.

The Commission on Accreditation for Marriage and Family Therapy Education (2017) accreditation standards call for the evaluation of student performance but do not address the processes or criteria for evaluation in graduate training programs. The standards also reference a code of conduct but do not require programs to have one. The definition in the glossary is "Codes of Conduct are shared statements regarding a commitment to ethical, legal and professional beliefs, values, and behavior that serve as foundational standards for making decisions and taking actions" (p. 44). AAMFT-approved supervisor training standards (AAMFT, 2014) discuss the provision of supervision in significant detail and provide instruction on the processes for evaluating supervisees; managing difficulties in supervision, including remediation; and, when necessary, advising family therapy trainees out of the profession. However, not all faculty in family and relationship therapy programs are required to be approved supervisors, so they may not have training on these best practices.

State Regulatory Boards

Saccuzzo (1997) noted a similar dilemma across the regulations of state licensure boards, observing that licensure laws are vague in delineating the specific criteria for supervision and often fail to define standards for who is qualified to provide supervision in the clinical professions. One reason for this is that the majority of training and supervision occurs during the predegree period. Licensure boards establish minimal requirements for coursework in content areas and the quantity of supervised experience prior to graduation, with some offering more specific direction than others; however, state-level licensing bodies generally do not legislate detailed requirements within the academic realm. Licensure laws designate only the entry requirements of licensure applicants (e.g., the type and level of degree: master's or doctorate), single line descriptions of required courses, and slightly more detail about the conditions of practicum experiences. For specific information about individual state licensure requirements, access the following directories of regulatory boards:

- Counseling (https://www.counseling.org/knowledge-center/licensure-requirements/state-professional-counselor-licensure-boards)
- Psychology (www.asppb.net/?page=BdContactNewPG)
- Marriage and family therapy (https://www.aamft.org/iMIS15/AAMFT/Content/directories/MFT_licensing_boards.aspx)
- Social work (http://aswbsocialworkregulations.org/licensingWebsitesReportBuilder.jsp)

Regulatory boards are responsible for defining postdegree, prelicensure experience requirements in greater detail, including the gatekeeping responsibilities of postdegree clinical supervisors for monitoring, evaluating, and screening for problematic trainees to determine which applicants can appropriately enter the given profession. Like ethics codes, laws and rules for the same license vary across states and may differ across the four allied clinical professions within a state. The absence of detail regarding the process by which supervisors determine endorsement for licensure typically boils down to checking a box on a form as the final gate checkpoint affirming that a supervisee is or is not considered to be in good standing or has or has not met the minimum standards of performance in professional activities as measured against general prevailing peer performance, or similar wording that is ill defined and does not necessarily confirm whether any gatekeeping procedures occurred.

Some states require that postdegree supervisors complete minimal training requirements to become qualified or approved supervisors prior to supervising postdegree clinicians who are obtaining experience to meet licensure requirements. These states may offer or require supervision training workshops that include knowledge of supervisee assessment, understanding of jurisdictional expectations in terms of the amount and frequency of supervision, and expected content to be covered in supervisory meetings (such as a review of case files or recordings of sessions). State regulatory boards may also require licensed or certified supervisors to attend continuing education workshops on supervision at assigned intervals to maintain their status as supervisors of postdegree license seekers. Most state licensing bodies rely on standards of practice assumed to be known by the licensed supervisor through either predegree training or ethics education through his or her professional association.

It is recommended that both pre- and postdegree supervisors seek ongoing education, training, and consultation to enhance their skills as effective supervisors, which includes the role of gatekeeper. Seeking information and consultation is particularly helpful when determining whether to endorse a questionable trainee for continuation toward licensure. Professional associations, conferences, and the professional literature are sources for knowledge and collegial support for postdegree supervisors who hold membership in the given association. Some professional associations also have specialty divisions or interest groups for the study of clinical supervision, such as the Association for Counselor Education and Supervision (https://www.acesonline.net/), AAMFT's approved supervisor training program (https://dx5br1z4f6n0k.cloudfront.net/imis15/Documents/Approved_Supervisor_Handbook_2014.pdf), or APA's Clinical Supervision Essentials series of books and videos (www.apa.org/pubs/books/clinical-supervision.aspx).

Defining Competency

The health professions, including mental health, are increasingly being held accountable for practices that fulfill quality assurance expectations to protect the public or risk facing legal repercussions for improper supervision or training (Custer, 1994; Frame & Stevens-Smith, 1995; Hutchens, Block, & Young, 2013; Polychronis & Brown, 2016; Saccuzzo, 1997). Safeguarding clients from practitioners who do not meet minimal standards of professional competence is especially critical in the health professions because the consequences of poor practice can be life threatening and/or result in long-term psychological injury. For this reason, higher education has moved toward a competency-based approach to training that can be demonstrated through outcomes—the training of competent professionals (e.g., clinical mental health practitioners). (See sidebar, What Would You Do? 1.1.)

In 2002, APA initiated a multiyear effort and convened a task force to identify and gain consensus about essential competencies for clinical practice, define competencies as standards for training programs, and develop methodologies for evaluating competencies that fittingly define the profession of psychology (APA, 2006). No other clinical behavioral health profession has undertaken such a broad effort, although expectations and standards have been generated by the professional organizations of all clinical fields, such as training program accreditation standards, ethics codes, and a growing body of research and knowledge that includes competency assessment methods and models.

The task force identified specific competencies within three domains of training considered critical to the development of competent clinical practitioners:

1. Attainment of requisite *knowledge*, primarily through academic learning and clinical experience, that can be applied in a clinical setting
2. Acquisition of *clinical skills* based in empirical evidence as therapeutic, accompanied by the ability to apply those skills effectively and ethically as appropriate to the client situation or setting
3. The ability to develop and maintain *personal behavior and professional conduct* expected of clinicians in the practice of their profession

What Would You Do? 1.1

You work as a school counselor at a high school that hosts school counseling trainees from a local university. Your unit of four counselors works together as a team to supervise master's-level counseling interns in their last year of their graduate program. In other words, all four of you work together collectively supervising three school counseling interns. You notice that one of the students, Roy, is very engaged in the internship experience but spends a lot of time kidding with the high school students and giving advice instead of using counseling skills to understand their concerns and facilitate their personal development of problem solving. His relationship with the students is more social than clinical or professional, and the students view Roy as a buddy. You have a conversation with Roy about your concerns and the professional boundaries differentiating personal and professional relationships. He expresses understanding and appreciation for the feedback, but his interactions with the student clients do not change. You believe that he has some clinical skills but is not applying them and continues to be chummy with the teens with whom he works; thus, you are unable to assess his skill level and are concerned about his professionalism.

You express your concerns to the supervisory team. They acknowledge that they have also witnessed this behavior but seem less concerned. It is time for your team to complete Roy's midpoint evaluation. The other team members minimize your growing concerns about Roy's consistent avoidance of his professional role, failure to engage appropriately with clients, and minimal demonstration of counseling skills. You believe that this information should be not only reported to his faculty supervisor but reflected in the evaluation ratings of Roy's professional conduct and interpersonal behavior. Your colleagues brush you off, stating that they do not want to interfere with the completion of this last stage of Roy's degree.

What would you do?

What would you say to your colleagues about your understanding of gatekeeping?

What standards would you refer to in your discussion? What steps would you take if you could not convince your colleagues to fulfill their gatekeeping obligation?

These domains are analogous to a three-legged stool representing professional knowledge, skills, and conduct (see Figure 1.2). It is important to acknowledge these three domains as essential to the training process because other non-human-service-oriented academic fields (e.g., chemistry or history) only address the first two domains and do not address behavior as an academic or training standard. In the clinical health professions, particularly mental health, personal functioning and professional conduct are essential components of competent practice and, hence, degree completion. Personal and professional conduct requirements must be modeled, taught, assessed, and evaluated as acceptable in order for a trainee to be considered suitable for the clinical profession. Furthermore, all three domains are fundamental and interconnected; criteria not required of other non-human-service majors hold a vital, interlocked relationship in clinical work that needs to be conveyed to and supported at the administrative levels of institutions of higher learning.

Two of the three domains are more straightforward to evaluate using standardized procedures. Knowledge achievement is generally determined by educational institutions or their departments with oversight from accreditation bodies. Knowledge acquisition can be evaluated by multiple quantitative and widely acceptable qualitative methods that result in the assignment of grades and is measured by standardized exams required for licensure.

Essential clinical skills are described in terms of observable demonstration of proficiencies as well as through client outcomes. Although they are not as objectively defined as academic knowledge areas, there is a generally accepted consensus about the fundamental clinical skills required to demonstrate competence, many of which are supported by research and/or theory within the behavioral health professions (Barber, Sharpless, Klostermann, & McCarthy, 2007; Bernard & Goodyear, 2014; Hatcher et al., 2013; L'Abate, 2008; Perosa, 2010; Spruill, Rozensky,

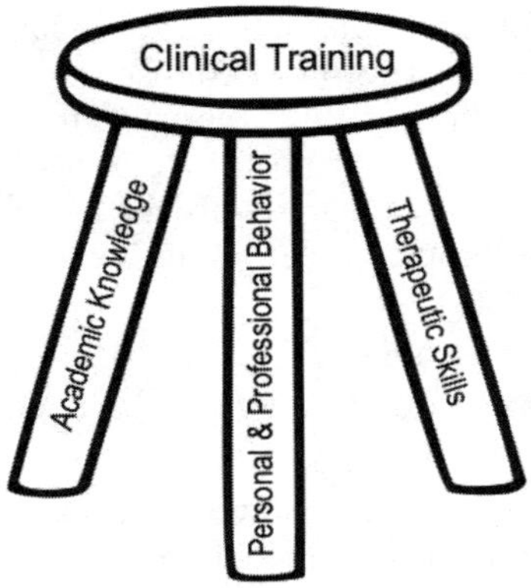

Figure 1.2 • Three Domains of Clinical Training

Stigall, Vasquez, & Bingham, 2004; Tweed, Graber, & Wang, 2010). Clinical skills are assessed using a range of standardized qualitative and quantitative instruments that are available to supervisors, several of which are discussed in Chapter 9. The relatively unambiguous establishment of criteria in these two domains—academic achievement and clinical skills—supports foundational training standards and provides clarity in the assessment of students and supervisees. Also, acquisition of knowledge and its application through skill demonstration are generally represented in most mental health fields of study.

Standards for the domain of personal behavior and professional conduct are, however, nebulous and must be gathered from multiple sources across each clinical profession—some professions identify many expectations, whereas other professions identify fewer expectations or use less definition. Despite the efforts of APA and other clinical professional associations to identify and define essential components of performance as a professional, expectations for personal and professional behavior remain vague, substantiated by limited empirical evidence, and lacking in broad consensus. This dilemma is due in part to the difficulty of identifying and defining common qualities expected of clinical trainees. Currently, training programs are expected to create their own criteria for professional behavior—a daunting task. In addition, the lack of a specific collection of personal and professional competencies hampers the construction of assessment instruments and evaluation processes that are reliable, valid, and widely accepted. The lack of consistent standards and measurement methods is the greatest challenge to the gatekeeping process and has long been lamented in the literature across the clinical professions. Several authors have described the problems created by the lack of a consistent, universal definition of gatekeeping and the related constructs that are the responsibility of the gatekeeper (Brear et al., 2008; Elman & Forrest, 2007; Forrest, Elman, Gizara, & Vacha-Haase, 1999; Homrich, 2009). Given that grounds for dismissing students from graduate programs lay primarily in the categories of ethical misconduct, emotional problems that impact professional behavior, and interpersonal skills deficits versus academic or clinical skills deficits (Crawford & Gilroy, 2012), defining gatekeeping criteria and developing assessment instruments that address these criteria should be considered a priority of the clinical professions.

Although not a recommended form of policymaking, many of the standards for trainee behavior developed within the mental health professions have been created in response to legal challenges that have forced the clarification of ethical standards, program policies, and the definitions of what constitutes academic requirements (Hutchens et al., 2013; *Keeton v. Anderson-Wiley*, 2011; McAdams, Foster, & Ward, 2007; *Ward v. Polite*, 2012), as discussed in Chapter 2. Learning from court rulings arising from vaguely defined criteria has contributed to clarifying professional benchmarks and procedures for responding to problematic behavior. Regrettably, amending practices by repairing errors, or allowing the courts to determine what defines gatekeeping practices, is risky and contributes to the continued avoidance of gatekeeping practices by faculty and supervisors (Wayne, 2004). Fortunately, the general history of case law up to the present demonstrates that courts prefer not to interfere with the academic judgment of faculty in evaluating behavior as part of academic performance when fair proceedings have occurred and due process principles have been followed (Gilfoyle, 2008). Essentially, case law supports faculty and supervisors in determining what is acceptable trainee performance, including personal behavior and professional conduct competencies (see On the Legal Side 1.2).

The APA Task Force report (APA, 2006) acknowledged that the profession of psychology, although at the forefront of the assessment of professional competence among the allied clinical professions, lags behind other health care professions such as medicine "in terms of the breadth and use of summative assessment approaches and in the extent to which multiple models of formative assessment has been standardized in professional education and training programs" (p. 88). This explains why Corey, Corey, Corey, and Callanan (2015) admonished professional organizations to

> develop specific guidelines pertaining to students' successful completion of a program: NASW for social worker students, AAMFT or [International Association of Marriage and Family Counselors] for students in marital and family therapy programs, APA for students in clinical and counseling psychology, and ACA for students in counselor education programs. Faculty in these respective professional training programs would then have the backing of their professional associations in determining evaluation procedures to be used when decisions regarding retaining or dismissing students are made. (p. 315)

This dilemma is due in part to the nature of training clinical mental health professionals: The process is multidimensional and iterative because it includes overlapping domains of academic development, clinical skill development, interpersonal functioning, and intrapersonal professional identity development (Gibson, Dollarhide, & Moss, 2010). Nonetheless, the lack of official standards for personal behavior and professional conduct creates challenges for supervisors and educators who uphold their obligations as gatekeepers. This is especially true when one is faced with a problematic supervisee who is academically competent and skilled yet lacking in interpersonal abilities or professional conduct. Models of gatekeeping from individual programs have been presented in the literature (Baldo, Softas-Nall, & Shaw, 1997; Bemak, Epp, & Keys, 1999; Frame & Stevens-Smith, 1995; Lamb et al., 1987; Lumadue & Duffey, 1999); however, they lack empirical validation, their efficacy has not been established in a definitive manner,

On the Legal Side 1.2

The primary legal issue pertinent to gatekeeping is due process. Due process is a right protected in the Fourteenth Amendment of the U.S. Constitution (Cobb, 1994; Knoff & Prout, 1985; Wayne, 2004), which holds states governable by the Bill of Rights; thus, denial of due process can be charged against institutions that receive federal or state funding (Gilfoyle, 2008).

Due process claims involving student dismissals have been interpreted at length by the courts (Gilfoyle, 2008; Olkin & Gaughen, 1991). Case law essentially serves as a guide for implementing due process rights. Of particular importance is the precedent of the court's respect for faculty expertise in determining academic decisions (Forrest et al., 1999; Frame & Stevens-Smith, 1995; Kerl, Garcia, McCullough, & Maxwell, 2002; Knoff & Prout, 1985; Lamb & Swerdlik, 2003; Olkin & Gaughen, 1991). In essence, Gilfoyle (2008) stated that the courts grant faculty "substantial leeway" in academic decisions regarding student evaluations and dismissals (p. 202).

A landmark legal case from the 1970s involving a medical student established the important precedent affirming the evaluation of clinical and interpersonal skills as an academic prerogative and has implications for gatekeeping in the clinical professions. In the case *Board of Curators of the University of Missouri v. Horowitz* (1978), Horowitz sued after being dismissed from medical school, despite high grades, because of poor interpersonal relationships with colleagues and patients, poor personal hygiene, and poor clinical skills. The case was eventually brought to the U.S. Supreme Court, which upheld the dismissal decision (Cole & Lewis, 1993; Enochs & Etzbach, 2004; Frame & Stevens-Smith, 1995; Gilfoyle, 2008; Kerl et al., 2002; Knoff & Prout, 1985; Wayne, 2004). Knoff and Prout (1985) summarized the importance of the *Horowitz* case as distinguishing the dismissal as academic in nature rather than disciplinary and upholding the evaluation of "students' interpersonal skills and attitudes within the academic domain" (p. 794); these conclusions regarding the importance of *Horowitz* were also emphasized by Cobb (1994) and Wayne (2004). For the mental health professions, the *Horowitz* case affirms the evaluation of personal and professional behavior as appropriate for academic purposes and hence within the purview of gatekeeping.

Three court cases directly involving counseling graduate programs also present important legal considerations for gatekeeping. The 1986 case *Harris v. Blake and the Board of Trustees of the University of Northern Colorado* involved a single faculty member in a counseling graduate program (Baldo et al., 1997; Bhat, 2005; Frame & Stevens-Smith, 1995; Lumadue & Duffey, 1999). The court upheld a dismissal decision over claims of denial of due process and discrimination after the dismissed student received a counseling degree from another institution. Lessons from this case applicable to gatekeeping include having a faculty committee responsible for remedial decisions rather than one faculty member deciding alone (Baldo et al., 1997; Bhat, 2005). Also, the case illustrates the value of having a

(Continued)

On the Legal Side 1.2 *(Continued)*

dismissal policy and procedure in place that defines problematic behaviors along with the importance of requiring signatures on any accompanying remediation documentation.

Another pertinent legal consideration for remediation is found in a court case against Louisiana Tech University (Baldo et al., 1997; Bhat, 2005; Custer, 1994; Enochs & Etzbach, 2004; Frame & Stevens-Smith, 1995; Kerl et al., 2002; Lumadue & Duffey, 1999) that alleged that the counseling program did not provide adequate training and was liable for graduating an impaired professional. The case was settled in 1994 for $1.7 million before Louisiana Tech University was included in the case as a defendant (Custer, 1994). This case shows the potential liability for graduate programs, highlighting the importance of actively addressing students with problematic behaviors and preventing the endorsement of problematic professionals (Enochs & Etzbach, 2004; Frame & Stevens-Smith, 1995; Kerl et al., 2002; Lumadue & Duffey, 1999).

A final court case that involved remediation was examined by McAdams et al. (2007). In the 2005 case *Plaintiff v. Rector and Board of Visitors of The College of William and Mary*, a student sued for being dismissed from the counseling program. Prior to the student's dismissal, remediation had been attempted. In this case, the faculty were charged by the plaintiff with due process violations and conspiracy, among a total of six charges. After 3 years in litigation, the case against the college was dismissed, and the dismissal was upheld on appeal. Many lessons from this experience were articulated by McAdams et al. and expanded on by McAdams and Foster (2007), including the following: using an assessment tool that clearly defines deficient behaviors, specifying remedial interventions in behavioral terms, holding regular meetings with students, documenting the occurrence of meetings, and requiring signatures on all remediation documentation.

An additional court case involved Southwest Texas State University. In 1998, the counselor education faculty at Southwest Texas State University were sued by a student attempting to force enrollment in an advanced fieldwork course. The student had not fulfilled the requirements of a remediation plan (Kerl et al., 2002). Prior to the lawsuit, the faculty had implemented the program's review policy, called the Professional Counseling Performance Evaluation, to address the student's problematic behaviors. The court ruled in the university's favor on all counts, indicating that due process had been afforded to the student and that faculty had followed established policies and procedures consistent with professional standards, a ruling that Kerl et al. (2002) directly attributed to the implementation of the Professional Counseling Performance Evaluation. Enochs and Etzbach (2004) also noted the role in this case of having a formal policy in place regarding student expectations and remediation and dismissal procedures about which students are informed on admission to a program.

and they have not been generalized across programs. Fortunately, the resources offered in the past and current professional literature provide a critical foundation that has moved the profession forward in terms of becoming more skilled at fulfilling the gatekeeping mandate. However, there is still much for clinical professions to do to create uniform definitions and standards, effective evaluation instruments, and enforcement practices to fulfill gatekeeping mandates.

Striving for Proficiency in Gatekeeping

The goal of this book, despite or because of the challenges identified here, is to encourage and support faculty and supervisors in developing or strengthening their confidence and skill in effectively addressing the third domain of trainee development: interpersonal behavior, intrapersonal functioning, and professional conduct as clinical professionals. The allied mental health professions continue to strive to develop an official or widely accepted body of clearly defined professional performance standards for trainees. Previous scholars have offered resources and tools as they have begun elucidating and implementing gatekeeping practices. These resources are at the forefront of establishing a foundation for gatekeeping best practices, and such research and shared knowledge must continue in order for the practice of gatekeeping to advance.

In the future, the clinical professions need to engage in careful study and deliberation to formulate national standards that will support the gatekeeping efforts of respondeat superiors—those members of the profession who engage most often in the quality control mechanisms of gatekeeping. Bringing definition and clarity to standards for professional conduct and personal behavior, obtaining consensus within and ideally across clinical professions, and developing evidence-based evaluation measures will enrich the credibility of the clinical professions on multiple levels. These measures will also assist those most actively involved in training the next generation of practitioners. Professional leadership efforts such as the APA Task Force or similar organizations such as the Association for Counselor Education and Supervision would benefit all constituencies participating in or affected by gatekeeping processes.

Another strategy for strengthening and ensuring the appropriate practice of gatekeeping is preparing future supervisors and faculty members. Constructing intentional curricular and experiential opportunities for doctoral students and individuals outside of academia who are moving into supervisory roles to learn gatekeeping strategies will support the development of proficiency among those who are expected to gatekeep as a part of their future career development. As Sowbel (2012) observed, unclear criteria, conflicting roles, and a lack of guidelines leads to ambivalence in gatekeeping. Because most clinicians supervise less experienced members of the profession at some time in their career, all clinicians could benefit from training in supervision and gatekeeping. Training in the practice of supervision, typically offered only at the doctoral level, should also be considered at the master's degree level. Usually a course in supervision is offered in doctoral programs, the training ground for future faculty and supervisors; however, the processes and outcomes of gatekeeping procedures may not be a deliberate component of the curriculum in those courses. Some doctoral programs have begun to develop training programs in gatekeeping that include assessing gatekeeping knowledge and self-efficacy, educating students about gatekeeping procedures, and completing experiential learning opportunities (Freeman, Coll, Juhnke, & Martinez, 2017; Rapp, Moody, & Stewart, 2017). The intention of these efforts is to demystify the gatekeeping process, prepare doctoral students for the gatekeeping role inherent in the responsibilities of a faculty member or supervisor, and assist these students in developing a gatekeeping identity as professionals.

An added challenge for faculty teaching in clinical fields is the need to educate colleagues in institutions of higher education, particularly administrators, about the integral necessity of the third domain essential in clinical training. Although personal behavior and professional conduct may not be considered an elemental aspect of the educational process in other majors, such as anthropology or business, graduating master's and doctoral students who are unable to demonstrate mastery of professional behavior according to the standards of the clinical profession has the potential to endanger others. In fact, a clinical training program was held accountable as part of a lawsuit alleging the graduation and endorsement of an incompetent clinician (Custer, 1994). Clinical educators must be familiar with standards defining the gatekeeping mandate in order to advocate for student evaluation methods and gatekeeping practices that may not be familiar to administrators or institution officials, such as deans, provosts, or risk management administrators. Proactive education of shareholders about the gatekeeping mandate in the profession is highly recommended and is addressed further in Chapter 6.

Conclusion

This book aims to be a guide for supporting clinical training programs, both pre- and postdegree programs, in the development of gatekeeping policies accompanied by practical suggestions for gatekeeping practices based on the literature of the clinical professions. Although this volume brings together current expectations for the gatekeeping process, it is only a start to the much-needed establishment of profession-wide standards. Just as ethics codes are aspirational guidelines that encourage practitioners to meet the highest standards of their profession (APA,

2017c), evidence-based findings identifying necessary parameters for the personal behavior and professional conduct of trainees as they affect therapy outcomes will contribute to a uniform or common understanding of expectations for trainees, support the development of valid and reliable assessment instruments, justify the adoption of gatekeeping standards by program shareholders, and provide the basis for defendable enforcement when gatekeeping practices are challenged formally or informally. The profession has accomplished this in other areas of practice, such as standards for supervision (AAMFT, 2014; APA, 2014; Center for Credentialing and Education, 2016) and can do so for this area of professional functioning, increasing the proficiency of gatekeeping in training settings.

This book is an accumulation of the literature from across the clinical mental health professions, collected in one place and organized intentionally for application to real situations encountered in the field of clinical education and supervision. This work specifically addresses the challenges confronted by respondeat superiors working with students and supervisees exhibiting problematic interpersonal behavior, intrapersonal behavior, and professional conduct. The hope is that equipped with information, standards of practice, and useful strategies, supervisors and faculty—and those seeking to attain these roles in the future—will be empowered to fulfill their role as gatekeepers for their profession. See Notes From the Field 1.1 for additional insights.

Key Points and Best Practices

- Gatekeeping is the process of monitoring student/supervisee development throughout the pre- and postdegree training process, evaluating trainee progress at predetermined checkpoints (gates) to substantiate appropriate progress, and intervening when problematic behaviors arise.
- The two primary purposes of gatekeeping are (a) to protect current and future clients from being harmed by incompetent clinicians and (b) to protect the integrity of the clinical professions.
- Gatekeeping processes are mandated by ethics codes, accreditation standards, and regulatory laws and rules governed by licensure boards.
- Gatekeepers are respondeat superiors, senior members of a clinical profession that influence the development of clinical knowledge, skills, and professionalism in novice members of the profession. Respondeat superiors are responsible for the actions of their trainees.
- Gatekeepers are typically faculty members and clinical supervisors, or doctoral students and supervisors-in-training, responsible for overseeing the gatekeeping process to assess trainee development at their institution or agency.

- Gatekeepers monitor three domains of training: (a) the acquisition of and ability to apply knowledge of clinical practices; (b) the development of clinical skills and the ability to apply those skills appropriately in work with clients; and (c) consistent demonstration of appropriate interpersonal, intrapersonal, and professional behavior expected of clinicians in the practice of their profession.
- Gatekeepers design, implement, and follow policies and procedures in their institutions and agencies in keeping with the standards of the profession they represent.

Notes From the Field 1.1

My first introduction to gatekeeping came as a new department chair in a counselor education program. One Friday afternoon, a student called me on my personal cell phone. I did not know her well and was surprised to receive the call. She was upset about an event that had transpired at her field site, which she recounted in the conversation. As she reported the situation, her anger increased. I chose to listen quietly, knowing that she likely needed to vent and was not asking for guidance. I was also trying to calm my own reaction as I attempted to track her report of the discriminatory events she experienced at her site. I was concerned about the student, her reactions, and what she was describing. My immediate thoughts were also influenced by a recent meeting with the university's risk management director (who happened to hold a graduate degree in counseling), during which I had been informed that as department chair I was an agent of the institution and had to be aware of my responsibilities of representing the university and not just caring about students' feelings. That responsibility was on my mind as I listened to the student because I was aware that she had a reputation for being combative, especially with those representing authority. I also knew that I was hearing one side of the whole story; I trusted what this student was telling me, but I did not know the site, her supervisors, or the context of the situation.

As the call came to a close, I affirmed her reactions and calmly expressed my concern and agreement that what had happened was unjust. The student responded that she was going to sue the site, regardless of whether the university or I liked it. That statement surprised me, as it sounded threatening, but I attributed it to her justifiably strong emotions. I immediately consulted with faculty colleagues. On their advice, I asked her to bring information about her site, particularly any antidiscrimination policies, to a meeting with her faculty supervisor and me the following business day. Concerns arose when she arrived to the meeting and accused me of having a hidden agenda. In trying to clarify her concerns, her level of anger escalated. I explained that I did not know her well but assured her that I had been very disturbed by the events at her site and wanted to understand the situation better so I could know how to take action. The meeting ended with the student angrily walking out. The senior faculty with whom I consulted provided support for my confusion and suggested that I ask the student to meet again to attempt to resolve her misunderstanding. The intention of the meeting was to understand her outrage at me and the department, to provide support for her experience, and to determine what action the program may need to take. Another faculty member, with whom she had a good relationship, and her faculty clinical supervisor joined us to help the student feel more comfortable. Unfortunately, her attacks and anger continued.

At this point the core faculty decided that the student's behavior had moved from an appropriate, yet strong reaction in the face of a discriminatory situation to the realm of being problematic. She was emotionally reactive, was unable to monitor her interpersonal responses, and was acting

(Continued)

Notes From the Field 1.1 *(Continued)*

unprofessionally. As a faculty, we became concerned about her ability to control herself with others, particularly with future clients who might provoke her strong beliefs. Her refusal to engage in a discussion with me was also troubling, as she blocked any attempt at conflict resolution.

This encounter was challenging, as I was trying to support the student, evaluate her behavior, and uphold my expected responsibilities as department chair. I was also considering the implication of ethical standards and the potential impact the student may have on the welfare of future clients.

The scenario had a positive outcome. My colleagues appropriately took leadership of the situation by conducting a formal meeting with the student, allowing me to step out because my role seemed to antagonize her. As a group, they expressed their concerns about her reactive emotional responses, provided feedback about her professional behavior, and identified the implications for her future effectiveness as a clinician. They constructed and implemented a remediation plan with a timeline and contingencies. The student followed the plan, reported back to the faculty according to the timeline, and was able to demonstrate her ability to control her emotions and conduct herself professionally for the remainder of her internship. The colleagues at her site evaluated her highly and were particularly enthusiastic about her clinical skills. She graduated and has been successful as a professional.

I learned a lot about the multiple roles and functions of being a gatekeeper and how to handle conflict while maintaining my professional responsibilities. I have dealt with many gatekeeping dilemmas since, minor and major, and each presents a unique set of circumstances requiring a distinctive response. I also discovered that there was much more to learn about the process of gatekeeping, as I realized that resources providing guidance to faculty and supervisors were disappointingly sparse. That first incident, encountering a student challenged with the process of becoming a mental health professional, began my journey of learning about the gatekeeping process. It also inspired me to create a source of information, in the form of this book, to support other gatekeepers in developing their own process of instituting best practices to fulfill this important professional mandate.

Chapter 2

Critical Terminology in Gatekeeping

Kyle D. Baldwin

Clinical gatekeepers (e.g., educators, faculty supervisors, and site supervisors) are responsible for protecting the integrity of the allied mental health professions by ensuring that supervisees are suitable for professional practice, thus protecting potential future clients from the harm that may occur from services provided by unskilled clinicians (Brear, Dorrian, & Luscri, 2008; Homrich, DeLorenzi, Bloom, & Godbee, 2014). Gatekeepers within the clinical professions (e.g., psychology; mental health counseling; and the related fields of social work, marriage and family therapy, rehabilitation, college counseling, and school counseling) may find the actual process of gatekeeping challenging and emotionally stressful. This concern is often due in part to a lack of clearly defined universal standards of conduct required for graduate students and supervisees during clinical training (Brear et al., 2008; Forrest, Elman, Gizara, & Vacha-Haase, 1999; Homrich, 2009; Homrich et al., 2014). In addition, gatekeepers encounter shifting terminology and descriptors, some of which are deemed preferable while others are considered poor or dangerous choices in the context of applying or describing gatekeeping practices.

The purpose of this chapter is to identify a gatekeeping lexicon that is currently considered preferable and representative of appropriate terminology, especially in the legal arena. The goal is to encourage professional dialogue on the importance of identifying specific terminology and definitions that could or should be utilized consistently within the clinical professions when identifying and evaluating standards of conduct for students and supervisees.

One of the main difficulties encountered in creating a set of standards of conduct for trainees is the wide range of terminology that has been used over time by the various clinical professions and professional organizations to describe problematic behaviors (Elman & Forrest, 2007; Forrest et al., 1999; Homrich, 2009; Homrich et al., 2014; Wayne, 2004). A review of the literature on the evaluation of trainee professional conduct indicates a lack of consistency regarding a clear and shared language for describing categories and types of problematic behaviors, which has been an issue since the early 1980s (Forrest et al., 1999). This is due in part to the use of an evolving collection of terms that change when a specific descriptor is discovered to be confusing or ambiguous, especially when tested by legal challenges. An additional problem with terminology has been that some terms have been defined in multiple ways depending on the source (e.g., professional organizations, textbooks, or journal articles).

Defining Gatekeeping

An example of concerns regarding terminology can be illustrated by the core term at the heart of this book: ***gatekeeping.*** Since the 1980s, a clear definition of this word has been elusive, with references that include discerning admissions processes, ethical responsibilities of supervisors and/or the clinical training process, or oversight of supervisees (Brear et al., 2008). Koerin and Miller (1995) defined gatekeeping as "preventing the graduation of students who are not equipped with the requisite knowledge, skills, and values for professional practice" (p. 247). Homrich (2009) defined gatekeeping as "a metaphor that identifies the process of monitoring progression through a series of stages via critical points of entry or passage" (p. 1). The *ACA Code of Ethics* (American Counseling Association [ACA], 2014a) defines gatekeeping as "the initial and ongoing academic, skill, and dispositional assessment of students' competency for professional practice, including remediation and termination as appropriate" (p. 20). Gatekeeping entails all of these perspectives and practices and much more, as described in this book and in particular as introduced in Chapter 1.

The issue regarding terminology can become even more confusing and complicated when the terms being used by clinical mental health professionals in the gatekeeping process are also being utilized in other professions, such as the legal field, with different definitions (Brear et al., 2008; Homrich et al., 2014). An example of this is the term ***impairment,*** which has been used in conjunction with students with problematic behaviors in the gatekeeping process and yet is also a term used in the Americans with Disabilities Act Amendments Act of 2008 (ADAAA) when defining a disability (Falender, Collins, & Shafranske, 2009).

Homrich et al. (2014) stated that gatekeepers in the clinical professions would "benefit from a set of clearly defined, observable, and measurable criteria for trainee behaviors that are widely agreed upon and uniformly acknowledged as minimal expectations across clinical disciplines" (p. 129) as the basis for evaluation and gatekeeping action. A preliminary step in this direction would include agreement on and standardization of terms frequently utilized in the gatekeeping process by clinical educators and supervisors at the global professional level. The lexicon discussed in this chapter is proposed as a starting point in this endeavor. This chapter reviews selected terminologies that have been identified in the literature relevant to the gatekeeping process. The focus is on suggestions for a recommended lexicon related to behavior, standards, and evaluation for trainees. In addition, controversial and ambiguous terms that have led to misinterpretation or legal challenge are acknowledged along with reasons to avoid their use. Ethical and legal definitions relevant to the gatekeeping process are also discussed.

Defining Trainee Behavior and Standards for Conduct

Behavior

There has been a lack of agreement in the counseling and psychology literatures about the appropriate terminology for describing concerning conduct or behavior of students and supervisees throughout the course of the clinical training process. The mental health profession and related professions have frequently described trainees as *distressed, deficient, inadequate, incompetent, impaired, problematic, psychologically unfit, unsuitable*, and *unsatisfactory* (Bernard & Goodyear, 2014; Brear et al., 2008; Goodrich & Luke, 2012; Goodrich & Shin, 2012; Homrich, 2009; Oliver, Bernstein, Anderson, Blashfield, & Roberts, 2004; Wilkerson, 2006). Current literature supports the use of the term ***problematic*** to make a clear distinction between trainee behaviors and disabilities (Elman & Forrest, 2007; Goodrich & Luke, 2012; Homrich, 2009; Wilkerson, 2006). Examples of problematic behaviors exhibited by clinical trainees have included demonstrations of unethical behavior, difficulties with professional conduct, deficiencies in interpersonal relations, and the inability to self-regulate intrapersonal functions (Forrest et al., 1999; Goodrich & Luke, 2012; Goodrich & Shin, 2012).

Educators and supervisors in the professions of mental health counseling and related fields (school, rehabilitation, and college counseling), along with social work, psychology, and marriage and family therapy, need benchmarks to be able to assess student progress and differentiate behaviors that may be chronically problematic from those that are typical of trainee developmental processes, such as expanding the capacity for empathy, the ability to regulate emotions appropriately across situations, or the development of a professional identity (Homrich et al., 2014).

Professional Behavior

The ***professional identity*** of clinical helping professionals includes the training process of assimilating knowledge, skills, standards of practice, behaviors, and attitudes leading ultimately to one's view of self in the role as a professional practitioner. For example, in the case of the counseling profession, counselor professional identity is commonly defined as the integration of professional training with personal attributes in the context of a professional community (Nugent & Jones, 2009). In "A Vision for the Future of Counseling: The 20/20 Principles for Unifying and Strengthening the Profession," 31 organizations representing the counseling profession agreed that the number one goal by the year 2020 was "sharing a common professional identity is critical for counselors," which is critical not only for counselors but also for the general public and legislators as well (Kaplan & Gladding, 2011, p. 372). This principle is likely considered important for all of the clinical professions.

Professional identity development has been described as a co-occurring process among clinical trainees that includes both ***intrapersonal processes*** (e.g., internalizing knowledge while identifying personal strengths and academic growth, increasing self-awareness and insight) and ***interpersonal processes*** (e.g., becoming immersed in the professional community and developing skills to relate clinically to colleagues and clients; Gibson, Dollarhide, & Moss, 2010; Limberg et al., 2013). The professional identity development of trainees consists of examining personal values, morals, and perceptions in relationship to the profession's values, ethics, standards, and expectations and integrating both to determine how one will conduct oneself in the professional workplace. The development of a professional identity, with feedback from the professional community (e.g., educators and clinical supervisors), is extremely important in ethical practice as graduate students transition from being supervisees to becoming practitioners (Gibson et al., 2010; Limberg et al., 2013). Students in graduate mental health counseling and related programs are responsible for exhibiting behaviors consistent with the ethical standards of their designated professional associations as part of their professional identity development. Thus, educators and supervisors must "appropriately monitor and evaluate behaviors and attributes that are clinical and interpersonal in nature" (Kelly, 2011, p. 112) in tandem with students' acquisition of academic knowledge and clinical skills. Trainees who do not develop a clear sense of professional identity or who do not integrate fully into the professional culture may be at greater risk for unethical practice as a professional (Gibson et al., 2010).

Professional standards are defined as specific levels of quality or attainment that are the expectation of a professional, institution, or program (Homrich, 2009). For example, best practice standards are guidelines that reflect a general consensus of expected behavior for those engaged in a professional endeavor and that serve as a model of the most effective process for achieving a specific objective or outcome (American Psychological Association [APA], 2015a). Ethics codes established by professional associations are examples of professional standards. Other groups that set standards may be regulatory bodies, legislatures, accreditation bodies, state or federal departments of education, or the institutions or programs that implement the standards within their operations. Standards are the foundation for policies and procedures pertaining to recruitment, retention, evaluation, remediation, and gatekeeping and thus should be the benchmark against which performance is evaluated. In the case of an educational or clinical training program, standards or expectations for trainees published in student handbooks, graduate catalogs, agency policy manuals, and related media such as websites are the professional standards that trainees are expected to fulfill within the context of that particular setting, although they should reflect the standards of the profession they represent. Standards should be easily accessible to both prospective applicants and current graduate students or supervisees because they are the criteria for providing informed consent for participation in a training program (Homrich et al., 2014; Hutchens, Block, & Young, 2013).

Descriptions of trainee performance standards (i.e., competencies, professional dispositions, behaviors, and conduct) should be clearly defined by educators and supervisors because these observable behaviors may be otherwise difficult to identify. ***Competencies*** have been defined as components of performance that can be assessed, measured, and evaluated against standards (W. B. Johnson, Porter, Campbell, & Kupko, 2005; Kaslow et al., 2007). The teacher preparation field first used the word ***dispositions*** to describe virtue ethics, or positive, observable professional behaviors of student teachers guided by values, beliefs, commitments, and professional ethics that support the operationalized standards reflecting the conceptual framework of a profession's or organization's mission. Identification of dispositions allows for systematic assessment of an individual as well as systemic evaluation of training program effectiveness to determine continuous improvement of the teacher candidate and educational program. Assessing dispositions also allows programs to flag deficient students at identified checkpoints in the teacher training process (McKnight, 2004). In its 2016 accreditation standards, the Council for Accreditation of Counseling and Related Educational Programs (2015) adopted and defined the term ***professional dispositions*** as "the commitments, characteristics, values, beliefs, interpersonal functioning, and behaviors that influence the counselor's professional growth and interactions with clients and colleagues" (p. 47).

In general, the term ***behavior*** refers to acts, responses, reactions, and processes that are measurable (Reber, Allen, & Reber, 2009) in relation to or interaction with one's environment. Behaviors can also be observed and measured, which is critical when considering trainee developmental processes and evaluation procedures. ***Conduct*** is more specifically defined as the way in which an individual behaves in a particular place or situation. Both behavior and conduct are dynamic and can vary or change over time. For example, a student's behavior may be measured as consistent or erratic in comparison to stated expectations or standards. Conduct may be termed professional or unprofessional in relationship to ethical guidelines, commonly held norms of the profession, or published expectations of the training program. Because educators and supervisors (and clinicians in general) cannot know what is going on in a person's mind, despite being trained in the emotional and cognitive aspects of psychology, the only truly quantifiable or assessable function of a trainee is observed behavior or outcomes. Thus, expectations for student or supervisee behavior will ideally be formulated into a set of standards that fulfill the definitions of behavior or conduct in that they are observable, measurable, and consistent with the expectations of the profession as stated in ethical, legal, and other related guiding principles.

Although previous literature has identified behaviors, conduct, dispositions, and qualities expected of graduate students in clinical programs, there is an ongoing need for the clinical professions to establish a comprehensive set of commonly held standards for the professional and personal conduct of clinical trainees (Homrich et al., 2014). Establishing a baseline set of behavioral standards or guidelines endorsed by the individual clinical profession beyond the limited mention in ethics codes is important for consistently evaluating trainee conduct across the clinical professions. This effort would enable gatekeepers to enforce behaviors that are not typically expected of students in other academic disciplines. Common professional training guidelines would assist gatekeepers in their ethical and legal responsibility to identify problematic trainees and determine the appropriate course of action to take when trainees are unable or unwilling to meet performance expectations (Wayne, 2004). These standards also are necessary to assist students and mental health trainees in understanding the criteria for "acceptable professional, interpersonal, and intrapersonal counselor conduct . . . and . . . how these standards are applied in evaluation processes" (Homrich et al., 2014, p. 139).

Chapter 8 reviews the literature that informs the construction of standards for the behavior and professional conduct of clinical trainees. It is important for educators and supervisors in the mental health professions to understand that it is essential to establish terminology and define expectations for each category of conduct prior to the onset of enrollment in a training program or engagement in a supervisory relationship. Clarity of expectations and appropriate terminology or definition will form the basis for a joint understanding of expectations between faculty and students and between supervisors and supervisees from the outset of the training relationship.

Measuring the Behavior and Conduct of Students and Supervisees

Student performance can be evaluated in terms of academic accomplishment and the demonstration of competence in both clinical and professional areas. Observational procedures for the informal assessment of student progress by educators and supervisors should be reliable and accurate (Falender et al., 2009). ***Informal evaluations*** occur throughout the graduate training and supervision experience (e.g., when students are evaluated in terms of how they conduct themselves in classes and complete their courses, during interpersonal interactions with peers and faculty, during clinical and field experiences when providing direct services, as well as during routine interactions; Homrich, 2009). When behaviors or conduct of concern arise during informal observations and interactions, educators and supervisors can address minor issues directly with graduate students and supervisees by teaching new behaviors via modeling, shaping, confronting, and providing feedback (ACA, 2009; Elman & Forrest, 2007; Homrich, 2009; Ivey, Ivey, & Zalaquett, 2014; Reber et al., 2009):

Modeling: The trainee learns by observing and imitating the supervisor, peer colleagues, or other professionals whose behavior is acknowledged by the supervisor or instructor as appropriate or noteworthy.

Shaping: The trainee's target behavior is rewarded as soon as it is observed through acknowledgment, typically praise or encouragement.

Confronting: The trainee's inappropriate conduct is acknowledged as incongruent with expected professional performance or conduct through an assertion by the supervisor or instructor.

Feedback: The trainee is provided with information regarding his or her behavior or performance, either positive or negative, which may be accompanied by a review of future expectations for functioning.

If behavior or performance continues to be substandard after ample training, supervision, and use of the interventions described here, gatekeepers typically move from informal to progressively more ***formal evaluation*** processes (e.g., providing organized feedback to students in writing or face-to-face meetings). Formal evaluations address specific concerns and review agency or program standards for conduct. This level of encounter is followed up with a plan for tracking and monitoring student progress. If problematic behavior continues, a faculty committee may be formed to construct a student performance plan or written remediation plan that further details expected behaviors, methods of evaluation, and deadlines for expected change (Wayne, 2004). Details of how to operationalize the evaluation process are described in Chapter 9.

Remediation, as defined by Dufrene and Henderson (2009), is "a documented, procedural process that addresses observed inabilities in trainees' performance with the intent to provide trainees with specific means to remedy their inabilities" (p. 151). Homrich (2009) referred to the process of remediation as being "a curative action that restores desired functioning, which . . . is the personal and professional performance of counseling students" (p. 15). Accreditation standards (e.g., Council for Accreditation of Counseling and Related Educational Programs standards) and ethics codes of professional associations (e.g., the *ACA Code of Ethics* [ACA, 2014a]) present guidelines for addressing personal or professional performance issues in supervisees and provide "definitive principles supporting the gatekeeping process" (Homrich, 2009, p. 8).

Evaluation and remediation processes and procedures are discussed in detail in subsequent chapters; however, it is important to understand that there is a distinct behavioral aspect involved in addressing the problematic performance of a student or supervisee. There are many points and approaches for intervention across the process of facilitating successful student development, beginning with those illustrated in Figure 1.1 in Chapter 1. The remediation process also involves prioritizing observable behavior as the point of measure for interpersonal, intrapersonal, and professional conduct or functioning. In general, the goal of remediation is to remedy problematic performance and support a trainee in achieving the expected standards designated by the program, institution, and clinical profession (Dufrene & Henderson, 2009).

Controversial Terminology and Recommended Language in Gatekeeping

Four specific terms have been identified as controversial terminology in defining the behavior of trainees in the gatekeeping process for psychology, counseling, social work, and marriage and family therapy graduate programs of study. The terms *impairment*, *competence*, *psychological fitness*, and *nonacademic factors* have had multiple or conflicting definitions throughout the years that have emerged from a variety of sources, including professional textbooks, journals, ethics of professional associations, legal advice, and/or legislation. This section provides a brief review of each term along with recommended alternative terminology for risk management considerations.

Impairment

The medical profession was a forerunner in using the term ***impaired*** when referring to practitioners of concern in the early 1970s when it established rehabilitative programs to assist impaired physicians. Research studies conducted by the medical profession identified alcoholism, drug dependency, or major psychiatric illness as the source of impairment and noted that high impairment rates in physicians were due to the stresses associated with their profession and the "omnipotent role of the professional" (Laliotis & Grayson, 1985, p. 85), which often discouraged professionals from seeking help.

A review of the literature traces the introduction of the concept of impairment to the mental health professions to psychologists, who in 1981 utilized it in a psychological training forum of APA (Forrest et al., 1999). At that time, impairment was associated with psychological problems, such as mental illness, substance abuse, physical and emotional limitations, or having an inappropriate relationship with a client (such as sexual intimacy; Falender et al., 2009). Impairment was broadly defined as the "interference in professional functioning due to chemical dependency, mental illness, or personal conflict" (Laliotis & Grayson, 1985, p. 85). Additional definitions have included references to depression, psychosis, suicidal ideation, and alcoholism.

Lamb et al. (1987) proposed that the term impairment be considered "one end of a continuum, competency at the other end, and 'problems' at a different point along the continuum" (pp. 598–599). The term ***problems*** can encompass an intern's attitudes, behaviors, or characteristics that require remediation. From this proposed perspective, if an intern were unable to meet the standards of professional competency required, then the term impairment would be applied.

Numerous definitions for the term impairment have been utilized throughout the years by the mental health professions, but, attempts to identify one clear definition have not been successful (Falender et al., 2009): Since the early 1980s, the terms impairment or impaired have been used by supervisors to describe problematic behavior in interns or to "characterize the root cause of patterns of substandard performance" (p. 240), yet the use of these terms now carries legal risks. In a legal context, these terms may raise serious conflicts when considered in relation to the ADAAA and the final rule interpreting the ADAAA, which both protect individuals who are not actually disabled but who are regarded as disabled (Constangy, Brooks, Smith, & Prophete, 2008).

An impairment under ADAAA is defined as a condition that significantly limits one major life activity, such as working; however, the condition does not need to limit other major life activities in order to be defined as a disability. An impairment substantially limits working when it limits an individual's ability to perform or meet the qualification for a specific type of work (Constangy et al., 2008). Wheeler and Bertram (2015) stated that mental health professionals may wish to take note that "an impairment that is episodic or in remission meets the definition of disability if it would substantially limit a major life activity when active . . . and includes episodic impairments such as bipolar disorder and schizophrenia" (p. 249). The ADAAA makes it easier for an individual seeking protection under the Americans with Disabilities Act (ADA) to establish a disability within the interpretation of the statute ("Regulations to Implement," 2011).

Use of the terms impairment or impaired in mental health settings may give rise to significant legal concerns now that "the ADA has appropriated the term impairment as part of its definition of disability"

(Falender et al., 2009, p. 241, italics in the original). It is important to note that the term impairment is currently being utilized and/or defined in various ways by textbooks on professional counseling, articles, and professional mental health organizations and associations when discussing ethical principles or codes of conduct relative to professional functioning. For example, the ACA Code of Ethics (ACA, 2014a) defines impairment as "a significantly diminished capacity to perform professional functions" (p. 20) and in Section F.5.b. addresses the need for counselors, students, and supervisees to "monitor themselves for signs of impairment from their own physical, mental, or emotional problems." Furthermore, Section F.6.d. advises supervisors not to endorse supervisees who are "impaired in any way that would interfere with the performance of the duties associated with the endorsement."

APA's (2017c) *Ethical Principles of Psychologists and Code of Conduct* utilizes the term *impairment* in the Section 3.05(a), Multiple Relationships, which states that "multiple relationships that would not reasonably be expected to cause impairment or risk exploitation or harm are not unethical." The *NASW Code of Ethics* (National Association of Social Workers [NASW], 2017) discusses impairment in regard to self and colleagues. Standard 2.08 addresses the impairment of colleagues "due to personal problems, psychosocial distress, substance abuse, or mental health difficulties . . . that interferes with practice effectiveness." Standard 4.05 addresses impairment as "personal problems, psychosocial distress, legal problems, substance abuse, or mental health difficulties . . . that interfere with . . . professional judgment and performance." The American Association for Marriage and Family Therapy (AAMFT) *Code of Ethics* (AAMFT, 2015), in Standard III (Professional Competence and Integrity), states that "marriage and family therapists seek appropriate professional assistance for issues that may impair work performance or clinical judgment" (Standard 3.3) and that they may be in violation of Standard 3.12.f. if they "continue to practice marriage and family therapy while no longer competent to do so because they are impaired by physical or mental causes or the abuse of alcohol or other substances." Thus, impairment is used broadly in professional ethics codes, promoting the use of the term in training programs when describing the performance of students and supervisees and complicating the definition as used by the ADA legislation.

An additional concern about clinical mental health professionals' use of the term impairment arises from the inference that it is a diagnosis of cognitive, intellectual, personality, or other functioning resulting from an assessment and assignment of a clinical mental diagnosis. Because supervisors and educators are also clinicians trained in the practice of diagnosing mental disorders, a determination of "impaired" by a diagnostic expert could be construed to imply that a formal diagnosis of a trainee's functioning has been made by a mental health clinician (the supervisor or educator). The inference of a clinical diagnosis by a supervisor or educator who is also a licensed clinician would implicate the supervisor or faculty member in the practice of boundary violation and engaging in an inappropriate dual/multiple relationship based on standards contained in professional ethics codes, such as the *ACA Code of Ethics* (ACA, 2014a, Section F). Alternatively, interventions that address performance concerns could be challenged with the argument that assigning the label of impaired to describe trainee functioning was done without appropriate formal clinical consideration, despite the intention of using the term informally. This confounds the already complicated situation regarding the use of impairment in ethics codes, licensure law descriptions, and ADA terminology.

Given the difficulty of providing one specific definition for the term impairment, and to avoid potential conflict with the current ADA disability legislation, clinical supervisors and educators are advised to refrain from using the word impairment when addressing the professional competence of trainees and to only utilize the term in conjunction with diagnosed disabilities (Falender et al., 2009; Homrich, 2009; Kaslow et al., 2007).

Problematic

The term ***problematic*** has been recommended in recent years as the preferred term for describing observed behaviors of concern in clinical trainees that interfere with academic functioning, clinical skills functioning, or professional conduct. Current literature supports the movement in the mental health professions to favor the term problematic to describe trainee behavior while also fulfilling the legal and ethical responsibilities of educators during the gatekeeping process (Bernard & Goodyear, 2014; Homrich, 2009) and making a clear distinction between student behaviors and disabilities (Goodrich & Luke, 2012; Homrich, 2009; Wilkerson, 2006). In their analysis of the literature on and history of terminology, Elman and Forrest (2007) recommended using the term problems or problematic "over other possible terms (e.g., insufficient, deficient, inadequate, unsatisfactory, unqualified) because problematic is inclusive, captures an array of difficulties, and can be assessed by qualitative as well as quantitative means" (p. 505). This term focuses on student behaviors without labeling a student as *incompetent* or *impaired* (Homrich, 2009; Rosenberg, Getzelman, Arcinue, & Oren, 2005) or inferring that a diagnostic assessment has been made.

Problematic behaviors may occur at any time throughout the graduate program or internship experience, interfere with academic and/or therapeutic skills functioning, or be exhibited in professional conduct and/or personal behavior and require the attention of training program professionals (Homrich, 2009). Language also needs to be established by behavioral health professionals to clarify the degree of the problematic behavior and whether the student is unable or unwilling to perform at an acceptable level, whether his or her functioning is temporary or chronic, and whether previously functional trainee behaviors have diminished or never existed in the first place (e.g., Forrest et al., 1999).

Some problematic behaviors, such as attitudes or personal conduct, may be initially expected of students or supervisees as they acclimate to the expectations of a newly entered profession or setting. As part of the professional identity development process, these actions typically prove to be transient or remedied with very limited intervention; they are thus often minor concerns for supervisors or educators that resolve on their own. There is a wide range of potential problematic behavior, from immature behavior in the classroom to extreme unethical practices in engaging with a client during clinical placement. Of course, there are many points along this continuum, and behavior is typically defined as highly problematic when it is not corrected and endures across settings. Constructing and defining a set of clear standards for expected interpersonal, intrapersonal, and professional behavior can be the starting point from which to benchmark problematic behavior.

Competence

In the realm of gatekeeping, supervisors and educators have been encouraged to use the lens of competence. In this context, ***competence*** is defined as successful attainment of the learning, skills, and conduct expected of a mental health professional. Bernard and Goodyear (2014) suggested evaluating the performance or behavior of students and interns from the perspective of competence attainment.

This term emerged in the early 1970s with a focus not only on the quality of professional education programs but also on the competence of the graduates who applied for licensure and entered the behavioral health profession. In the 1980s, there was an increased focus on program accreditation, credentialing, and the outcomes of education known as the assessment movement in higher education (P. D. Nelson, 2007). There was also recognition during this time that professional education and training programs needed to come to an agreement regarding the meaning and assessment of competence (P. D. Nelson, 2007). This focus on the assessment of competence was valuable to the health care professions in terms of fostering learning, identifying effective curriculum and training programs, advancing the profession, and protecting the public (Kaslow, 2004; Kaslow et al., 2009).

The term competence has been defined in multiple ways and can differ across groups or experts. Competence refers to a global capacity to perform as a professional (Kaslow et al., 2009). Some of the professional functions that make up competence have been identified as professional judgment, scientific-mindedness, relationship skills, clinical reasoning, critical thinking and analysis, self-awareness, openness to learning, and commitment to professional growth (Kaslow et al., 2007).

The term ***competencies*** refers to the "demonstrable elements or components of performance (knowledge, skills, and attitudes and their integration) that make up competence" (Kaslow et al., 2009, p. S34) and is used interchangeably with the term ***standards,*** which specifies an adopted set of competencies indicating a level of expected quality or attainment that is used in the comparative evaluation process. Standards are used to measure a supervisee's expected level of performance via benchmarks and, according to Kaslow et al. (2009), are generally assessed at three stages of professional development: "readiness for practicum, readiness for internship, readiness for entry level to practice" (p. S34). The extent to which a supervisee can improve performance, generate new knowledge, and adapt his or her skills is referred to as ***capability*** (e.g., Fraser & Greenhalgh, 2001; Kaslow et al., 2007). The literature across the mental health professions identifies additional competencies and standards, as do legislative wording related to licensure standards, accreditation bodies, professional specialization areas and/or certification programs, as well as individual graduate training programs.

Problems with trainee competence can occur within many domains, such as basic, functional competencies demonstrated in comparison to expected levels of knowledge, skills, and attitudes. Alternatively, problems of personal and professional competence are generally outside the realm of academic functioning and may be specific (e.g., substance abuse) or general (e.g., interpersonal problems and difficulties receiving supervisory feedback and direction; Kaslow et al., 2007). Competence problems may be categorized in several ways: based on situational circumstances, based on ongoing developmental issues, or by their degree of severity and the potential for remediation. Students or supervisees may demonstrate chronic problems with competence by repeating the same mistakes or failing to meet required standards of performance in professional functioning despite support and remediation efforts (Kaslow et al., 2007).

Professional associations and organizations address competence in their ethics codes. For example, the AAMFT *Code of Ethics* (AAMFT, 2015) addresses the oversight of supervisee competence and states that "marriage and family therapists do not permit students or supervisees to perform or to hold themselves out as competent to perform professional services beyond their training, level of experience, and competence" (Standard 4.4). The *NASW Code of Ethics* (NASW, 2017) addresses competence and incompetence in Standard 4.01(a) ("Social workers should accept responsibility or employment only on the basis of existing competence or the intention to acquire the necessary competence") and Standard 2.09(b) ("Social workers who believe that a social work colleague is incompetent and has not taken adequate steps to address the incompetence should take action through appropriate channels established by employers, agencies, NASW, licensing and regulatory bodies, and other professional organizations"). These examples parallel the mandates of other clinical professions, such as ACA.

Competence may also be addressed in state laws that govern clinical practice. The Florida Board of Clinical Social Work, Marriage & Family Therapy and Mental Health Counseling governs the practice of clinicians in the three master's-level professions, addressing expectations for both licensed professional and registered interns through laws and rules. It addresses the issue of competence and states that the board may impose, fines, probation, or the suspension of a license based on an individual

> being unable to practice the profession for which one is licensed under Chapter 491, [Florida Statute], with reasonable skill and competence as a result of any mental or physical condition or by reason of illness; drunkenness; or excessive use of drugs, narcotics, chemicals, or any other substance. (2016, Rule 64B4-5.001[p])

Most legislative bodies have similar mandates, general or specific, that set minimal standards for competent performance on the part of mental health practitioners enforceable by disciplinary action as authorized by the legislature or approved governing body.

Professional Competence

A review of the literature reflects a move away from the single term competence when discussing the evaluation of supervisees in favor of prefacing the term with specifiers such as *professional* to express standards of performance (Elman & Forrest, 2007). ***Professional competence*** has been defined as the "cognitive, integrative, relational, affective/moral, and habits of the mind dimensions" (Kaslow et al., 2009, p. S34), the "ability to carry out certain tasks appropriately and effectively" (W. B. Johnson et al., 2008, p. 590), and "intellectual ability, personality traits, motivation, attitudes, and values" (Elman & Forrest, 2007, p. 505). Epstein and Hundert's (2002) definition of professional competence is also phrased positively as "the habitual and judicious use of communication, knowledge, technical skills, clinical reasoning, emotions, values, and reflection in daily practice for the benefit of the individual and community being served" (p. 227).

Evaluating the professional competence of supervisees can be difficult because of the perceived subjective nature of the term *competence* and becomes especially problematic when there is a lack of consensus around the specific constructs and behaviors encompassed by this global categorization (Homrich, 2009). Despite this concern, the term *competence* is used within ethics codes to identify an assumed, inexplicit set of behaviors. For example, the *Ethical Principles of Psychologists and Code of Conduct* (APA, 2017c) states that "Psychologists provide services, teach, and conduct research with populations and in areas only within the boundaries of their competence, based on their education, training, supervised experience, consultation, study, or professional experience" (Standard 2.01[a]). P. D. Nelson (2007) reported that criteria need to be established to distinguish the various levels of competence required for each stage of the professional development and training process (e.g., a novice or supervisee vs. an expert such as a licensed clinician). Other examples of the vague directive of this term are noted in the National Association of School Psychologists (2010) *Principles for Professional Ethics*, which states in Section II (Professional Competence and Responsibility) that "school psychologists must practice within the boundaries of their competence" (p. 6). The *ASCA Ethical Standards for School Counselors* (American School Counselor Association, 2016) states that "school counselors seek physical or mental health support when needed to ensure professional competence" (p. 7). Such references are targeted to clinical knowledge and interventions and are inadequate when it comes to monitoring professional behavior and conduct, especially in the case of clinical trainees. Nebulous language does little to support gatekeepers who are obligated to evaluate the competence of future clinicians and monitor those who enter into professional practice without clear guidelines for the personal and professional behaviors that affect the determination of competence or lack thereof.

The terms ***professional competence problems*** and ***problems of professional competence*** are also important to this discussion (Bernard & Goodyear, 2014; Elman & Forrest, 2007; W. B. Johnson et al., 2008; Shen-Miller, Forrest, & Elman, 2009) and offer three essential components necessary to define professional competence: "(a) the inclusion of the concept that there is a problem with performance, (b) a professional standard, and (c) a focus on competence" (Elman & Forrest, 2007, p. 505). Additional related terms used in the professional mental health literature include ***students and trainees with problematic professional competencies*** (Bodner, 2012) and ***trainees identified with problems of professional competence*** (Forrest, Shen Miller, & Elman, 2008), which have both been utilized when referring to problematic students and supervisees. Of these four interchangeable terms present in professional writing, the most common is problems of professional competence, which may include difficulties with moral character or psychological fitness, according to Elman and Forrest (2007).

Moral character includes traits such as caring and integrity and "refers to the honesty and integrity with which a person deals with others and is . . . relevant to maintaining public trust" (W. B. Johnson et al., 2008, p. 590). The concept of moral character is inferred in legislation and ethics codes, which extend not only to practitioners but also to trainees. Again, this is a vague term that represents norms and assumptions about expected behavior but in itself is unclear and ill defined. Chapter 8 provides guidance on how to develop clearer standards or expectations for behavior and conduct.

En masse, the terms competence, professional competence, competencies, and professional standards refer to the general classification of specific qualities, characteristics, and behaviors of functioning or expectations for professional conduct. They denote performance expectations that should be distinctly identified and defined for trainees and supervisees by clinical educators and supervisors in advance of engagement in a training relationship. Standards of competence and professional competencies are the criteria that define and motivate the development of expected behavior for both emerging and practicing professionals. They are also the comparison against which to assess acceptable performance at various points in the clinician development process as well as in ongoing professional functioning after licensure.

W. B. Johnson and Campbell (2002) proposed that greater attention be given to screening graduate students and licensure applicants on both character and appropriate psychological functioning, based on criteria specific to the profession of professional psychology. Although a deterioration in psychological functioning can occur at any time during a professional's career, such as through phase-of-life problems or adjustment disorders, W. B. Johnson et al. (2005) "hypothesized that pre-licensure indicators of character and fitness concern would predict later ethical and professional transgressions" (p. 656), an important note for training faculty and supervisors as they serve in their role as gatekeepers. Thus, attending to the lexicon is important when designing program or agency standards, and definitions of terms may be a helpful accompaniment.

Psychological Fitness

The term ***psychological fitness*** refers to the psychological health of a professional (e.g., his or her emotional and mental stability) and his or her ability to practice in the profession safely and effectively (W. B. Johnson et al., 2008). The term psychological fitness has been identified as a problematic phrase in terms of gatekeeping because it has been connected in the professional literature to other questionable terminology, such as impairment and competence (W. B. Johnson et al., 2005). Psychological fitness may be evaluated by the presence of effective personal functioning and adjustment; the absence of psychological problems that interfere with professional practice; and the consistent and appropriate ability to meet standards of performance interpersonally, intrapersonally, and professionally in terms of conduct (W. B. Johnson et al., 2005, 2008). Psychological fitness has been considered one of the "essential foundational characteristics or qualities required for executing the duties of the profession" (W. B. Johnson et al., 2005, p. 655). It is a phrase utilized by professional psychologists when discussing the importance of moral character and personal fitness (W. B. Johnson & Campbell, 2002). Educators and supervisors in the training of professional psychologists consider psychological fitness, character, and competence important factors in the gatekeeping process (W. B. Johnson et al., 2008).

The term psychological fitness is commonly used in the military and refers to the mental or emotional stability of an individual as it extends to his or her ability to practice a professional skill safely and effectively (W. B. Johnson & Campbell, 2004). A review of research conducted with psychologists indicated that from 1983 through 2001, the "most common reasons for disciplinary action against licensed psychologists . . . could reasonably be related to both moral character and psychological fitness problems, e.g., sexual relationships with clients, unprofessional conduct, conviction of crimes, fraudulent acts, impairment" (W. B. Johnson et al., 2005, p. 656). The term psychological fitness can be viewed as conclusory, implying that diagnostic criteria have served as the basis for a decision, which casts this term in the same troubling category as impairment or incompetence.

As with all other constructs discussed in this chapter, the dilemma comes down to this: What do these terms mean? The answers may vary from one training program to the next, especially when one is using an outdated term such as *fitness.* Thus, the establishment by the field site or training program of very clearly defined terminology and criteria is imperative to creating a common understanding among all constituents affected—administrators, educators, supervisors, persons who serve as evaluators, affiliated staff, students, and supervisees.

Psychological Health

Psychological health has been defined as "a dynamic assembly of a person's psychic features that provides harmony between an individual's and a society's needs . . . to fulfill life tasks" (Sekach, Perelygina, & Zotova, 2013, p. 88) and the "preservation of inward and outward regulations" (p. 89). In the current literature within the clinical mental health professions, psychological fitness has recently been replaced with the preferred phase psychological health. Professionally speaking, psychological health is considered a foundational quality that characterizes the importance of maintaining the responsible psychological functioning necessary to attain professional performance (W. B. Johnson et al., 2005). The concept of psychological health is also referenced in the *Psychodynamic Diagnostic Manual,* which was developed by psychologists, to focus on the whole person and various stages of development (Gordon, 2010).

Bemak, Epp, and Keys (1999) identified attributes of psychological health that are vital to becoming a professional counselor. These attributes include interpersonal sensitivity; empathy and caring; a capacity for introspection; healthy interpersonal dynamics; and a commitment to personal growth, which includes a willingness to pursue personal counseling if needed. Some graduate training programs focus on the importance of addressing and facilitating psychological health through course requirements. Experiential classroom activities and assignments, such as self-reflection papers, small-group counseling experiences, peer-to-peer mentoring, and consultation with course professors, invite students to examine and address personal and professional issues. In addition, programs may require new students to complete a specific number of individual counseling sessions with a licensed mental health professional during their first year of academic study in order to enhance their own psychological health; to experience the counseling process as a client; and to facilitate personal awareness of their values, personal qualities, and motivations as they engage in their graduate studies in pursuit of their clinical profession of choice (Rollins College, 2017b).

Like much of the terminology described in this section, psychological health and psychological fitness are, in theory, important in the development of professional clinicians; however, when they remain undefined, without specific operationalized definitions that could support performance measurement or evaluation, these broad categorizations of desirable conduct and professional behavior expected of clinical trainees are of minimal use to faculty and supervisors in gatekeeping roles. Terminology used to describe the functioning of students and supervisees should ideally be consistent across the clinical professions. Common agreement would provide consistency and common ground, lending strength to the importance and value of monitoring professional performance to those within the profession as well as stakeholders and consumers of clinical services. Furthermore, identifying specific qualities, characteristics, and behaviors of functioning or expectations for professional conduct is ineffective to those responsible for gatekeeping—primarily faculty and supervisors but also peer colleagues—when terminology is not operationalized by specific behavioral descriptions that can be measured and evaluated (Homrich, 2009).

Nonacademic Versus Academic Factors

The term ***nonacademic factors*** has been used to describe program requirements that are not categorized as either traditional academic knowledge acquisition activities or the development and demonstration of clinical skill (Homrich et al., 2014). Terms and criteria for intrapersonal and interpersonal functioning and the professional behavior or conduct of a clinical trainee have often been conceptualized under the category of nonacademic factors for the purposes of gatekeeping (Koerin & Miller, 1995). This distinction implies that academic and nonacademic expectations are separate categories and that the latter is not valued as a requirement of academic performance under the purview of faculty, supervisors, or a credible endeavor within the domain of higher education. This categorical separation makes it difficult to evaluate and enforce standards for a student's behavior because of the presumed personal or subjective nature of identifying criteria (Hensley, Smith, & Thompson, 2003; Homrich, 2009).

Continued research on behavioral indicators of performance—interpersonal, intrapersonal, and professional—would be beneficial in establishing guidelines and procedures for clearly identifying, defining, and evaluating behaviors essential to achievement as a clinician and the academic training of future clinicians. The profession-wide adoption of such guidelines would assist supervisors and inform supervisees of the parameters of behavioral performance that are assessed throughout the gatekeeping process (Bernard & Goodyear, 2014; Li, Lampe, Trusty, & Lin, 2009). For example, the forming of effective interpersonal relationships and openness to self-examination have been referred to as *nonacademic standards* (e.g., Bernard & Goodyear, 2014; Duba, Paez, & Kindsvatter, 2010); however, the legal and ethical expectation that these personal qualities are essential for professional functioning makes them compulsory for clinicians (and clinicians-in-training) and allocates them as requirements for professional training and thus as criteria addressed and evaluated under the academic umbrella.

The parsing of academic and nonacademic criteria risks negating qualities expected of students and supervisees that are and should be requirements of those enrolled in a professional training program. Demonstration of functional interpersonal and intrapersonal behaviors and professional conduct is expected of clinical practitioners and should thus be expected during the training period. These qualities are also taught in graduate programs as directed by ethics codes and mandated in licensure laws. They are the expected outcomes of the professional identity development process that occurs within the academic arena of a training program and are thus subject like all other aspects of the educational and field experience milieu to the gatekeeping mandate (Knoff & Prout, 1985; Wayne, 2004). It is recommended that all expectations of a clinical training program be classified as academic requirements and not categorized separately.

Legal Implications of Nonacademic Terminology

The inclusion of personal and professional behavior in academic standards is somewhat unique to the fields of mental health counseling, psychology, social work, and marriage and family therapy but also extends to other medical professions. The expectations for professional conduct may be in contrast to those of other graduate education programs in the arts and sciences that are generally not concerned about evaluating the personal and professional behavior of students as a condition of completing an academic program. Thus, if students are required to meet standards of personal and professional behavior to complete a graduate program, it is critical that this conduct be evaluated as a component of mandatory competencies and therefore considered an ***academic factor.***

The term *nonacademic factors* and related descriptors (e.g., *nonacademic traits, nonacademic standards,* and *nonacademic behaviors*) have also been implicated as problematic language in the gatekeeping process (Bernard & Goodyear, 2014; Knoff & Prout, 1985; Wayne, 2004) in litigation cases when students and supervisees have been dismissed from clinical programs because of interpersonal, intrapersonal, and professional conduct when remediation efforts have been unsuccessful. Flanders (2008) noted that courts typically grant judicial deference to institutions of higher education by upholding dismissals based on disciplinary concerns such as student behaviors or standards of professionalism expected in the academic setting. Thus, "appropriate professional behavior is an academic requirement rather than a misconduct issue" (Cobb & Jordan, 1989, p. 90). Medicine, also a clinical training profession, has established case law that supports student remediation and dismissal for professional and personal behavior as part of the academic requirements of a training program. Knoff and Prout (1985) cited a 1975 court decision that supported interpersonal skills, attitudes, and professional character as appropriately included under the umbrella of academic performance in the case of a medical school dismissal involving program faculty. These authors went on to state that

> the inclusion of professionally related interpersonal skills within the academic domain provides a firm rationale for the evaluation and, if necessary, dismissal of psychology graduate students because of problems in this area as well as problems in the more traditional academic knowledge and skill performance areas. (1985, p. 792)

Some attorneys have also recommended refraining from using the phrase *academic versus nonacademic* when evaluating the competencies of supervisees because the term *nonacademic* may be defined or viewed differently by the courts and by jury members and may be a point of legal contention for a student dismissed from a graduate program (Bernard & Goodyear, 2014; Forrest et al., 1999; Homrich, 2009; Knoff & Prout, 1985; Wayne, 2004). The recommendation from the legal community is that if criteria are required for graduation from a program or for the advancement of a supervisee into the profession, such as for licensure, then they are academic factors. Forrest el al. (1999) recommended use of the term professional in place of academic and nonacademic when evaluating trainee competencies (Homrich, 2009). Use of the term professional when discussing competencies can serve as a reminder of the ethical behavior that is expected of educators, supervisors, and supervisees. At the minimum, the current literature recommends that the term nonacademic be eliminated from the lexicon of gatekeeping, from graduate catalogs, and from published program requirements.

Ethical and Legal Terminology in Gatekeeping

Defining ethical and legal terminology relevant to gatekeeping can be challenging, especially for mental health professionals or supervisors who do not have extensive legal training or who are not attorneys (Wheeler & Bertram, 2015). Professional associations develop ethics codes for their professional members to define guidelines of ***ethical behavior*** (i.e., moral or good behavior), for "member decision making and, when necessary, [to] provide a basis for regulating member behavior" (Bernard & Goodyear, 2014, p. 253). Ethics codes and standards of conduct are constructed with careful and continuous vetting by members of professional associations. Codes of ethics set forth conditions for membership and provide guidelines and standards that "serve as the basis for processing inquiries and ethical complaints" (Wheeler & Bertram, 2015, p. 49). The term ***law*** is defined "as a set of rules, enacted by a legislative body, that governs a particular activity within society" (Wheeler & Bertram, 2015, p. 6).

The professional codes of conduct and standards for practice for psychology, mental health counseling, and related professions, along with accreditation standards, provide the foundation for addressing problems of professional competency. In the clinical professions, ethics codes are constructed to protect and promote the best interests of clientele engaged in services, research participants, trainees engaged in learning and supervision, and the profession itself by inspiring members of professional organizations to perform to the level of best practice. Ethics codes of professional organizations are the "standards adopted . . . to govern the definitions of ethical behavior for their members" (Welfel, 2006, p. 17) and are utilized in many graduate programs as standards against which to qualitatively assess the professional competency of students. Clinical educators and supervisors are mandated by ethics codes to respond and "take action in situations of personal or professional performance concerns" (Homrich, 2009, p. 8) in their role as gatekeepers. Students and supervisees who are knowledgeable about the professional values and ethical commitments required by their professional organizations are expected to have a better understanding of personal and professional competence.

Professional ethics codes speak to interpersonal, intrapersonal, and professional conduct and behaviors, but only generally. Gatekeeping expectations are not addressed in the same level of detail across ethics codes. Depending on the specific behavior expected of trainees and practicing clinicians, ethics codes address some topics in detail and others, not at all. In addition, the ethical standards adopted and the depth to which they are defined vary significantly across the clinical profession, as the following examples show. The *ACA Code of Ethics* (ACA, 2014a) addresses ethical standards of behavior throughout the code. In Section F (Supervision, Training, and Teaching), counseling supervisors are obligated to monitor the services that are provided by supervisees, review their work, and "help them become prepared to serve a range of diverse clients" (Section F.1.a.). Section F.6.b. specifically addresses gatekeeping and remediation in terms of reviewing the requirements of ongoing evaluation of supervisees, securing remedial assistance for supervisees when needed, and seeking consultation and documenting decisions to dismiss or refer supervisees for assistance. Section F.7.i., addressing field placements, discusses appropriate field placement and clinical experiences, and Section F.9. on evaluation and remediation discusses competency concerns. Alternatively, the AAMFT *Code of Ethics* (AAMFT, 2015) addresses professional competence and integrity in Standard III and responsibility to students and supervisees in Standard IV yet does not specifically address gatekeeping. The *NASW Code of Ethics* (NASW, 2017) states that although "a code of ethics cannot guarantee ethical behavior," it can set forth "values, ethical principles, and ethical standards to which professionals aspire and by which their actions can be judged" (p. 3), again without an explicit directive for gatekeeping.

In the United States, clinical licensing laws vary from state to state because individual legislatures have enacted statutes that provide definitions specific to the provision of mental health services called *practice acts.* These state-level statutory definitions determine what is legal clinical practice in each mental health specialty area and what clinical practitioners can (and cannot) do in terms of their scope of professional practice (Wheeler & Bertram, 2015). Although laws define the requirements for graduate education and postdegree supervision prior to independent licensure (Wheeler & Bertram, 2015), they typically do not dictate student professional performance, nor do they define how educational institutions design their academic programs. Educators and supervisors involved in the gatekeeping process should review guidelines pertaining to graduate education requirements and postdegree supervision requirements for the mental health professions on a state-by-state basis, as "an increasing number of state licensure boards are . . . beginning to address the roles and responsibilities of supervisors in their regulations" (Wheeler & Bertram, 2015, p. 84).

Individuals reading this book need to be attuned to the ethics codes of their particular profession as well as the specific licensure regulatory requirements in their state that govern not only their particular professional license but also the practice of their students and supervisees. This is especially important if a supervisee is seeking a professional license that is in a different profession from that of the supervisor (e.g., if a psychologist is supervising a mental health counselor). Legal terminology, when not clear, should be interpreted in consultation with staff of the licensure board or an attorney who specializes in health law. (See Notes From the Field 2.1.)

Notes From the Field 2.1

While testifying in a jury trial that resulted from dismissing a student for problematic interpersonal behavior, unprofessional conduct, and failure to participate in a remediation plan, faculty members were questioned by the plaintiff's attorney about their alleged premeditated decision to dismiss the student on the arbitrary grounds that they did not like her personality or professional style. The plaintiff was convinced that the faculty members did not like her and was attempting to prove that they had conspired to capriciously terminate her enrollment prior to providing her with the opportunity to change her behavior, denying her due process. The university's case was supported by careful documentation procedures implemented by the program faculty. In one particular situation that had occurred prior to her dismissal, the student was being especially uncooperative about setting up a meeting with faculty intended to give her a forum to report on her fulfillment of a remediation plan assigned several months prior. A chain of eight e-mail messages from the department chair contradicted the student's claims. The messages recounted the agreement made during the remediation meeting to schedule a follow-up meeting during the fall semester and review the problem areas the student was supposed to have actively addressed in order to determine her readiness to continue in the graduate program. The correspondence offered multiple alternative dates for a meeting to allow the student to provide evidence of her participation in the remediation plan and change in behavior. The correspondence also clearly indicated that there was a deadline for the meeting because the faculty wanted to evaluate the student's completion of remediation requirements in order to place her for practicum the following semester. Thanks to the clear and deliberate documentation of intention and multiple efforts on the part of the faculty to provide opportunities to meet, the case was decided by a jury decision in favor of the university and program faculty.

Sources of Legal Mandates

Legal terms that may be relevant to the gatekeeping process include *statutory law*, *common law*, *criminal law*, *civil law*, *administrative law*, and *respondeat superior*. ***Statutory law*** refers to laws (statutes) created by a legislative body, whereas ***common law*** refers to "precedent set by cases in which judges make decisions" (Wheeler & Bertram, 2015, p. 6). Common law is sometimes referred to as ***case law.***

Two major categories of legal oversight are criminal law and civil law. ***Criminal law*** refers to "acts that are prosecuted by the government, not by private individuals" (Wheeler & Bertram, 2015, p. 44), and ***civil law*** "generally includes everything that is not criminal in nature concerning the civil rights of individuals or other bodies" (p. 44). Also of importance to mental health professionals is the term ***administrative law,*** which is

> created (usually by a process of *rulemaking*) by government administrative agencies charged with the task of developing regulations to help define the laws, or statutes, that are passed by Congress or a state legislative body. (p. 45, italics in the original)

Administrative law is typically under the purview of professional licensing boards that have been given the authority by legislative bodies, such as state legislatures, to make rules that further clarify laws within a narrowly defined scope or delineated area. For example, a regulatory board composed of representatives of the profession is charged with the responsibility of further defining, clarifying, and operationalizing criteria for practice, discipline, and licensing of professionals based on statutes that have generally provided the framework for each of these categories. Boards also hold the responsibility of enforcing the rules and related laws of the profession within their state.

Gatekeepers need to understand legal terminology to protect their practice and should have an awareness of the potential legal risks of negligence or malpractice action claims. This is particularly important for clinical supervisors who could face legal action that arises from the actions of interns or supervisees who exhibit problems of professional competence. Hutchens et al. (2013) stated that "exposing a client to a counselor who is unable or unwilling to integrate ethical standards into his or her practice could result in a negligence lawsuit" (p. 85).

Awareness of legal terminology and potential risks that apply to employment is beneficial for field site supervisors who provide clinical supervision to graduate student interns and/or postdegree supervisees seeking licensure. Employment contracts have various types of clauses that pertain to liability and lawsuits that may include two theories of law: (a) "The counselor is acting as the agent for his or her supervisor or employer" (Wheeler & Bertram, 2015, p. 239) or (b) the notion of ***respondeat superior***, a Latin phrase meaning "let the master respond," in which the "employer is responsible for his or her subordinate" (p. 238; see Chapter 1). These "two theories of law permit employers of counseling professionals to be held liable for the negligent acts of their employees" (p. 238). This same premise holds true, even more strongly, for supervisors assigned to have oversight of and responsibility for the clinical work of supervisees.

Due Process

Problematic trainees who have difficulties with academic performance, clinical skills, ethical behavior, and interpersonal abilities and who are unable to demonstrate improvement during the remediation process may need to be dismissed from the clinical training program (Forrest et al., 1999; Wayne, 2004). Faculty and supervisors involved in the gatekeeping process have an obligation to act fairly and follow published procedures that protect the rights of students and supervisees.

Educators and clinical supervisors may be at risk ethically, legally, and professionally if they do not provide due process when dismissing individual students or supervisees from a training program.

Due process is a provision in the Fourteenth Amendment of the U.S. Constitution that protects citizens from being deprived of life, liberty, or property ("The Constitution," 1886). It consists of procedural and substantive elements that are applicable to the gatekeeping procedures of clinical educators and supervisors. ***Procedural due process*** is "a person's right to receive notice and the opportunity for a hearing prior to being deprived of a liberty or property interest" (Kerl, Garcia, McCullough, & Maxwell, 2002, p. 326). Wayne (2004) noted that this includes "a right to be heard by an unbiased decision maker, and a right of appeal" (p. 404). ***Substantive due process*** is defined as "the protection of such liberty and property rights from arbitrary and capricious interference, particularly by those acting as agents of the state" (Kerl et al., 2002, p. 326) and means that standards and procedures in graduate training programs must be applied consistently and fairly to all trainees or supervisees without prejudicial treatment by the program (Gilfoyle, 2008; Homrich, 2009; Knoff & Prout, 1985).

When issues pertaining to problematic behavior or performance arise in clinical trainees, whether they be students or supervisees, "every stage of the process, from informed consent, evaluation, notifications of problems, exchanges of communication, remediation plans, and dismissal procedures should be documented in detail by all representatives of the institution" (Homrich, 2009, p. 4). In the spirit of due process, students and supervisees must be given the right to explain or defend their actions as well as the opportunity to remedy their behavior and demonstrate achievement of an acceptable level of performance prior to being dismissed from a training program or deprived of the opportunity to obtain a professional license.

Under substantive due process, ***arbitrary*** and ***capricious*** action means that an individual or institution has used (or abused) its possession of power without cause or a reasonable basis and/or with bias or inadequate consideration of the circumstances. This applies to cases that lack a rational connection between the facts and actions taken (Knoff & Prout, 1985). This might include unexplained dismissal or inconsistent application of policies or disciplinary procedures across trainees by clinical educators, supervisors, and/or related administrators and institutions. In order to avoid charges of arbitrary and capricious acts, educators and supervisors must maintain meticulous and consistent procedural standards "in order to be protected legally when taking disciplinary action for students' interpersonal performance or psychological competence" (Homrich, 2009, p. 4). To mitigate charges of arbitrary and capricious action, clinical training programs are advised to publish formal policy statements and procedures addressing the conditions that constitute problematic performance, accompanied by clearly described remedial procedures and consequences that the program or supervisor will utilize when encountering and supporting change in a problematic student (Homrich, 2009). Knoff and Prout (1985) cited legal cases that highlight the critical importance of notifying or informing trainees of problematic behavior, and in circumstances "regarding termination, evaluation, and due process, professional programs must provide specific feedback in any form to the endangered student prior to termination" (p. 794). (See On the Legal Side 2.1.)

Conclusion

In conclusion, the wide range of terminology used to describe problematic behavior in students and supervisees—and the inconsistency with which these terms are applied from program to program, supervisor to supervisor, and profession to profession—has made it difficult to establish universal standards of conduct across the clinical professions. This variation increases the risk of legal reprisal for faculty and respondeat superiors in the gatekeeping process, especially when institutional policies neglect to observe due process rights. Developing a shared, consistent lexicon to describe categories of professional conduct and specific behavioral expectations would be beneficial in creating a foundation for a universally recognized gatekeeping lexicon and would benefit not only the mental health professions but also those engaging in legal processes. Once this is accomplished, fair and accurate assessment strategies for evaluating trainee professional com-

On the Legal Side 2.1

In her article about legal guidelines for dismissing students for poor performance in social work, Wayne (2004) discussed several seminal legal cases that provide guidance to faculty and supervisors on applying due process procedures in gatekeeping situations. The key components of procedural due process include the following:

- The trainee should receive notice of the concerns and possible consequences if the behavior does not change.
- The trainee should receive the opportunity to be heard before a decision is made.
- The trainee should be given information about his or her right to appeal an adverse decision.

It is important to incorporate these criteria into departmental or agency policy guidelines for responding to problematic trainees. Wayne included additional recommendations in her article for articulating program policies to avoid violating students' and supervisees' legal rights as well as case examples.

petency and performance and standardized procedures for addressing problematic behavior can be implemented. These efforts will assist in ensuring that administrators, educators, supervisors, and students are aware of the professional expectations integral to graduate studies, clinical training, and postgraduate training, ultimately strengthening the universal regard for and implementation of gatekeeping as a professional commitment with a common language across professions. (See What Would You Do? 2.1.)

Key Points and Best Practices

- Utilize the current professional literature to construct defined terms for developing gatekeeping policies and procedures.
- Consider constructing a glossary of key terms related to the gatekeeping process for the benefit of students, supervisors, and administrators. This effort will also support the faculty, particularly new faculty, in being consistent when interpreting policy and making determinations.
- Realize that expectations for gatekeeping are not addressed in the same level of detail in all ethics codes. Consider referencing ethics or professional literature from allied mental health professions that have extensively developed gatekeeping directives and guidelines.

What Would You Do? 2.1

A new student in your psychology doctoral program is enrolled in your introductory course. Frances is frequently late for class and occasionally leaves early. In addition, you notice that Frances's clothing is unlaundered, wrinkled, and at times has an adverse odor. This is more typical than not for this student, and you notice that the other students are avoiding interactions with Frances, who does not seem to notice or care. This same comportment is noticed by other faculty members as the semester continues. Despite this, Frances's grades are excellent, and assignments are turned in at or in advance of the deadline. This adds to your reluctance to approach this student about concerns of a personal nature.

What would you do?

Given Frances's excellent academic performance, what leverage do you have to comment on or complain about her personal care practices?

How would you approach this topic with a student?

Would your approach be different if you were the same gender as Frances?

Would your approach be different if you were a different gender than Frances?

How would you respond to a student who suggests that you have no right to comment on his or her personal choices and that doing so is overstepping your bounds as a professor?

- Investigating the recommended practices of other professions in this realm, especially counseling and psychology, not only provides additional information but demonstrates an effort to determine best practices in gatekeeping, which is especially important in cases of highly problematic students or supervisees.
- Stay attuned to the ethics codes, licensure laws, regulatory decisions, and legal trends that govern your specific profession, and educate colleagues, students and supervisees accordingly.
- Legal terminology and interpretation, when not clear, should occur in consultation with an attorney that specializes in health law or the regulatory board that enforces the statutes and rules of your profession.
- The wide range of terminology used to describe problematic behavior in students and supervisees and the inconsistency with which they are applied from program to program, supervisor to supervisor, and profession to profession have made it difficult to establish universal standards of conduct across the clinical professions. This variation increases the risk of legal reprisal for faculty and respondeat supervisors in the gatekeeping process.
- Developing a shared, consistent lexicon to describe appropriate categories of professional conduct and specific behavioral expectations would be beneficial in creating a foundation for universally recognized standards of conduct of clinical trainees, ideally among the allied mental health professions.

Chapter 3

Challenges and Strategies in Addressing Problematic Trainees

Leigh D. DeLorenzi

The Transformative Nature of Training

Students across the helping fields enter their training with a brave face and a caring heart, clothed in a desire to help people and make the world a better place. However, becoming an effective helper demands far more than attending class, reading books, listening to lectures, and passing exams. It requires a willingness to *trust the process* inherent in engaging in experiential learning and to personally approach the sealed, dark rooms of one's inner emotional world to discover oneself in order to better assist a future client who must do the same. Despite clinical educators' and supervisors' best efforts to prepare them for this experience, students may not anticipate the curriculum's propensity to elicit strong emotional reactions.

Clinicians-in-training are not just learning about mental illness and human suffering through an academic lens that partially desensitizes them to painful case scenarios and teaches them how to effectively help; they are also embarking on a journey that will necessitate intense introspective questioning about their personal beliefs, biases, and convictions. This can be life changing, deeply meaningful, and at times terrifying for students. For some, this process requires a deconstruction and rebuilding of the self and a close examination of one's innermost values, anguish, fears, regrets, prejudices, and traumas.

Facing their beliefs and experiences can cause people to feel like they are swimming against the riptides of their survival instincts that are protectively yanking them in the opposite direction.

One of the leading battle cries aimed at gatekeepers—*do no harm*—is most frequently interpreted as the primary ethical mandate to protect the public from an individual who has failed to meet the minimum competence requirements. A caricature of the nightmare trainee often emerges in one's mind, evoking images of a boundary-less, advice-giving, judgmental, self-centered, incompetent, unethical, predatory, overpriced, and undertrained practitioner. As gatekeepers, clinical educators and supervisors are told to keep their eyes peeled, to join ranks, to "Man the gates!" and remain alert for any harmful individuals trying to squeak through and contaminate the helping field with incompetent practice. However, gatekeepers are more than just witch hunters seeking to block the passage of delinquent trainees. Instead, gatekeeping is best viewed as an opportunity for enhanced training, assessment, nurturing, and support for all students—including the sometimes slow-to-develop or vulnerable trainee.

Consider, for example, trainees who arrive to their graduate programs with a personal history of severe and chronic trauma. These well-meaning students may be pushing themselves, in the name of professionalism, to report to a classroom environment that continuously evokes deep negative emotional and psychological experiences. As gatekeepers, educators and supervisors should have policies in place to assist in monitoring, slowing down, and supporting vulnerable trainees who are attempting to push through dangerous and destabilizing triggers. For some students, that danger takes the form of harmful coping styles, like an addiction relapse; for others, severe, terrifying, and/or disruptive episodes of reexperiencing or dissociation. The destabilizing impact of these repeated and intense trauma triggers can also usher in depression, panic attacks or other anxiety reactions, and/or suicidal thoughts, to name a few of the more severe responses. Thus, gatekeeping policies should be designed to protect *all* parties—not just future clients but also the struggling trainee and all other students sharing the training environment.

The most rewarding part about training future helpers is also the most challenging. Educators and supervisors are charged with engaging adult learners in a manner that simultaneously celebrates and confronts a boundless diversity of ideas, norms, cultures, trauma histories, moral centers, political beliefs, gender expectations, and values. In order to support the learning and emotional well-being of trainees, educators must master a dual awareness: paying careful attention to the functioning of each individual student while simultaneously monitoring the interaction of the whole group. This chapter discusses the first task of all gatekeepers: the mandate to support, encourage, and educate the struggling trainee while also enforcing fair and equitable remedial opportunities for all students. Gatekeeping does not occur before diligent efforts to support student learning and development have been exhausted.

Trainees as Developmental Beings

Chapter 9 emphasizes the importance of selecting and utilizing gatekeeping assessments that consider important developmental characteristics of trainees. When gatekeepers are able to view students' development as an evolving, progressive process that might be responsive to intervention (Kegan, 1982), they move away from the conceptualization that trainees are permanently stuck with fixed, inflexible traits and instead are able to focus on their ability to improve trainees' evolving capacities for becoming effective clinicians. For a more detailed discussion of trainee development, please refer to Chapter 4.

Conflicting Philosophies and the Gatekeeping Mandate

Gatekeeping requires faculty to balance the student's rights with client protection issues and institutional pressures—a time-consuming effort that may still boil down to the student's viewpoint against the trainer's perspective (Bemak, Epp, & Keys, 1999). Laws, ethics codes, and researchers across the helping professions all recognize formalized student review procedures as necessary and helpful for decreasing the number of problematic trainees in the field (Gaubatz & Vera, 2006), yet gatekeepers struggle with how best to intervene and remediate struggling trainees. Furthermore, programs in related fields within the helping professions have different needs and priorities, which has led to inconsistent (and sometimes nonexistent) policies for addressing problematic professional behavior (Hensley, Smith, & Thompson, 2003).

The American Psychological Association's (2017c) *Ethical Principles of Psychologists and Code of Conduct* highlights the gatekeeping mandate in Principle C, with Standards 7.06, 1.05, 2.06, 3.04, and 3.08 being most relevant to gatekeeping obligations. Similarly, the *ACA Code of Ethics* (American Counseling Association, 2014a) states that educators and supervisors must not endorse trainees whom they believe to be impaired in any way. Moreover, for doctoral students seeking to become counselor educators, the Council for Accreditation of Counseling and Related Educational Programs (2015) Standards require future counselor educators in doctoral training programs accredited by this body to receive training in the detection of problem competence, along with how to provide useful and corrective feedback. These doctoral programs must demonstrate how Standards 2.i and 3.f are covered in the doctoral curriculum. Specifically, counselor educators must receive training on "evaluation, remediation, and gatekeeping in clinical supervision" (p. 34) as well as "screening, remediation, and gatekeeping functions relevant to teaching" (p. 35).

However, some researchers argue that as mentoring bonds strengthen between trainer and trainee, gatekeepers encounter a conflict between their roles as nurturing professional advocate and evaluator (W. B. Johnson, 2007; Le Maistre, Boudreau, & Pare, 2006; Lichtenberg et al., 2007). W. B. Johnson and colleagues (2008) discussed the role conflict, definitional ambiguity, and anxiety that emerge for many gatekeepers responding to trainee competence problems. For example, the authors asserted that "it is often quite difficult to actively foster growth and development, to be compassionate, to be supportive, and to engage students as a mentor while simultaneously rendering objective and accurate summative evaluations" (p. 591). Furthermore, rather than working collaboratively to address problems of trainee competence, educators, field supervisors, and credentialing boards play a game of hot potato with problematic trainees—all assigning the responsibility and blame to one another with little sense of shared responsibility (p. 590).

In their article on gatekeeping in counselor education, Glance, Fanning, Schoepke, Soto, and Williams (2012) further expanded on the emotionally vulnerable and, at times, painful process of gatekeeping. They highlighted the naturally empathic nature of faculty and supervisors whose desire to help usurps their decision to pursue dismissal. In some cases, gatekeepers continue to advance incompetent trainees because of how far they have come in their training, hoping deficiencies will dissipate or be screened out at the credentialing stage (W. B. Johnson et al., 2008). Also, training directors and supervisors may adopt different gatekeeping philosophies altogether. For example, faculty within the same department may hold opposing views about what actually constitutes incompetence (Forrest, Elman, Gizara, & Vacha-Haase, 1999; Kaslow et al., 2007). A body of research identifies factors associated with miscarried gatekeeping, including writing inflated letters of recommendation, allowing likeability to influence grading (R. K. Miller & Van Rybroek, 1988; Tabachnick, Keith-Spiegel, & Pope, 1991), not fully revealing competence shortcomings to licensing boards, and/or failing to admit when remediation efforts are unsuccessful (W. B. Johnson & Campbell, 2004). Other research shows how untenured faculty might avoid gatekeeping for fear it will lead to unflattering teaching evaluations (Gaubatz & Vera, 2002).

Gatekeeping avoidance leads not only to greater impairment in a troubled student but also to greater liability faced by the institution (Glance et al., 2012) educating, supervising, or employing the trainee. For example, programs that graduate a student who does not meet the minimum competence requirements may be held responsible for injuries or damages to a client who was harmed by that student (Enochs & Etzbach, 2004; Polychronis & Brown, 2016; Saccuzzo, 1997). Thus, incorporating a standardized process for identifying, discussing, evaluating, and reporting students of concern and creating opportunities for faculty and supervisors to share trainee observations and experiences with one another is essential. These discussions should be built into regular faculty meetings, retreats, annual student reviews, and site visits with supervisors rather than only emerging on an as-needed, reactive basis. Also, openly discussing common threats to successful gatekeeping can prevent instances of gateslipping and of unqualified trainees progressing to the next checkpoint. The following list summarizes common themes that may contribute to gateslipping.

Gatekeeper Guilt Leads to Leniency/Hesitation

- The student spent a large amount of money in the program and/or has or is connected to someone in a position of power or influence.
- The student is close to graduation.
- The student is in personal crisis, and faculty want to help or support the student.

Gatekeeper Fears Lead to Avoidance

- Fear of poor student evaluations
- Fear of the student due to intimidation or threats
- Fear of the complications that gatekeeping processes entail, which leads to avoidance of development of program standards for personal behavior and professional conduct
- Fear of legal action/lawsuits against the faculty member, department, college, or university
- Fear of reduced student retention, which results in financial hardships for the program and scrutiny by administrators

Gatekeeper Confusion Leads to Avoidance

- Uncertainty as to whether behavior is developmentally appropriate or a sign of impairment
- Uncertainty as to whether a student is exercising his or her spiritual/religious beliefs in a manner that imposes on clients
- Uncertainty as to whether a student is exercising free speech
- Uncertainty due to inconsistent departmental enforcement (i.e., the department allowed other students to behave in a similar way without remediation)
- Hopefulness that inconsistent unprofessional behavior will become more consistently appropriate on its own

Timing Challenges, Due Process Violations, or Gatekeeper Negligence

- Busy schedules or negligence prevents remediation action in a reasonable timeframe.
- Busy schedules or negligence causes faculty to forget to follow up with a problematic student.
- Time and attention must be dedicated to more pressing departmental matters.

- Faculty and/or site supervisors found out about problematic behavior after the student had already graduated.
- Faculty fail to provide the student with formal feedback early enough in the program.
- Faculty fail to provide the student with the opportunity to improve or change problematic behavior.
- Faculty and/or site supervisors are not monitoring the student closely enough to have a solid understanding of his or her behavior.

Policy or Administration-Related Barriers

- Faculty attempt to remove a student, but the administration overturns the student's dismissal because of lack of understanding of or regard for the profession's standards and ethics.
- The department does not have support from the administration to exercise gatekeeping (i.e., the administration frowns on efforts to remove students for reasons other than academic failure because of pressures related to student retention and/or avoidance of legal action).
- The department does not have or use established or formalized gatekeeping procedures.

Due Process and Gatekeeping Procedures

Hutchens, Block, and Young (2013) discussed critical considerations encountered by clinical educators when developing gatekeeping procedures. First, all gatekeeping efforts should be anchored in the program's responsibility to support and educate its students. In addition, gatekeepers should recognize the subjective nature of supervision while keeping consideration for future client welfare at the forefront during student evaluations. Last, gatekeeping procedures must provide students with the opportunity respond to formal feedback and, in many cases, allow adequate time and occasion for students to address the feedback and demonstrate change. Therefore, all gatekeeping procedures should be designed with due process in mind. Abiding by due process procedures ensures that programs make decisions based on thoughtful evaluative guidelines that are not arbitrary or personal (Lamb et al., 1987).

What Is Due Process?

Due process encompasses a set of practices and procedures that are aimed at protecting students' rights as consumers of education. The Foundation for Individual Rights in Education's (2016) *Guide to Due Process and Campus Justice* traces due process back to medieval England and describes its evolution over centuries as a way to ensure that accusatory proceedings lead to accurate and truthful results. This legal doctrine is emphasized as a necessary part of remediation across ethics codes in the helping profession (e.g., American Counseling Association, 2014a, Standard F.9.b.).

The relevant gatekeeping literature discusses both substantive and procedural due process as necessitating (a) notification to the student, usually in writing, of the decision to remediate or dismiss; (b) the opportunity for the student to respond to the decision; and (c) a means afforded to the student of appealing the decision (Forrest et al., 1999; Gilfoyle, 2008; Henderson, 2010; Kerl, Garcia, McCullough, & Maxwell, 2002; Knoff & Prout, 1985; Lumadue & Duffey, 1999; McAdams & Foster, 2007; Wayne, 2004). Wilkerson (2006) further suggested the application of a therapeutic process model for training, in which commonly accepted components found in the therapeutic process are applied to gatekeeping procedures. Accordingly, components such as informed consent, intake and assessment, evaluation, treatment planning and follow-up, and termination are reflected in remediation efforts to address problematic students. Although Chapter 10 discusses a step-by-step process for designing remediation procedures in line with due process requirements, the following sections provide a helpful overview.

Step 1: Communicate Concerns Early, Clearly, and Consistently

As mentioned in Chapter 9, programs should publish policies that clearly explain program standards and expectations for conduct in graduate catalogs, student handbooks, and published codes of conduct. This information is communicated at the preadmissions phase and made available to prospective and matriculated students through preapplication information sessions; at the point of applicant acceptance of an offer to enroll in the program; in new student orientations; and through program literature, marketing materials, and websites. Program literature and resources should inform students of the gatekeeping mandate and the specific times and methods by which each student will be evaluated.

Furthermore, Cole (1991) pointed out that courts tend to support program decisions related to admissions or dismissal as long as the program standards are reasonable, fair, and not arbitrary or capricious. Therefore, programs should make every attempt to link published program standards to relevant ethical and conduct standards in the field and to fairly and consistently apply these standards to all trainees. When concerns arise, faculty should endeavor to communicate their concerns early, clearly, and in relation to the published standards. Thorough, accurate, and timely documentation of notification content and procedures is crucial for providing evidence of adequate due process at every stage of the student feedback process and is discussed at length in Chapter 11.

Beyond informing students through documented policies, gatekeepers should reflect on how their direct interactions with trainees might help (or harm) an outcome. When a student goofs off in a benign way during class or at his or her clinical site, how might the gatekeeper intervene to support student learning while nurturing a positive relationship? Of greater concern, what does a student hear or experience through direct interactions with his or her instructor or supervisor when that student has violated a more serious behavioral standard(or standards)? Consider the real example of classroom misconduct described in "What Would You Do? 3.1" (the details of this case have been modified to obscure the identity of the student and to protect privacy).

Tips to Consider for Interacting With Trainees

The following list includes ways a gatekeeper might intervene in a manner that (a) nurture a positive relationship, (b) educate the student on behavioral standards and expectations, and (c) hold the student accountable:

What Would You Do? 3.1

Caroline is a 23-year-old student who was accepted into a master's-level training program shortly after she graduated with her bachelor's degree in psychology. On several occasions, you have witnessed unprofessional behavior in the classroom that you attribute to a lack of maturity. For instance, when students are taking their final exam, Caroline finishes early and begins talking and laughing with a peer in a manner that disrupts other test takers. As her volume escalates, you make the following announcement to the class: "Students, please remember to refrain from talking until all test takers are finished." A few minutes later, Caroline erupts in distracting giggles as you witness her passing a note to her friend several seats away. You say, "Caroline, I'm going to have to ask you to either sit quietly in your chair or leave the classroom." Caroline becomes tearful and shouts, "Are you kidding me?" She then stands up, slams her book on the table, aggressively shoves her chair out of the way, and runs out of the room. After class, you ask to speak to Caroline privately. Tearfully, she says, "You didn't have to shush me like I was in grade school. You embarrassed me in front of everyone!"

What would you do?

What are the problematic student behaviors you observed in this case scenario?

Have you ever witnessed similar behavior as either a peer graduate student, an instructor, a supervisor, a professor, or an advisor?

What did you do?

What are your thoughts on how the situation was handled in this example?

What would you have said or done differently?

What are other ways one might address a student who consistently demonstrates benign yet disruptive behaviors in the classroom?

1. *Practice what you preach—use active listening.* "I can see that you're feeling embarrassed and upset by what happened in class tonight. I want to give you the opportunity to tell me what happened from your perspective."
2. *Educate and inform the student about behavioral expectations.* "Caroline, our profession outlines very specific expectations for professional behavior. It's important for you to understand that our classroom is considered a professional arena. As I mentioned on the first night of class, and as described in the syllabus, students are evaluated on dimensions of professional competence, including their capacity for professionalism in the classroom. Things like classroom outbursts, disrespectful exchanges, showing up late on a regular basis—these are all examples of behaviors that fall below our behavioral standards and expectations. How you conduct yourself in the classroom is important to us because it might also indicate how you will conduct yourself in other professional settings, like at your training site or in session with clients." The instructor can take it a step further and point out specific standards of conduct as described in the student handbook, ethics codes, and/or syllabus.
3. *Hold the student accountable.* "Clinicians-in-training need to demonstrate an ability to engage thoughtfully and professionally in the classroom at all times. This shows us that you can maintain appropriate interpersonal boundaries—a skill that is crucial for interacting with future clients. Because I've witnessed this pattern of conduct in the classroom with you several times before, I think it's time we come up with a plan to monitor your professional classroom behavior as well as help you improve in this area. Being mindful of your impact on the learning environment, regulating emotional outbursts, and maintaining respectful boundaries in the classroom are things I'm going to be watching more closely as we progress this semester. In addition, I wonder if there's anything I can do to support you to be successful in this aspect of your professional growth." Depending on the student's response, it may also be necessary to talk specifically about consequences for not meeting the stated expectations, both verbally and in writing.

Step 2: Provide Students With Time and a Forum to Address Concerns

When a trainee is identified as violating a behavioral standard, it can be helpful to call an initial meeting with the problematic trainee to (a) clearly outline the concern(s) to the student; (b) provide an opportunity for the student to give his or her side of the story; (c) educate the student about specific ethics codes, laws, and program policies that relate to the issue; and (d) determine whether the student is open to learning about ways to improve. Although it is always possible that a student may not be interested in working with faculty through remediation, it is essential that faculty at least offer the student the opportunity to learn and improve. It is also important that a student be informed of the potential consequences of not addressing the identified problems (Forrest et al., 1999).

Researchers strongly emphasize the need for programs to provide assistance to problematic students to remedy any identified problems (Glance et al., 2012; Hutchens et al., 2013). This is at the heart of why remediation plans were invented—to help *remedy* an identified problem. Accordingly, in order for students to accomplish outlined tasks or action plans associated with remediation plans, they need sufficient time to work on resolving the issue and providing a track record of demonstrating that their performance meets standards. There are no legal definitions of exactly what constitutes a reasonable amount of time, and therefore timelines will vary according to the nature of the issue. Furthermore, timelines are usually decided by program faculty but also agreed on with the student prior to the enforcement of remedial requirements.

In addition, students need a forum for addressing problems. For example, if the plan outlines a requirement for personal counseling, they may need appropriate referrals as well as information on whether a signed release will be needed to allow faculty to communicate with the therapist. In another example, if additional training is required to address the behavior or concern (e.g., workshops on ethical behavior or book reading requirements), the trainee may need assistance connecting to appropriate resources associated with these requirements. Or it is possible that the student needs regular access to mentoring with faculty members to help deepen his or her understanding of the dilemma and the changes in performance expected and allow the faculty member close contact to monitor the student's progress.

Step 3: Provide Students With a Means of Appeal

Checking in with a student during the course of the remediation process is necessary to assess whether he or she needs additional direction, support, or adjustments to the original plan. It is only *after* the plan is not satisfactorily followed that a committee should make decisions related to a problematic student's standing in the program. Students who are dismissed as a result of unsatisfactory remediation outcomes should receive information about the available appeals process, such as formal communication with the department chair, dean, or other members of the administration within the institution (Frame & Stevens-Smith, 1995; Kerl et al., 2002; Ziomek-Daigle & Christensen, 2010). Information on student appeals should be discussed, formalized, and published by faculty and the administration and made available to all students through program handbooks and policy standards. These policies should also be explicitly included in correspondence related to remediation and dismissal. See Appendix B for a sample published appeals process in counselor education.

Upholding Ethics While Minimizing Litigation

More and more, college and university decisions are being challenged in court, which requires that both faculty and administrators study, understand, and follow case law affecting admissions or dismissal decisions. Institutions and students have contractual relationships. Contract theory states that an institution must honor its published criteria, which can lead to challenges when applied to university–student relations if gatekeeping policies are not published and made explicit. Although caution should be exercised when relying solely on the fiduciary relationship to inform dismissal decisions related to gatekeeping (Cole, 1991), this further highlights the need for gatekeeping processes and procedures to be published and disseminated to all applicants and matriculated students. Making expectations known in advance to applicants and students is particularly critical for training programs in the mental health professions, as well as other clinical vocations, because of the additional expectations for performance. Specifically, in addition to the expectations for academic achievement typical of all students regardless of discipline, clinical training includes a specific skill set. Furthermore, this clinical skill set is based on interpersonal capabilities and professional conduct as defined by ethics, laws, and administrative codes unique to the practice of therapeutic services. A lack of necessary interpersonal, intrapersonal, and professional skills can harm individuals seeking mental health services. Given the challenge that universities face in justifying changes in the implied contract between students and institutions, training departments should not only publish but also regularly examine and revise their gatekeeping policies and procedures for accuracy. These periodic reviews should include consideration of faculty fidelity in following and executing the standards (Hutchens et al., 2013). Furthermore, admissions and/or gatekeeping standards must not discriminate on the basis of race, sex, age, handicap, or citizenship, which is a basic requirement of equal protection under the law. Supervisors and educators should also know that documentation must be maintained to comply with the provisions of the Family Educational Rights and Privacy Act of 1974 (Cole, 1991).

As decided in the 1986 federal court case *Phelps v. Washburn University of Topeka*,

> admission into a training program is considered not a constitutional right but a privilege. To that end, professional programs are allowed to define special behavioral criteria or requirements by which applicants and students are deemed suitable as long as they are relevant to the lawful mission of the program and are applied equally to all students.

In addition to publishing and disseminating performance standards and gatekeeping procedures, the following list summarizes helpful tips for reducing liability in professional training:

1. *Nurture positive relationships.* Harmonious relationships between faculty and students are associated with reduced liability risks. Pollock and Poteet (1983) found that nursing students were less likely to sue a program if they believed that they were treated fairly and impartially and if decisions were made with careful deliberation of known criteria.
2. *Maintain thorough and accurate documentation.* As discussed in Chapter 11, maintaining routine documentation with dates, times, locations, names, signatures, and an outlined basis for concern can be powerful evidence of due process validation in court. Two separate court cases, *Keeton v. Anderson-Wiley* (2011) and *Ward v. Wilbanks* (2010), demonstrated how incorporating documentation can help show how standards are communicated to students, such as having them sign statements acknowledging that they have read relevant program rules and handbooks (McAdams & Foster, 2007).
3. *Standardize and follow gatekeeping procedures.* In the same court cases listed previously, faculty did not act on troubling behavior when it appeared in the classroom. As a result, the court did not support some of the actions taken by program faculty. Therefore, Kerl et al. (2002) and McAdams and Foster (2007) recommend standardizing procedures for responding to problematic student behavior wherever possible throughout the student's experience in the program.

Conclusion

In conclusion, gatekeeping is a long and dynamic process that is most effective when implemented as a team approach rather than a series of tasks in isolation. Depending on the student or scenario, gatekeeping often requires considerable endurance from faculty and site supervisors who are juggling a long list of additional responsibilities, including observing, communicating with, teaching, and evaluating every trainee from his or her first step into the helping profession to graduation and beyond. Because of its complexity and intensity, gatekeeping can be an easy process to avoid; however, well-executed gatekeeping yields benefits for students, supervisees, programs, and the community that far outweigh the challenges.

Key Points and Best Practices

- Educators and supervisors are charged with engaging adult learners in a manner that simultaneously celebrates and confronts a boundless diversity of ideas, norms, cultures, trauma histories, moral centers, political beliefs, gender expectations, and values.

The first task of all gatekeepers is the mandate to support, encourage, and educate the struggling trainee while also enforcing fair and equitable remedial opportunities for all students in clinical mental health training programs.

- Gatekeeping decisions are not made before diligent efforts to support student learning and development have been exhausted.
- Because professional training programs are capable of eliciting a transformational crisis for students, faculty members and supervisors must be able to tell the difference between a developmentally expected response to a stressful training environment and one that requires remediation or dismissal.
- Despite a clear ethical mandate to engage in fair, consistent gatekeeping procedures, many programs fail to exercise proper gatekeeping because of conflicting philosophies, priorities, and practices across trainers. To decrease these instances, gatekeepers should design and implement gatekeeping procedures that uphold due process requirements.
- Standardizing gatekeeping procedures while regularly revising program policies for accuracy helps reduce the risk of liability faced by programs that need to dismiss a student with problematic behavior.

Chapter 4

Trainee Development and Factors Affecting Behavior

Page L. Thanasiu

I often tell students that it would be wonderful if we could teach them to be mental health professionals in only a semester or two; however, there is a time-intensive process of development that each must undergo. This developmental process pertains partly to students acquiring the knowledge that will inform concepts such as their professional identities, perceptions of helping skills, and insight into legal and ethical guidelines. Comprehension of these concepts can usually be measured academically; however, other processes taking place (e.g., along the continuums of personal growth and professional identity development) are more difficult to quantify and thus challenging to use as the basis for advancing students. Supervisees' abilities to comprehend and respect cultural diversity, develop cognitive complexity, and attain personal insight into their own values and triggers are every bit as important as their academic knowledge. When students enter a training program, they are not expected to already be highly self-aware, nonjudgmental, and professional in demeanor. It is, however, expected that they will make great strides toward acquiring these attitudes while in training and then continue to grow after graduation throughout subsequent supervisee roles.

A common underlying belief within the helping professions is that all people are capable of growth and positive change. This value keeps us as mental health professionals in business and allows us to believe in our clients and encourage them to achieve the goals they set for themselves. This same value is reflected in how faculty and supervisors approach trainees with competency concerns: in the spirit of believing in the developmental process and positive growth. Consequently, some faculty experience an inherent values conflict when the process of gatekeeping ultimately involves preventing problematic trainees from achieving their professional goals. Despite this perspective, gatekeeping must be a priority within training programs if educators and supervisors are to protect the profession's reputation and the well-being of current and future clients.

As faculty and supervisors serve as gatekeepers monitoring student behavior during the learning and training process, it is important that they keep in mind the space and time needed for a student to develop into a clinical professional. In this chapter, you are reminded of the developmental processes that students and supervisees will undertake while in training. Some practices are explored that can help the supervisor or faculty member maintain a positive and proactive relationship while supporting a supervisee struggling to attain professional proficiency. It is important to remember that students should not become the enemy during their remediation process. At the same time, supervisors and educators must remain firmly planted in their given roles and avoid the slippery slope that can lead to crossing boundaries and counseling students who are struggling. Finally, contextual factors are examined in this chapter that can influence supervisees' behaviors as they navigate their training and development. To begin, let us consider what normal development looks like within the helping professions.

A Developmental Perspective

Cognitive Complexity

When considering the developmental stages of students and supervisees in the helping professions, it is important to recognize that no model will capture the experience of all individuals. Even so, research indicates that a helping professional's developmental process can often be broadly predictable along multiple continuums. Perry's (1970) cognitive development theory is applied to college students and provides the understanding that one begins with a highly dualistic, right/wrong conceptualization when learning a new field. During this dualistic stage, students in the helping professions believe that there must be one right way to approach a client, to respond to an ethical challenge, or to fulfill the counseling role. Students begin their early semesters needing a high degree of structure in assignments and the overall learning environment. At this early stage, they also tend to benefit from a more prescriptive approach to advising in which the faculty advisor helps them to organize their program of study, gives them resources and checklists, and answers their questions very specifically (Granello, 2006). Students are looking for factual knowledge and specific skills, and this concrete beginning stage for mental health professionals in training also applies to students who begin training at a later stage/age in life. Granello (2002) found that gains in cognitive complexity for counseling students were not related to grade point average, gender, age, or previous experience in the helping professions. Because graduate programs in the clinical professions enroll students with a wide range of ages, personal experiences, and intellectual abilities, it is important for faculty and supervisors to maintain some flexibility in expectations regarding the cognitive capacity and complexity of their trainees.

Loevinger's (1998) model of social–cognitive development, when applied to graduate counseling students, also describes an evolution over time toward more complex levels of meaning making, impulse control, interpersonal relations, and intrapersonal congruence (Cohn & Westenberg, 2004; Duys & Hedstrom, 2000). Mental health professionals with higher levels of cognitive complexity have been found to do the following:

- Formulate better clinical hypotheses (Holloway & Wampold, 1986; Holloway & Wolleat, 1980)
- Have stronger case conceptualizations and sophisticated client descriptions (Borders, 1989; Borders, Fong, & Neimeyer, 1986; Fong, Borders, Ethington, & Pitts, 1997; J. Martin, Slemon, Hiebert, Hallberg, & Cummings, 1989)
- Demonstrate less anxiety and self-focus (Birk & Mahalik, 1996)
- Exhibit greater flexibility (Holloway & Wampold, 1983; Stoppard & Miller, 1985)
- Make greater use of empathy in the client–counselor relationship (Lovell, 1999; Lyons & Hazier, 2002)
- Have a better understanding of the client–counselor relationship (Borders et al., 1986)

Consequently, facilitating supervisees' growth in cognitive complexity (e.g., through the inclusion of supervised experiential-rehearsal activities in the classroom) is a desired goal of those educating and supervising mental health professionals.

When Granello (2002) and Fong et al. (1997) applied these models of cognitive development to counseling students, they found that although students made small incremental gains throughout their educational programs, they experienced the most significant growth after their practicum class. In fact, Granello (2002) discovered that students at the end of practicum and at graduation are often best described by Perry's (1970) second developmental stage, which he termed *multiplistic*. In this stage, helping professionals have moved away from seeking one right answer or method for approaching a client and are aware that there may, in fact, be many right approaches or ways of responding. The confusion for a person in this stage of cognitive complexity stems from an inability to distinguish between approaches that may be more appropriate and other viable options. Supervisees can become overwhelmed by the multitude of possibilities and unable to form a hierarchy to help them decide their best course of action. An awareness of developmental appropriateness at this stage of training can assist faculty who are evaluating the progression of students in graduate programs. Developmental models can also be useful guides in determining further evaluation or a direction for remediation for students who have not demonstrated an expected level of cognitive development professionally (in the realm of clinical skill or content) or personally (in the contexts of interpersonal, intrapersonal, or professional behavior).

Once helping professionals graduate from their respective training programs, they typically become supervisees functioning in a professional capacity as they begin to work toward licensure. Cognitive development continues to progress long after graduation, with most clinicians believing that a significant amount of their learning and integration occurred more than 10 years after they had begun to practice (Skovholt & Ronnestad, 1992). Perry's (1970) final stage of relativistic thinking finds practitioners who are able to take multiple perspectives, discriminate among a vast array of reasonable options, synthesize large amounts of information, and use creativity to actively engage clients in a collaborative pursuit for personal solutions. These developmental stages, although linear in their order of achievement, are not necessarily permanent. To the contrary, even after attaining multiplistic and relativistic complexity within a particular realm, supervisees will naturally regress to a dualistic perspective when confronted with crises or high levels of stress (Tracey, Ellickson, & Sherry, 1989) and/or when encountering new categories of information, such as learning a new practice specialty or encountering unfamiliar clientele. This later stage of professional and personal development in the context of clinical training is more challenging for a supervisor to evaluate; however, the most important criteria to measure are supervisees' abilities to progressively expand their cognitive conceptualization of their clinical and interpersonal practice skills and advance their clinical judgment. As trainees gain experience, their clinical practice and conduct should reflect deepening cognitive complexity in relation to their personal and professional behaviors within the clinical setting.

Competency and Expertise

The field of psychology has focused on the stages of development that result in expertise while conceptualizing competency assessments for supervisees. The Competency Assessment Toolkit for Professional

Psychology (www.apa.org/ed/graduate/competency.aspx; see Kaslow et al., 2009) serves as a valuable collection of best practice resources for psychology programs and licensing boards to use to assess competence as students and practitioners develop professional knowledge, skills, and attitudes. The toolkit targets functional domains of competence, which include the development of professionalism, reflective practice, scientific knowledge and methods, relationships, individual and cultural diversity, ethical and legal standards and policy, and interdisciplinary systems. In conjunction with these domains, functional competencies are evaluated, which include assessment, intervention, consultation, research/evaluation, supervision, teaching, administration, and advocacy. Using the toolkit, supervisors are given an avenue to look for essential components and behavioral anchors that indicate whether the supervisee is demonstrating professional competence at a level of readiness for practicum, internship, or entry-level practice.

The level of readiness takes into consideration the fact that supervisees often progress through qualitatively distinct phases as they develop expertise (Alexander, 2004; Dreyfus & Dreyfus, 1986). Hatcher and Lassiter (2007) modified earlier category descriptions in order to make them more specific to the helping professions. At a novice level, students have little to no ability to analyze client problems or to understand and implement intervention skills. They have difficulty recognizing patterns or seeing the distinction between important and unimportant aspects of the client's story. They are best served by breaking down concepts and domains into elements that students with no experience can understand. Students reach the next level, intermediate, once they have continued through their coursework and experienced at least some level of practice and supervision. Hatcher and Lassiter emphasized that, prior to beginning practicum, students should be able to successfully demonstrate baseline competencies as they pertain to the following:

- *Interpersonal skills:* effective nonverbal and verbal communication, empathy and respect for others, openness to feedback
- *Cognitive skills:* intellectual curiosity, flexibility, problem solving, critical thinking, organized reasoning
- *Affective skills:* the ability to tolerate varying affects, interpersonal conflict, ambiguity or uncertainty
- *Personality/attitudes:* a desire to help others, openness to new ideas, honesty and integrity, personal courage, the ability to value ethical behavior
- *Expressive skills:* the capacity to communicate ideas, feelings, and information in verbal, nonverbal, and written form
- *Reflective skills:* the capacity to consider one's effect on others and to examine one's own motives, attitudes, and behaviors
- *Personal skills:* personal organization, hygiene, appropriate dress

At an intermediate level, helping professionals are able to recognize recurring domain features and conceptualize their client cases at a deeper level than surface level. Although they may be able to select appropriate interventions for a particular client, there is still a limited ability to generalize diagnostic and intervention skills to other situations. These trainees must rely on their supervisors to provide guidance in their practice. In fact, supervisees may, for a period of time during their development, conceptualize themselves as becoming "we" with the supervisor (Lent, Hackett, & Brown, 1998). This joining with the supervisor highlights the interactive nature of supervision and may also allow the trainee to experience a boost in perceived abilities not unlike utilizing training wheels while learning to ride a bicycle. The supervisor–trainee relational dynamic also reminds supervisors of the impact they have on supervisees as role models for the development of interpersonal and professional behavior.

Once supervisees achieve the advanced level, they are able to demonstrate integrated knowledge, including knowledge of research literature that supports their understanding of individual competency domains. They can fluently recognize patterns in client presentation and select appropriate intervention strategies. These supervisees are able to take into account multiple domains at the same time in order to conceptualize a case and use this integrated knowledge to recognize potential diagnoses that can guide their actions. For instance, the mental health professional becomes able to discriminate among subtypes of depression by identifying different patterns of client experiences, affect, and behaviors associated with diagnostic criteria. Advanced helpers also enjoy a higher level of confidence in their professional abilities and develop the capability to self-supervise. This confidence continues to build as practitioners move into the higher developmental levels known as proficient and expert (Dreyfus & Dreyfus, 1986). During these stages, the helper no longer needs to consciously analyze the situation and instead finds that plans or perspectives come to mind almost automatically. As an expert, he or she also finds that there is almost instant knowledge of how to implement a client-related plan without calculating or comparing alternatives.

Integrated Developmental Model of Supervision

Currently, the integrated developmental model (Stoltenberg & Delworth, 1987; Stoltenberg & McNeill, 2010) is one of the most widely used models of clinical supervision (Bernard & Goodyear, 2014). Integrated developmental model theory proposes that supervisees in clinical practice progress through four levels of development with distinct characteristics based on changes in awareness of self and others, motivation, and autonomy (Stoltenberg & McNeill, 2010):

Level 1

- Has high levels of anxiety and insecurity that may or may not be well managed
- Is very dependent on the supervisor
- Has little ability for insight
- Is focused on own behaviors, thoughts, and emotions
- Is highly motivated

Level 2

- Experiences conflict between dependence and autonomy
- At times, increased understanding and empathy increases motivation
- At other times, more confusion and frustration decreases motivation
- Still relies on the supervisor for guidance but strives for independence
- Uses the supervisor as an advisor
- Is client focused but less aware of countertransference (self)

Level 3

- A higher sense of self-confidence and professional identity increases motivation
- Is more tolerant of others with opposing views
- Has a greater ability to empathize
- Is able to conceptualize the client from a broader context
- Reflects on the client–counselor relationship
- Can have moments of both client focus and self-focus

Level 3—Integrated

- Has insightful awareness regarding self and others
- Is able to integrate and move smoothly among different domains of clinical practice (e.g., assessment, conceptualization, goals, interventions)
- Has a stronger awareness of limitations
- Is able to confront personal/professional issues
- Uses a peer supervision context

Notice that most of the characteristics and qualities identified at the various levels are interpersonal, intrapersonal, and professional behaviors critical to the development of clinicians beyond the traditional realms of academic achievement and clinical skills.

Although it has been found that supervisees progress through these levels in a linear fashion, they can also function within multiple stages of development at a given time when it comes to separate domains of practice (Stoltenberg, 2005). A supervisee's movement through the stages is heavily dependent on the amount of experience he or she has, so a helper who primarily works with individual clients and has very little group counseling experience may, in fact, be at a beginning Level 3 stage when counseling individuals and a Level 1 stage when providing group counseling. Because a supervisee at one particular stage of development will have different supervisory needs than someone at another stage, the supervisor in this example may need to provide very direct and specific guidance and skills when discussing group counseling and then become more nondirective, encouraging reflection, while conferring about individual counseling clients. In addition, Tracey et al. (1989) found that both beginning and advanced trainees preferred more structured supervision (which is specific to Level 1) when discussing content that was especially anxiety provoking (e.g., client suicidality).

Outside of clinical skill development, supervisors may also find that trainees can operate interpersonally or professionally from two different stages at the same time. For example, a student may be experiencing interpersonal and/or intrapersonal difficulty as evidenced in part by consistently heightened anxiety. The trainee may have awareness of and insight into personal struggles with anxiety and be actively engaged in attempts to manage these anxiety reactions; however, the trainee may still be experiencing unmanageable anxiety symptoms during interactions that cloud clinical judgment and functioning, especially during sessions with clients. Trainees may also experience varying levels of integration and awareness at different times depending on the surrounding circumstances. For instance, a student may respond to many situations with a highly judgmental position that seems to reflect insecurity or a need for dominating others, yet in other situations or when personal reactivity settles down, the student may exhibit high levels of awareness and empathy. Consequently, there may be times in which a supervisor must modify the level of structure provided for supervision depending on the level from which the supervisee is primarily operating at the time.

Although the majority of students/supervisees progress through these stages without incident, some trainees encounter difficulties in developing an acceptable standard of personal and professional functioning that require intervention and additional guidance by faculty and/or supervisors. From a developmental perspective, the manner in which the intervention and/or remediation processes are perceived and carried out can impact how successful the trainee will ultimately be in demonstrating appropriate change. The approach by the faculty member(s) or supervisor(s) in supporting trainee development may also influence perceptions of fairness regarding the actions taken in response to the trainee's behavior.

Upholding the Dignity of the Supervisee

Maintaining the Relationship

Clients grow best in an accepting and supportive environment that includes the establishment of an effective working relationship, and students/supervisees are no different. When faculty and supervisors first encounter a trainee who requires extra developmental guidance or support, it should be seen as an opportunity to set the tone for how the interactional process of implementing program standards will occur. As mental health professionals, supervisors and faculty are already equipped with an assortment of clinical skills that are effective across a range of life and work roles designed to assist people in navigating and coping through very difficult life events. Learning that he or she is not developing professionally as expected qualifies as a difficult life event for a trainee. Consider the perspective of supervisees for just a moment by stepping into their shoes:

> You have dreamed for years of becoming a mental health professional, but you have also always been afraid that you couldn't actually do it. You were pleasantly surprised when you were accepted into a training program, and you've spent a large sum of money on enrollment fees, books, lost wages, and so on, so far. You figure it will be worth all of the debt. You're taking steps to achieve something that will make you and others proud. Perhaps you've struggled with the opinions that others have of you or found it difficult to feel "good enough." Being in a graduate program has boosted your self-perception some, and you see the impressed looks on others' faces when you say you're getting a graduate degree. You feel better about yourself than you can remember feeling in the past. Suddenly it's brought to your attention that you aren't doing quite as well as you should be. Your professor points things out that you didn't even realize you were doing incorrectly. You really thought that becoming a helper was going to feel more natural, and that familiar fear that you can't actually do this grows to loom larger than ever before. You know you're catastrophizing, but you just can't help it. Even though nobody has yet said that you're going to be excused from the program, terrible thoughts begin to run rapidly through your mind: "I'm going to prove to my family that I'm the failure they've always thought I was. They were just starting to change their opinion. And it's going to be so humiliating. . . . How will I tell my friends that I couldn't pass my program? I knew I wasn't as good as the other students, but now they'll know it too for sure. And all of my student loans! Oh, God, how will I ever pay them off when I don't even know what I'll be if I can't become a helper? I've never had a plan B!"

In the beginning moments of remediation, when the trainee is experiencing a high level of anxiety, fear, and possibly anger, the faculty member or supervisor has the opportunity to portray a supportive, strengths-based perspective that lays the groundwork for maintaining a positive working relationship with the supervisee. The blending of both supportive and evaluative roles by supervisors can be an understandable challenge. In fact, some training programs attempt to separate out the evaluative piece in order to protect the supportive element when possible (Homrich, 2009). In such cases, one or more faculty members will meet with the student/supervisee to discuss the problematic behavior and present the remediation plan while another faculty member with whom the student has previously established a supportive guidance-oriented relationship will remove himself or herself from the proceedings or solely adopt a listening or witnessing role in discussions. This faculty member is thus able to more effectively serve as a support for the student as he or she seeks to understand the situation and navigates the remediation process to meet the changes in behavior called for by the program's standards. When this arrangement is not feasible, how does one person manage both roles in such a way that the student/supervisee can be open to feedback and change? Maintaining connection and trust with those needing remediation is of utmost importance in order to foster resolution of the identified issues. The supervisor's responsibility is to attend respectfully to the relationship between the trainee and gatekeeper, especially when there is a high level of emotional reactivity on the part of the trainee. Not only do harmonious faculty–student relationships help students feel supported and valued throughout remediation efforts, but Cole (1991) asserted that these relationships are also highly effective at reducing a program's risk of liability. Using reflective skills while also providing clear and direct, yet empathic, communication is an essential way of nurturing the relationship even while delivering difficult feedback or confronting a lack of developmental progress. During all interactions throughout a training program, students and supervisees deserve to be treated with respect and dignity and to be acknowledged as individuals with unique qualities of value, even (and especially) during the difficult circumstance of challenging unprofessional or developmentally inappropriate conduct.

Providing Supportive Communication

In the early stages of training, it is critical that faculty maintain an ongoing informal and formal assessment of students' interpersonal, intrapersonal, and professional behaviors that occur in and are connected to the classroom setting (Homrich, 2009), as discussed in detail in Chapter 9. Discovering areas that need improvement gives faculty members an opportunity to initiate a concrete discussion with students about what is expected and also provides students with immediate feedback and guidance in a supportive manner, both of which are necessary for the continued growth and development of students and supervisees. For instance, students in the early stage of training and professional development may display a judgmental attitude and a lack of awareness of the impact their comments have on others. Consider the case of Linda: In one of her first-semester graduate courses, Linda made mildly judgmental comments to a guest speaker who came into class. Although the professor knew it was common to encounter these attitudes in beginning students and assumed that Linda would gain insight and become more accepting in time, she addressed the issue with the following comments included on Linda's related written assignment:

> Nicely done, Linda! You've applied the theories of Erikson, Kohlberg, and Fowler to the guest speaker's presentation in a systematic and empirically supported manner. I would also like to give you some feedback regarding your interaction with the guest speaker that I hope you'll be able to further utilize during this next semester in your skills class. One of the goals for students during this program is to become aware of the tendency one may have to quickly judge others. We can refer to your student handbook for a reminder of specific expectations of graduate counseling students, if needed. The first step is to become aware of when you are being judgmental, then to explore what is being triggered within you to cause the judgment. It is also important as a professional to have control over your resulting behavior, your actions and words, reflecting your judgment toward others. While questioning the guest speaker about his life, I noticed that at times it seemed as though you believed he was answering questions in a less than desirable way. Later, the guest speaker made a comment to me that confirmed he also felt what I had perceived as your judgment toward him. For now, it's just something for you to begin to notice during your daily exchanges with others. When you feel frustrated toward others, consider what you think it may be related to. Consider whether your reactions should be expressed, and, if so, what is the best way to share your experience of the situation. We have to manage our reactions and thought expression constantly when working with clients. We'll all be talking much more in depth about these concepts during your skills class.

This feedback was developmentally appropriate and, because it was delivered via an online grading platform, also provided documentation of Linda's judgmental behavior and the guidance that was provided. This approach connected Linda's reactions in class to the program's standards for academic performance as well as professional behavior expectations for students. The following semester, Linda was in the same professor's counseling skills course. When they met individually to discuss the professor's final assessment of Linda's counseling skills, Linda shared that she had felt guilty about judging the guest speaker the previous semester and had worked very hard to become more self-aware of her judgmental tendencies. The professor had noticed that Linda was becoming much more accepting and thoughtful in her comments to others in class and was pleased to share this observation.

Other examples of common behaviors of concern seen early in a helping professional's training and development include the voicing of biases toward groups of people stemming from a lack of understanding or exposure, limited self-awareness of one's impact on others, high levels of anxiety that can get in the way of learning helping skills, and insufficient self-care and coping strategies. Some educators are hesitant to formally address these kinds of behaviors, especially so early in the person's training, because they assume that the trainee will develop beyond these constraints with informal discussion. The professor or advisor may additionally be motivated by the desire to avoid intimidating the student or damaging the developing relationship by initiating a more formalized process of providing feedback or entering into a remediation process. However, students who become gatekeeping concerns at a later point in their program often revealed problematic interpersonal and intrapersonal behaviors much earlier in their training (Henderson & Dufrene, 2013), and subsequently it will likely become necessary to demonstrate that there were patterns of problematic behavior prior to formal intervention. An example of establishing documentation after an impromptu discussion while also being supportive could be to follow up the informal exchange with an e-mail stating something similar like this:

> I just wanted to check in with you regarding the conversation we had about (e.g., your confusion as to whether you would be able to refer lesbian, gay, bisexual, and transgender clients based on religious beliefs). I realize that what we discussed was a lot of information to take in. I also want to acknowledge that you said you wanted to take some time to examine your values in relation to the ethical expectations of the counseling profession, a decision I support. I thought I'd see if you have any further questions I can help with at this point.

Following up in this manner respectfully honors the developmental process of the individual to integrate new information while also documenting the fact that opportunity and encouragement to grow and change was provided early in the student or supervisee's course of training. This is consistent not only with humanistic values of counseling but also with the intent of due process.

When customary educational techniques and supervision methods are not effective with a trainee, it may become necessary to escalate to a more formalized process. As discussed in Chapter 10, creating a written remediation plan that is concrete and tangible, such as Dufrene and Henderson's (2009) individual remediation plan, can serve to reduce supervisee anxiety and lessen catastrophizing. The student or supervisee's development as a counselor should always be considered in the construction of a remedial intervention of any kind; the goal is to provide feedback or prescribe a plan that will advance the student from a position of deficit in functioning to an acceptable level of personal and professional performance. The way in which formal feedback and/or remediation procedures are explained is an integral part of this process and can foster either a more supportive or an offensive tone from the student. At the outset, students can misinterpret the term *remediation* to indicate that the faculty's goal is to dismiss them from the program. Although the early clinical training literature focused more heavily on models for student dismissal within gatekeeping, there has been a recent shift in emphasis toward exploring methods of monitoring, intervening, and remediating as a part of the trainee development process (Dufrene & Henderson, 2009; Elman & Forrest, 2004; Kaslow et al., 2007; Kress & Protivnak, 2009; McAdams & Foster, 2007). Consequently, it is important to operationally define what the supervisor or training program means by remediation and to publish this explanation in multiple locations (e.g., the supervision contract, the student handbook, syllabi, the written remediation plan). For example, remediation may be conceptualized from a strengths-based perspective and defined in student publications as a structured process of defined interventions through which a struggling supervisee has the opportunity to demonstrate competence. The ultimate goal of attending to the developmental process of trainees is to avoid, if possible, having to enact gatekeeping processes that result in truncating students' pursuit of their goal of becoming helpers.

There are other opportunities to influence the reaction that a supervisee may experience to standards and expectations by way of supportive communication. The manner in which the remediation guidelines are communicated to a student in writing provides another opening to express a respectfully direct yet empathic position. A sample letter that demonstrates an attempt to balance these two dimensions is included in Appendix C. Yet another occasion presents itself the first time a student meets with a faculty member, advisor, or supervisor during the remediation process. It is recommended that the supervisor and student/supervisee sign or otherwise acknowledge (e.g., via e-mail) documentation of each step (Dugger & Francis, 2014), as noted in Chapter 11. Collecting signatures from both the student and advisor on a written summary that describes a required meeting between the two can provide proof, from a legal standpoint, that the program has followed procedural due process law (McAdams, Foster, & Ward, 2007); however, if the request for a student signature is conveyed as a means of protecting the program, the student will likely feel less supported and more defensive. If, instead, the supervisor introduces cosignatures with "I've written up a brief summary of our meeting, and I ask that we both sign it to confirm what we've covered today. I'll also give you a copy each time so that you can keep an ongoing record of the progress you're making," the student may perceive a higher level of respect and react with cooperation rather than defensiveness. As with the other examples in this chapter, a respectful trainee-centered approach with the intention of providing the opportunity and support for a student or supervisee to demonstrate change and behave appropriately—interpersonally, intrapersonally, and professionally—is the ultimate goal of the remediation process.

Respecting the Supervisee's Values

Another process of development that helping professionals undertake has, at times, been referred to as "cognitive development in the moral domain" (Neukrug, Lovell, & Parker, 1996, p. 104). Along with learning codes of ethics, decision-making models, and laws that pertain to the clinical professions, trainees embark on a journey of self-discovery that includes a deeper understanding of their own motivations and values. Professional helpers are not supposed to be bias free; however, they are expected to engage in a process of self-examination and evaluation and ultimately reconcile their biases with the standards of the profession (Mintz et al., 2009). When a student or supervisee requires remediation because of behaviors related to the personal values that inform his or her beliefs, the supervisor must be careful to respect the individual trainee's right to hold differing values-informed perspectives. The goal is not to change the supervisee's values but instead to assist in the process of decision making and ethical bracketing. Kocet and Herlihy (2014) explained that

> ethical bracketing (EB) is defined as the intentional separating of a counselor's personal values from his or her professional values or the intentional setting aside of the counselor's personal values in order to provide ethical and appropriate counseling to all clients, especially those whose worldviews, values, belief systems, and decisions differ significantly from those of the counselor. (p. 182)

Handelsman, Gottlieb, and Knapp (2005) described four strategies that trainees use over the course of their training as they become acquainted with the values of the profession, integrate professional ethics with personal values, and develop the ability to set their personal values aside in deference to the client's process. *Marginalization* describes a strategy used by an individual with a low level of insight into his or her personal values and no real knowledge of the ethics codes and values of the mental health professions. This might be a new trainee who says that she would not work with members of a particular religion (unaware that this is considered unethical by the American Counseling Association [ACA]) because she thinks she would be uncomfortable for some reason (and has yet to examine her values to understand where the conflict actually lies).

The next strategy, *separation* (Handelsman et al., 2005), is used by somebody who has a better developed sense of his or her personal values but who does not identify with the values of the profession. An example would be a trainee who is quite aware of her feminist personal beliefs (e.g., has felt marginalized by members of the identified religion, disagrees with the value that women are less than men as she understands the religion to promote) yet is not influenced by the profession's ethical principles (e.g., counselors may not refuse a client based on a values conflict, do no harm) and makes her decision about counseling members of a religion that embraces traditional gender roles purely based on her personal beliefs.

As the trainee becomes more aware of ethical and/or legal expectations of counselors and continues to examine her own beliefs, she might reverse her perspective and adopt the *assimilation* strategy (Handelsman et al., 2005), wherein she would completely forfeit her own personal values in order to fully adopt the agreed-on values of the helping profession. Therefore, she would likely choose to counsel members of the specified religion because the professional values direct her to avoid discriminating against clients and to refrain from withholding valuable services from whole groups of people. She would disregard or suppress her previously held beliefs gleaned from earlier experience as well as her disagreement with the perceived gender hierarchy when making clinical decisions.

Finally, *integration* (Handelsman et al., 2005) is a favorable strategy for helpers, during which the trainee would develop the capacity to utilize the profession's values while also holding on to important aspects of her personal belief system. She would not experience a conflict because she would be able to set aside, but maintain, her own beliefs about gender equality while also behaving in a way that is consistent with the standards and principles of the profession. The ability to successfully engage in ethical bracketing is usually a developmental process for clinical trainees that needs to be evaluated for stage appropriateness as they progress through their training program.

Learning how to negotiate and incorporate their personal values into their ethical decision making is a critical element in mental health trainees' training. This requires opportunities for practice with support (and oversight) from faculty and supervisors as students and supervisees undergo the cognitive transition from either/or to more flexible both/and thinking. Ametrano (2014) suggested strategies such as having students write an ethics autobiography at the beginning of an ethics course during which they answer questions to explore their own personal values, beliefs, and cultural background in an effort to foster personal awareness. Students can then revisit these questions at the end of the course with an additional focus on the integration of professional values and guidelines learned throughout the semester. In their article, Kocet and Herlihy (2014) suggested helping conflicted supervisees navigate a process they called the counselor values-based conflict model, which may include immersion, education, consultation, supervision, and personal counseling. These valuable strategies can be used both in the initial training and in the remediation of mental health supervisees. Regardless of the strategies used to help students move forward in their development, supervisors are advised to use their reflecting skills to explore their trainees' values and developmental juncture and to refrain from communicating intolerance. Respecting the supervisee's right to have differing values and focusing on the required behaviors and dispositions expected of all student trainees will provide the supervisee with concrete goals to achieve.

Factors That Influence Supervisees' Behavior

The human element of supervisees ensures that many personal factors will influence their behavior as they adapt to demonstrating standards of professional conduct. (See On the Legal Side 4.1.) Supervisees' personal development and maturity level, individual style differences,

On the Legal Side 4.1

As students develop into helping professionals, they undergo a process of examining their personal values and beliefs. It is critical that students understand the limited role their values are permitted to play in their process of counseling others. This limitation is determined by a combination of state and federal laws along with the profession's codes of ethics. Although studies have found that counselor educators give mixed messages on the subject of referring clients based on values conflicts (Burkholder & Hall, 2014; Burkholder, Hall, & Burkholder, 2014), ACA and the Council for Accreditation of Counseling and Related Educational Programs are firm in their positions that the personal values and opinions of counselors and counselors-in-training must not affect their willingness to counsel protected client populations, with the sole exception of terminally ill clients wishing to consider options for hastening their death (Kaplan, 2014). In the legal cases of *Ward v. Wilbanks* (2010) and *Keeton v. Anderson-Wiley* (2010) the gatekeeping abilities of universities were challenged by students who were dismissed from their counselor education programs after declining to counsel lesbian, gay, bisexual, and transgender clients based on religious values (Kocet & Herlihy, 2014). In *Keeton v. Anderson-Wiley* (2011) a federal appellate court upheld the university's decision. In *Ward v. Wilbanks,* the court initially granted a summary judgment in favor of the university, and a settlement was later reached outside of court after the student's appeal. ACA's chief professional officer, Dr. David Kaplan, provided expert testimony during *Ward v. Wilbanks* and at the outcome of the case reconfirmed ACA's position:

- Professional counselors may not deny counseling services to a homosexual person (or an individual belonging to any other protected class of clients) on the basis of the counselor's values.
- Referrals are to be made on the basis of skill-based competency, not values.
- To avoid abandonment, referral is an option of last resort.
- The counselor's ethical obligations to an individual start at first contact or assignment, not at the first session. (Kaplan, 2014, p. 146)

The National Association of Social Workers (NASW) takes a slightly different approach to some portions of this mandate. Consistent with ACA's stance (Whitman, Glosoff, Kocet, & Tarvydas, 2013), NASW has been very specific about its position, which strongly rejects any form of *sexual orientation change efforts*—an umbrella term for conversion therapy, reparative therapy, and transformational ministries—by social workers (NASW, 2015). In addition, social workers are expected not to "practice, condone, facilitate, or collaborate with any form of discrimination on the basis of race, ethnicity, national origin, color, sex, sexual orientation, gender identity or expression, age, marital status, political belief, religion, immigration status, or mental or physical disability" (NASW, 2017, p. 16). NASW expects its members to seek supervision or another form of consultation in an effort to resolve any values conflicts that may arise between them and their clients. Nevertheless, it is recognized that consultation may

(Continued)

On the Legal Side 4.1 *(Continued)*

always successfully resolve the conflict. Dawn Hobdy, director of the NASW Office of Ethics and Professional Review, explains:

> In addition to respecting the dignity and worth of a person and not discriminating, social workers are also required to be aware of any conflicts of interest that interfere with the exercise of professional discretion and impartial judgment. A sincerely held value or belief "could" present such a conflict. According to the Code, social workers should inform clients when a real or potential conflict of interest arises and take reasonable steps to resolve the issue in a manner that makes the clients' interests primary and protects clients' interests to the greatest extent possible. In some cases, protecting clients' interests may require termination of the professional relationship with proper referral of the client. (D. Hobdy, personal communication, November 18, 2016)

APA (2015b) asserts that "the core responsibility of all professional psychologists and their supervised trainees is to provide competent service to the public based on the knowledge, skills, and awareness to work effectively with individuals from a wide range of backgrounds" (para. 4). A separate statement on the APA website provides guidance for professional psychologists whose religious beliefs or worldviews conflict with the profession's commitment to offering culturally sensitive services to all clients, especially to those from marginalized populations. APA prohibits the discrimination of client populations and expects professional psychologists to engage in competency training that ultimately allows them to integrate their personal values with the standards of professional conduct. When a professional psychologist is unable to provide competent, ethical, and noninjurious services, the decisive consideration must always be the welfare of the client. APA defers to the policies of the practicing agency when considering the option of client referral. The statement recognizes that some institutional policies may prohibit a psychologist from refusing services to any client; however, it is emphasized that when allowed, referrals must be made in a compassionate and caring manner that puts the interests of the client at the forefront.

APA Working Group on Restrictions Affecting Diversity Training in Graduate Education (2013) also provides guidance for psychology training programs as they address trainees with worldviews, religious values, or beliefs that conflict with the professional standards of psychology. It acknowledges the need for a supportive training environment that recognizes the developmental process that students experience. Trainees are expected to learn about and practice providing services to all client populations regardless of values and beliefs. During this time, educators are encouraged to help trainees learn strategies for upholding their personal beliefs while also providing diversity-sensitive psychology services to their clients. If this is not possible, trainers are expected to put the client's welfare ahead of the student's and reassign clients when necessary. The need for client reassignment should be followed by remediation for the trainee. APA is firm in its position that trainees may not make the decision to reassign

(Continued)

On the Legal Side 4.1 *(Continued)*

clients and may not refuse to provide services to a client population while in training.

Along with abiding by the code of ethics specific to their mental health field, supervisees and supervisors alike must remain up to date in their knowledge of state and federal laws that affect the role that values may play in their treatment of clients. Multiple states have attempted and/or succeeded in putting forth legislation based on the conscience clause, laws that allow health care providers to opt out of activities because of conflicts with personal religious beliefs and values. Depending on the state, these laws may apply to mental health professionals and/or training institutions and students.

cultural perspectives and experiences, social identities, and personal history and/or the presence of disabilities are all factors that will likely prove significant when one is considering the trainee in context.

Individual Style Differences

Individuals may engage in the clinical training process in multiple ways that are influenced by many personal variables. One's inherent view of the world, previous personal and professional experiences, personality traits, and perceptual learning style are examples of characteristics that cumulatively result in individual style differences that affect the way in which one feels, thinks, and acts—the unique qualities of the individual. An individual's personal distinctiveness is also a result of the influence of the contexts in which he or she grew up or currently lives. Add another layer of individualism as students come to training programs accompanied by their personal identities, which may be especially salient if, for example, they are members of one or more marginalized groups. The result is a trainee with an individual style and unique ways of perceiving, reacting to, and interacting in the world. Faculty and supervisors must respect, value, and work with students, understanding their individual ways of operating within a training context and how they meet the standards of conduct devised by the profession and the training program.

An example of how individual differences might affect supervisor–supervisee interactions has to do with the way in which a trainee responds to being approached with feedback requiring changes in behavior and/or introduction to a remediation plan. The response, of course, will vary from one student to the next. One student might appreciate the opportunity to change and take the initiative to do so, whereas another trainee may perceive feedback as threatening his or her self-concept or compromising future career plans and become defensive and combative during the process. It would perhaps be ideal if, on hearing that he or she is not meeting developmental expectations, a supervisee would respond confidently and with an open mind, thanking the supervisor for the feedback as he or she pulls a pen and notebook out and asks, "How can I best achieve this growth you speak of?" Yet this response is rarely if ever seen! Henderson and Dufrene (2012) found that difficulty receiving and ultimately integrating feedback emerged as two themes of challenging student behavior within the literature associated with remediation. Some trainees externalize their disappointment, directing negative thoughts and/or emotions toward the supervisor or professor. Resulting behaviors may be overt (e.g., scowling, verbal denial, blaming, or justifying the problematic behavior) or delivered passive aggressively (e.g., telling other students not to trust the faculty member because he or she uses personal information against students, disparaging the program, and/or becoming uncooperative in other training-related settings). Some recipients interpret the feedback as threatening to their egos and internalize it with fear, guilt, embarrassment, and/or shame. Select students/supervisees react with a desire to flee the conversation initially and may need to be given some time to organize their thoughts and calm down their immediate reactions.

Depending on their past personal histories, still other supervisees may have the tendency to use dissociation when confronted with critical feedback intended to be constructive, seeming to disconnect from the experience and have difficulty following the conversation and responding clearly. For this reason, it is beneficial to follow up face-to-face discussions that include feedback requiring change with a detailed written summary or e-mail, as discussed earlier, describing the concern and expected adjustments in conduct in the event that the supervisee may not clearly recall what was said. Even without the experience of dissociation, a trainee's increased anxiety can hinder comprehension in the moment because of emotional flooding.

As with clients, it can be helpful to conceptualize student reactions as the defense mechanisms that they truly are. With this frame of thought, the supervisor may be uniquely positioned to assist students/supervisees in lowering their defenses in order to hear what is being communicated. For example, a student/supervisee experiencing dissociation or otherwise feeling high anxiety in the remediation meeting may benefit from basic grounding techniques or guided breathing strategies in the moment. Even more important, the supervisee will benefit from experiencing a respectful and overall caring demeanor by the person delivering the negative feedback. Demonstrating professional behavior when encountering anger, outrage, or sadness from clients and refraining from taking another's emotions personally or responding from a place of countertransference is a positive stance to extend to students or supervisees who may feel momentarily cornered while attempting to manage their emotions. Modeling professional conduct is an important role of educators and supervisors in order to effectively guide students and supervisees in their growth and development.

Cultural Perspectives

Supervisors are responsible for distinguishing challenges that are specific to the supervisee from those that are intricately related to culture and/or ethnicity. For example, international students in training programs may have the additional hurdle of being less aware of American society's legal and ethical norms. As can be seen in the Notes From the Field 4.1, this lack of awareness can have vast implications for ethical practice that may not be related to goodness of fit with the profession. When there is a need for remediation, Forrest, Elman, Gizara, and Vacha-Haase (1999) maintained that

> trainees will be more responsive to acknowledging their limitations if cultural sensitivity is used in identifying the inadequate performance and that remediation plans will be more effective if cultural contexts and socialization experiences underlying the problematic behavior or performance are considered. (p. 671)

It is important for educators and supervisors to remember that an individual's cultural identity reflects a sum of customs, attitudes, meanings, hierarchies, beliefs, and values that distinguish the identity of one group of people from that of another. Culture is the accumulation of knowledge, experiences, meanings, rituals, sometimes language, roles, notions of time, concepts of the universe, and spiritual beliefs that are transmitted from one generation to the next. Culture is a system of being and knowing that is acquired and shared by a group of people over the course of generations through individual and group striving. Culture significantly influences a trainee's view of the world, just as personal history does (Baldwin, Faulkner, Hecht, & Lindsley, 2008), and supervisors, professors, students, and/or supervisees may not have a full awareness of these influences on their thinking, feeling, or behavioral reactions to a training situation.

The mental health professions arose from a European- and American-dominant culture perspective that was generally informed primarily by the influence of White men in positions of power in the medical professions during the late 19th and 20th centuries. Even though subsequent perspectives on mental wellness and mental illness have evolved, the worldviews of the mental health professions largely represent the values and beliefs of the dominant culture. With this foundational understanding, consider the perspective of students or supervisees from different cultures of experience and understanding, especially those who have not previously been influenced by exposure to the American White dominant culture, as in the case of international students.

For trainees from cultures other than the dominant culture, the meaning of concepts such as professional conduct or intrapersonal appropriateness may initially be incongruent with a profession's or program's expectations. For example, the Council for Accreditation

Notes From the Field 4.1

Akilah was an international student who had relocated from a Middle Eastern country in order to attend a counselor education program in the United States. She retained many of her cultural values and practices while studying in the States, including her desire not to drive a car and instead to be driven by her male family members. When Akilah was placed at a domestic violence shelter for her internship during the third year of her training, she was required by the site to sign a nondisclosure agreement and then list in writing who would be driving her. Akilah wrote only her brother's name as her driver, and this worked well for the first few months of her clinical experience. Then one evening, her brother was unavailable, so she asked her father, who was visiting from her country of origin, to drive her to her internship site. The site was unaware that somebody different had driven Akilah until her father mistakenly returned early to pick her up. Because he did not speak English, Akilah's father struggled at the security gate to communicate why he was there; when he became angry during the process, the police were called. Ultimately, Akilah's father was removed from his vehicle and held at gunpoint face down on the ground while authorities at the domestic violence shelter attempted to determine whether he was an aggressor of one of the women in residence.

Once it was determined that Akilah had broken confidentiality by disclosing the location of the domestic violence shelter to somebody other than the person on her list, the site immediately terminated her placement with them. This was the first example of problematic behavior by Akilah during her training. After extensive consideration, the program faculty determined a remediation plan that, among other things, included her writing a paper describing her cultural values and beliefs and how they had conflicted with American norms, thereby contributing to her predicament. When Akilah's advisor initially met with her to discuss what had happened at her site, Akilah did not understand why it was such a big deal for her to let her father know the location even though she had signed an agreement stating that she would not. During her remediation process, Akilah identified the United States as more litigious than her country and observed that most dealings involved putting things in writing. This was very different from her culture's norms, in which suing others was very rare and few things were documented in writing. She noted that although she had signed the nondisclosure agreement, she had interpreted her commitment as a promise not to do anything that would put the women at the shelter in danger. She believed very strongly that her father was not a threat to the women. Her family was also a patriarchal unit, and thus she did not question that her father could go anywhere she could go. Akilah was able to successfully complete her counseling program, and the remediation process allowed her to become more aware of the ways in which her cultural values and experiences influenced her legal and ethical understanding while practicing in the United States.

of Counseling and Related Educational Programs (2015) defined *professional dispositions* as "the commitments, characteristics, values, beliefs, interpersonal functioning, and behaviors that influence the counselor's professional growth and interactions with clients and colleagues" (p. 47). How this definition intersects with one's cultural character and professional identity must be considered in working with trainees navigating the development process of adapting differences between the two domains.

Social Identities

Students come into training programs already wearing multiple hats and identifying with different social roles and personal identities, and each of these can impact their personal and professional behaviors. For instance, a trainee may be the problem solver in his family system or a mother whose parenting role includes nurturing, judging, and directing the behavior of others. Students sometimes enter the helping professions after already having engaged in other careers, such as teaching or sales, for a number of years in which they may have served as employees, managers, or owners. These other career fields and related roles have defined professional ways of being that may differ from those of counseling, and direct discussion of role differences may need to occur in order for students to recognize the distinctions. Consider the case of Lance, a mental health student entering his training program after a successful 25-year career in pharmaceutical sales. Some of the tactics that had worked well for Lance in sales, such as heavily complimenting others and relying strongly on self-disclosure to find common ground for conversation, did not work as well for clinical training. In addition, faculty found his boundaries problematic at times. For example, when needing to meet with a professor, he would repeatedly suggest that he take the professor out to lunch. He also often engaged in conversations with faculty in which it seemed that he was trying to remove the power differential (e.g., mentioning how much younger the faculty member was than him, stating that he knew a person related to the faculty member and would be "keeping an eye on" her for the other person). It became necessary for Lance's advisor to talk with him directly about the differences in behavioral expectations and boundaries between the two fields and also how to better define the role of student at this stage in his life.

At the other end of the spectrum, trainees may enter their program very young and introverted, still developing their own identities and self-awareness. Although a student in this category may never dream of confronting others or asking them about their level of sexual satisfaction, the ability to facilitate these interventions with clients is necessary within the counseling realm. The social identity of a trainee can cause conflicts within the helper when it comes to embodying interpersonal, intrapersonal, and professional expectations.

There may be other areas of identity development that are particularly salient for individual trainees, and where trainees are in the development process can influence perceptions of self and others, thereby guiding interpersonal and intrapersonal experiences. For example, stage (Cass, 1979; McCarn & Fassinger, 1996; Savin-Williams, 1988; Troiden, 1979, 1988) and life-span (D'Augelli, 1994) theories attempt to describe the multifaceted process one may undergo during non-heterosexual identity development. Cass's (1979) model of gay and lesbian identity development describes a process that fits the experience of some sexual minority members. After many years of clinical work with this population, Cass posited six stages through which a person may broadly progress. In the beginning, there is identity confusion as one initially questions the assumed heterosexual identity and thus begins a journey from confusion, inner turmoil, and isolation to varying levels of self-acceptance and social integration. At Stage 6, the individual has found self-acceptance and identity synthesis and is able to reconcile personal and public identities and conceptualize sexual orientation as only one aspect of the self. Consider Vanessa, a trainee who identified as gay and appeared to be in Stage 6 of Cass's identity development model. She was found to have very strong interpersonal and intrapersonal skills and behaviors while in her training program. She reported having previously engaged in personal counseling while going through the process of discovering her sexual identity. Vanessa had subsequently become very involved in her local gay subculture, finding validation and true connections in her friendships. While in her training program, she also made strong connections with heterosexual peers and engaged in advocacy work for the lesbian, gay, bisexual, and transgender population. Vanessa chose to intern at a counseling center that specifically assisted and supported these youth. She modeled positive intrapersonal behaviors while serving at her site, such as self-acceptance and the use of mindfulness practices that helped her to manage stress. Consistent with her developmental stage, Vanessa also exhibited strong interpersonal behaviors that allowed her to facilitate calm and rational discussions when she encountered individuals with negative biases against her internship organization and/or clients. For instance, police officers who brought youth to her internship site sometimes voiced negative biases toward her clients, and in supervision she was able to separate these individuals from other more accepting heterosexual people. Her advanced stage of identity development allowed Vanessa to have a positive influence on her site through her professional, interpersonal, and intrapersonal behaviors.

Personal History

Instructors within the helping professions at times incorporate material during class that could potentially expose students to vicarious traumatization (Cunningham, 2004). Sometimes guest speakers talk about their own traumatic childhoods, or a video can take the viewer through the detailed experience of having a child who dies. A case study may recount the story of a client losing her sister to a serial killer's rampage. Some classroom activities are established with the intention of having students seriously examine their perceptions of humanity and understand the broad scope of human experience. Other curricular experiences are meant to expose trainees to likely client scenarios and desensitize them to difficult contact in advance of direct work with clients experiencing the same concerns. Although these types of activities can trigger students emotionally, there is the argument that it is better to initially experience and process the triggers during training than later while in session with a client.

Although all students may be vulnerable to vicarious traumatization when exposed to stories of human suffering, students with a past history of personal trauma are at a higher risk (Pearlman & Saakvitne, 1996) and may additionally be susceptible to experiencing triggers for posttraumatic stress response (Cunningham, 2003). The risk of these reactions may be reduced when the helper who has experienced personal trauma has previously sought effective therapy and expresses his or her emotions more freely (Khan, 1974). As Ellis (1972) and others have pointed out, some graduate students have a tendency to enter training with their own unresolved personal issues that then may be addressed through the informational and experiential portions of their rigorous training programs (Khan, 1974). Compared to students in some training programs in other professional realms, students of the helping professions are more likely to have experienced alcoholism and mental illness within their families of origin (Black, Jeffreys, & Hartley, 1993; Marsh, 1988; Rompf & Royce, 1994; Russel, Gill, Coyne, & Woody, 1993) and are more likely to report a history of early life traumatic experiences and sexual abuse (Black et al., 1993; Russel et al., 1993; Vincent, 1996). Taking into consideration that these early experiences can be risk factors for maladaptive adult functioning (Main, Kaplan, & Cassidy, 1985; van der Kolk, Hostetler, Herron, & Fisler, 1994), Regehr, Stalker, Jacobs, and Pelech (2001) asserted that "the implications for social work education are clear: social work students who have had difficult life experiences may require help to recognize, acknowledge and work through their feelings in order to avoid imposing their issues on clients" (p. 130).

These students are best served by experienced supervisors who are supportive while consistently maintaining clear professional boundaries and avoiding the counselor role. Furthermore, faculty and supervisors must constantly remain alert to problematic behavioral actions and reactions in trainees that may be rooted in trauma experiences that outwardly may appear to be inappropriate professional conduct. Examples include overt defiance or challenge to those in roles of authority, immature behavior in peer group interactions, avoidance of interpersonal engagement with others, defensiveness to feedback, and emotional reactions that occur out of proportion to the context or event. Consider the example of Faith. A professional from the community was delivering a guest presentation to Faith's class about the indicators and detrimental effects of childhood sexual abuse. About halfway through the presentation, Faith drew attention to herself by sighing loudly and beginning to complain verbally about the length of the presentation. The instructor asked Faith to leave the room with her to address her outburst, and during their discussion Faith disclosed that she had been sexually abused as a child. She was able to recognize that her triggered anger precluded her ability to behave professionally in the moment and decided that she wanted to return to personal counseling in order to work further on this issue.

Intense responses or overreactions in and of themselves must be addressed, especially if they occur in the context of offering feedback or remediation for another concern. If a trainee's response is rooted in personally historical trauma, it is critical that the individual find the resources to address the concern and resulting behavior with compassionate support from faculty or supervisors. Although personal in nature, intrusive history must be resolved in order to determine whether behavior change is possible and can be demonstrated in the context of the expected standards of a functional, effective mental health professional. If not, gatekeeping actions must be instituted.

Disabilities

Supervisees with disabilities have the same challenges related to professional growth that all trainees of the helping professions encounter but also face additional systemic and attitudinal barriers (Hauser, Maxwell-McCaw, Leigh, & Gutman, 2000). Lund, Andrews, and Holt (2014) found a high incidence of barriers and perceived discrimination among students with disabilities in psychology training programs, especially during graduate coursework prior to internship. Common ways in which discrimination may present itself include inaccessible training environments, uncomfortable comments, questions and assumptions by supervisors and peers, and inappropriate pressure to disclose one's disability to clients or potential clients (Andrews et al., 2013). Depending on factors such as whether his or her disability is apparent to others, one trainee may encounter greater or fewer biases from peers, instructors, supervisors, internship site staff, and clients than another disabled trainee experiences. Although individuals with disabilities are often skilled at helping others feel more comfortable around them (Gill, 2001), peer and supervisor discomfort can still lead to awkward communication and avoidance that feels like rejection or dismissiveness. In contrast, peers may shower the trainee with inappropriate concern and sympathy, which also leads to a feeling of uneasiness and difference. Furthermore, a trainee's disability status may incorrectly influence how others perceive that person's clinical skills (Levinson & Parritt, 2006). For example, peer trainees can be influenced by negative stereotypes that diminish their appraisal of the trainee's skills and competence, whereas others may incorrectly assume that a person with a disability would naturally be adept at counseling a client with a similar disability.

As students progress through their training programs, they are encouraged to explore each of the dimensions that make them who they are. This can be a stressful process as they learn about their own use of defense mechanisms and examine family dynamics and values they may not have realized they possessed. Students with disabilities experience these periods of confusion along with their peers but also have the additional task of examining their disability identity. Gill's (1997) stage-based disability identity development model suggests that disabled people may initially seek societal acceptance and attempt to make themselves fit in with the able-bodied population. Then they tend to move away from the dominant cultural values and instead connect more with disabled peers and begin to value the disabled self. Finally, there is a shift back in the direction of the mainstream society with a fully integrated disability identity. Gill (1997) described four distinct types of integration within disability identity development that encompass these tasks, which she termed (a) coming to feel we belong, (b) coming home, (c) coming together, and (d) coming out.

Although it may seem that propelling trainees with disabilities toward a more integrated identity would be beneficial, supervisors must be careful not to move into a personal counseling role. Instead, supervisors are advised to have knowledge of the identity development process in order to better understand their trainees while leaving the therapeutic work of addressing acceptance of or adjustment to their disability to the trainees' personal counseling sessions or other support services (Andrews et al., 2013).

Supervisors within the helping professions often have very little if any training in working with and supervising people with disabilities (Artman & Daniels, 2010; Hauser et al., 2000). This creates a gap in preparation that deserves much more attention. Because these trainees have a right to an accessible environment and an equal opportunity training experience, supervisors need to be knowledgeable about relevant legal and ethical standards. Furthermore, the supervisor will need to be prepared to address topics during supervision that relate to the trainee's professional experiences as a person with a disability. A comprehensive overview of these areas is beyond the scope of this chapter, but the following valuable resources do justice to these topics:

- Americans with Disabilities Act (Americans with Disabilities Act Amendments Act of 2008; Americans with Disabilities Act, 1990)
- Application of the Americans with Disabilities Act across clinical settings (Crewe, 1994; Klimoski & Palmer, 1994; Vande Kemp, Chen, Erickson, & Friesen, 2003)

- Barriers to accessibility (Pope, 2005)
- Disability culture (Gill, 1995)
- Issues of disability accessibility in psychology training and practice (http://kpope.com/)
- Provision of culturally competent supervision to trainees with disabilities (Andrews et al., 2013)

Supervisors must also make the time to examine their own biases regarding disabilities. If supervisors experience feelings of pity or discomfort in the presence of a person with a disability, or view the person in an overly positive or permissive light, these responses are indicators that supervisors need to address their own reactions through personal counseling or a form of supervision or consultation. If these steps are not taken, then supervisors will be more likely to inadvertently make comments or otherwise behave in ways that are offensive and/or oppressive to supervisees with disabilities (e.g., telling them that they are an inspiration, using insulting terminology; Andrews et al., 2013). In addition, some helpful suggestions made by Andrews et al. (2013) for supervisors of trainees with disabilities include the following:

- Consider disability an element of diversity. Help trainees understand and respond to client and family reactions to disability in a way that is both clinically appropriate and comfortable for the trainee.
- Interviewers may appropriately inquire how trainees would explain their disability to a client and what accommodations the intern would need to perform the essential functions of the position.
- Routinely inquire of all trainees whether any accommodations are required, regardless of whether a disability is apparent.
- Learn about various options and types of accommodations that could potentially benefit trainees, staff, and clients.
- Assist as an advocate in securing appropriate reasonable accommodations.
- Be aware of the boundary between supervision and psychotherapy.
- Make supervision an opportunity to discuss all trainees' diversity, including disability.
- Resist the medicalization of trainees with disabilities; it is not appropriate to ask trainees specific questions about their disability for the sake of curiosity.
- Be able to process and problem-solve reactions to disability with trainees in supervision.
- Facilitate opportunities for trainees to make contact with psychologists with disabilities for mentorship.
- Assist trainees with disabilities in developing their own style of coping with systemic and attitudinal barriers. (p. 236)

When contemplating the gatekeeping role with regard to trainees with disabilities, it is important to ultimately require the same standards of all students. As Andrews et al. (2013) stated, "The *spirit* of the [Americans with Disabilities Act] is to prevent people with disabilities from being excluded from training and employment opportunities and allowing for reasonable accommodations to level the playing field" (p. 237, italics in the original). Reasonable accommodations must be made so that the trainee has an equal opportunity to reach the required benchmarks. If required interpersonal, intrapersonal, and behavioral standards are not being met, it is important not to automatically assume that the trainee's disability is the cause of the struggle (Andrews et al., 2013). The supervisor is obligated to focus on what specifically needs to be achieved and approach the remediation process as he or she would with any trainee.

Assisting Trainees in Accepting Feedback

Creating a program climate that genuinely facilitates student growth and supports the gatekeeping responsibility of training programs lays the foundation for helping individual students successfully navigate critical feedback and remediation and may even potentially avoid litigation when efforts to improve trainee performance are not possible (Cole, 1991). Having consensus among faculty about the importance of the gatekeeper role helps students experience a consistent message and assume that competency assessment and remediation are important elements of helper development. It is imperative, both from a legal standpoint and in order for students to be most open to feedback, that all students experience equal and fair treatment throughout the program. If exceptions have been made of some trainees or the program has not explicitly followed its own stated policies at some point, a student's attorney can use this information compellingly in a court of law (Dugger & Francis, 2014). Because attorneys can potentially gain access to numerous sources of information (e.g., university e-mail accounts, university computer servers, other student and client files, faculty computers, text messages, past students who previously underwent a remediation process; Dugger & Francis, 2014) it can be next to impossible to portray an equitable culture if the application of standards is inconsistent.

Lent et al. (1998) stated that effective supervision inspires trainees' self-efficacy and gives considerable support and encouragement along with resources for managing anxiety and other emotions. Each of these practices is especially beneficial when students/supervisees have encountered difficulties in interpersonal, intrapersonal, or professional functioning and are engaging in the active effort of changing behavior. Although educators and supervisors can more directly assist in enhancing academic performance and clinical skill development when focusing directly on the specific details of a student's performance, becoming involved in the nuances of a trainee's personal functioning may risk crossing ethical and/or legal boundaries. In general, feedback about personal functioning, especially as related to professional conduct, can inspire or motivate trainees to engage in a process of self-reflection about their situation, which is hopefully followed by a resolve and plan to change behavior. In many situations affecting trainees' interpersonal, intrapersonal, and professional functioning, personal history as well as multiple systemic contexts and social identities, as discussed previously, also are influencing factors in conduct. In examining the etiology of or rationale for behavior, faculty and supervisors should not enter into a diagnostic or therapeutic stance with their trainees, even as they attempt to support proactive change. The ethics codes for most mental health professional organizations support the practice recommendations that doing so is considered unethical. For example:

- *Standard IV. 4.2 Therapy With Students or Supervisees:* "Marriage and family therapists do not provide therapy to current students or supervisees" (American Association for Marriage and Family Therapy, 2015).
- *Standard F.10.e. Counseling Services:* "Counselor educators do not serve as counselors to students currently enrolled in a counseling or related program and over whom they have power and authority" (ACA, 2014a).
- *7.05(b) Mandatory Individual or Group Therapy:* "Faculty who are or are likely to be responsible for evaluating students' academic performance do not themselves provide that therapy" (American Psychological Association [APA], 2017c).

For these reasons, one of the most widely recommended components of trainee remediation is participation in personal therapy outside of the program of study (Russell & Peterson, 2003), a prescription that could potentially provide an opportunity to process personal triggers and learn resources for managing difficult emotions. Although multiple authors (Bemak, Epp, & Keys, 1999; Kaslow et al., 2007; Schoener, 1999; Vasquez, 1999) have expressed concern about requiring personal counseling as an element of remediation, others (Elman & Forrest, 2004; Gilfoyle, 2008) have presented guidelines for encouraging the requirement to be more transparent and ethically sound. Even though students/supervisees requiring remediation are training to serve others in a counseling capacity, they still may hold negative personal biases about attending counseling themselves. Some students, especially early in training, express apprehension that becoming a client means that they lack the mental stability needed to become a mental health professional. If personal counseling is a suggested or recommended ingredient of the remediation plan, it can be advantageous to specifically assess for this belief when meeting with the trainee to discuss the remediation process. Furthermore, more than three quarters of practicing counselors have reported choosing to utilize personal counseling (Norcross, Strausser-

Kirtland, & Faltus, 1988), and knowing this may also help supervisees to feel more comfortable seeking it out themselves. Creating a program culture that communicates acceptance and professional appropriateness of attending personal therapy can assist all students with feeling more supported as they strive to enhance their personal coping skills and styles. This may be encouraged, for example, by including personal therapy as a program requirement for all students (Homrich, 2009) and/or by having faculty mention that they too attend personal counseling.

Conclusion

As faculty and supervisors evaluate the appropriateness of trainees' interpersonal, intrapersonal, and professional behaviors, an array of developmental considerations must also be acknowledged. Faculty and supervisors are better able to evaluate trainees when they are knowledgeable about what constitutes normal or typical professional developmental processes. Respondeat superiors must also realize that students and supervisees have individual differences and that degrees of variation will occur as trainees navigate new dimensions of growth and development in the professional realm. When having discussions or creating experiences meant to facilitate trainees' growth, effective evaluators also consider a multitude of contextual factors, including, but not limited to, cultural perspectives, social identities, personal histories, and the presence of disabilities or other challenges.

Although most trainees respond as anticipated to their training, moving through their personal and professional development more or less predictably, some others will require assistance or additional intervention on the part of faculty and supervisors to become effective helpers. Throughout this process, it is especially important to remember that regardless of how strong or how challenged a trainee may seem, all students and supervisees deserve to be treated with respect and dignity while being given the opportunity to prove their abilities. Engaging with a faculty member or supervisor who demonstrates empathy, honesty, respect for trainees' values, and direct communication will provide the best possible environment for building a strong working relationship. (See What Would You Do? 4.1 and 4.2.)

Key Points and Best Practices

- Supervisors and educators have the unique opportunity to develop positive working relationships that set the stage for the tone of feedback and remediation processes for students/supervisees.
- Trainees should be considered through a developmental lens.
- Trainees found to exhibit concerning interpersonal, intrapersonal, and professional behaviors often evidence early signs of this behavior near the beginning of their training. Addressing these concerning behaviors as early as possible provides the trainee with the best chance of successful development.

- Trainee behavior should be assessed from the very beginning of enrollment or engagement and supportive guidance and feedback provided whenever possible.
- It is educators' and supervisors' responsibility to demonstrate respect for and uphold the dignity of the supervisee in order to facilitate change and maintain a positive working relationship.
- Providing clear and direct, yet empathic, communication during interactions requiring either formal or informal feedback increases positive outcomes.
- Respect supervisees' right to have values that differ from those of the profession and the supervisor; help them learn how to bracket personal values and reconcile them with professional standards and behaviors.
- Consider contextual factors that influence trainee behavior, such as cultural perspectives, social identity, personal history, and disabilities, when assessing student performance and remediation.

What Would You Do? 4.1

At separate times over 3 days, two students come to your office individually to report that they are concerned about Emily, one of their peers and your advisee. Emily is in the middle of her third semester of your mental health graduate program. The two students, Courtney and Erin, are both reporting the same concern. They have become friends with Emily since the three women began the program at the same time. Each expresses feeling guilty for betraying Emily's confidence by coming to talk with you; however, they are upset by some of Emily's comments and worry about her goodness of fit for the program and the profession. Courtney says that Emily told her that she disagrees with the legal and ethical mandates to refrain from engaging in sexual relations with clients and that she is hoping to convince her current therapist to have sex with her. Erin reports the same conversation. Emily has been a strong student academically in her coursework thus far. However, you have noticed that Emily's discussion in class reveals a tendency to challenge rules, and her presentation during class (both her manner of dress and her demeanor) appears provocative. When the legal mandate was discussed in class last semester, Emily had seemed unconvinced that having sex with clients could be harmful to them, depending on the circumstances; however, she had eventually agreed that therapists should follow the laws and ethics codes.

What would you do?

Which baseline competencies are inadequate for Emily at this time, and how might her developmental level be affecting her behaviors?

What other factors may be influencing her behavior?

How would you address this situation?

What Would You Do? 4.2

You are a supervisor of Mary, a postgraduate supervisee who is working on gaining clinical experience toward licensure. Mary comes to supervision and tells you about an incident that occurred earlier in the week. Mary had been counseling a client, Lisa, for 6 weeks to address symptoms of depression and anxiety that were significantly impacting her ability to maintain employment. On Monday, Mary received an e-mail from Lisa in which Lisa expressed personal attraction for Mary. Lisa wrote that she was afraid to tell Mary in person, so she wanted to e-mail her and then talk about it when they next met. Mary was upset by the e-mail and the stated attraction and immediately wrote Lisa back stating that she was not a lesbian and explaining that Lisa's attraction would make a working relationship impossible. Mary explained via e-mail that she thought it would be best to give Lisa a list of referrals for other mental health professionals in the area. Lisa has not responded since. Mary did not contact you during or after this e-mail exchange and, although still emotionally upset by the situation, does not seem to believe that she did anything illegal or unethical.

What would you do?

What role did Mary's values play in her decision to counsel and/or refer Lisa?

How would you address Mary about this topic in a manner that respects her right to her own values yet upholds the values of the profession?

How should Mary have proceeded with her client given her level of discomfort?

What intervention or remediation procedures would you suggest for Mary?

What steps could you take to protect your supervisory relationship with Mary?

Chapter 5
Faculty and Supervisor Roles in Gatekeeping

Kyle D. Baldwin

The first line of gatekeepers in the clinical field are faculty members. Faculty impart knowledge, provide clinical skills training, model professional and personal conduct, and evaluate the professional judgment and personal dispositions of students and supervisees in order to determine whether they exhibit the qualities necessary to continue in the profession (Jackson-Cherry, 2006). Predegree supervisors, both faculty and site based (e.g., those in mental health agencies, hospitals, residential facilities, schools, and university counseling settings), are also gatekeepers because they play important roles in providing clinical supervision for graduate students during practicum and internship activities within the academic realm of the graduate program.

Postdegree supervisors are also as critical to the gatekeeping process, providing supervision beyond the academic arena of the postgraduation experience for degreed clinicians who are seeking licensure under the mandate of their state's licensure or regulatory board requirements. Postgraduation supervision may be provided by a qualified or an approved supervisor, depending on the definitions and requirements of the particular jurisdiction. Postgraduate trainees are recognized by a variety of titles, defined by the regulatory board, including *registered intern*, *clinical intern*, *associate*, *conditional*, or *provisional licensee*, or are postdoctoral trainees, all of whom are working toward licensure according to the requirements of their respective clinical professions.

This chapter first identifies and defines the roles of faculty and supervisors and addresses the importance of leadership and modeling regarding the gatekeeping process. Next, it explores seven categories of gatekeeping activities of significance for training programs and/or clinical settings. Gatekeeping activities addressed in this chapter pertain to the following areas: (a) providing support to trainees in their learning and development as clinicians; (b) preserving the safety and well-being of others, particularly the welfare of clients; (c) enlisting colleagues and coworkers to comply with policies and procedures; (d) providing students with opportunities to address concerns; (e) maintaining confidentiality; (f) intervening when injustices in the gatekeeping process are observed; and (g) managing liability risk.

Roles of Faculty and Supervisors

Clinical educators and supervisors are expected to take active roles in training, evaluation, and gatekeeping processes to ensure that supervisees receive appropriate educational experiences and clinical skills training (Kaslow et al., 2007). In clinical education, faculty members overseeing clinical activities and (pre- or postdegree) field supervisors are considered the respondeat superiors of a supervisee. This legal term identifies supervisors as having responsibility and vicarious liability for the actions of their trainees and thus "placing themselves at some risk every time they agree to provide supervision" as the ultimate responsible party (Wheeler & Bertram, 2015, p. 266). Polychronis and Brown (2016) observed that "strict liability leaves clinical supervisors responsible regardless of their rendering of exemplary, textbook clinical supervision" (p. 140) for the misconduct of their supervisees. (See On the Legal Side 5.1.)

Ethical definitions for standards for supervision and practice differ across the clinical professions, and legal requirements vary from state to state as defined in regulatory law. Those supervising pre- or postdegree trainees, whether faculty or agency based, need to be familiar with the ethical and legal mandates under which they practice supervisory oversight. This is especially important in the arenas of gatekeeping and endorsement. *Endorsement* is a critical aspect of gatekeeping, as it is a formal pledge by a supervisor or faculty member that a trainee is ready to proceed with advancement in the training or professional practice process (e.g., candidacy, practicum, internship, graduation, licensure, or certification in the case of a specialty area).

Professional organizations and certification bodies publish guidelines useful to supervisors that include guidance for gatekeeping. Useful resources are *Best Practices in Clinical Supervision* (Association for Counselor Education and Supervision, 2011), the NBCC *Code of Ethics* (National Board for Certified Counselors [NBCC], 2016), and *Best Practice Standards in Social Work Supervision* (National Association of Social Workers & Association of Social Work Boards [NASW & ASWB], 2013). These standards can be utilized and interpreted in legal proceedings or licensure board disciplinary hearings as the expectation

On the Legal Side 5.1

Polychronis and Brown (2016) reported that 27 of 51 jurisdictions in the United States use the strict liability standard to define the responsibility of clinical supervisors in overseeing the professional behavior of their supervisees:

> Strict liability holds clinical supervisors responsible for the actions of supervisees in a professional setting without having to demonstrate any negligence or wrongdoing on the part of the supervisors. Consequently, in those jurisdictions, clinical supervision is a particularly high-risk endeavor. (p. 145)

In light of this legal standard, supervisors should be conscientious about their supervisory practice and maintain careful oversight of their supervisees. Risk management strategies include providing as much supervision as possible in light of a supervisee's caseload and the chronicity of clients; asking questions of the supervisee to seek out as many details about his or her work with clients as possible—the more the better; consulting with other supervisors to gain collegial suggestions and perspectives if there are concerns about the supervisee; documenting supervision meetings, including all directives given to the supervisee; and viewing or listening to as many recorded client sessions as possible to get a sense of the supervisee's effectiveness with clients. Clinical supervisors have the right and responsibility to observe, listen to, and/or watch supervisees in clinical practice; supervisee self-report is not considered an adequate single source of information. Although the circumstances of litigation will necessarily question the supervisor's carelessness or negligence in fulfilling his or her supervisory duties, documenting the strategies listed here may help bolster evidence to the contrary.

for best practice standards within the clinical profession whether or not the supervisor is a member of those organizations. For example, the NBCC *Code of Ethics* (NBCC, 2016) states that supervision includes documentation of the goals and progress of supervisees and the requirement that supervisors should intervene when "supervisees are impaired or incompetent and thus place client(s) at risk" (p. 2). Other professional organizations express similar expectations in their ethics codes and standards, some of which are covered in other chapters in this book and in Appendix A.

Some of the characteristics necessary for supervisory competence include knowing about supervision models (Bernard & Goodyear, 2014), understanding the professional supervisory relationship, maintaining competence as a clinician, and obtaining a thorough understanding of "the ethical, legal, and regulatory dimensions of supervision" (Welfel, 2006, p. 295). Supervision during practicum and internship provides opportunities to address the issues or concerns of trainees, and supervisors can model professional and ethical behavior by doing so. Supervisors can also provide interventions that "range from information recommendations to more pointed suggestions bordering on directives for changes in behaviors" (Bemak, Epp, & Keys, 1999, p. 23) to support student development or remediation.

Supervisors from all clinical professions are responsible for maintaining supervisory skills, competence as defined by their jurisdiction of practice and their specific profession, and cross-cultural competence in working with clients and in the supervisory relationship. Inherent in this responsibility is the knowledge of and competence to appropriately institute gatekeeping skills, which include evaluation, remediation, and ethically and legally proper professional endorsement practices. To effectively demonstrate leadership skills and model professional and ethical behavior, clinicians are responsible for developing their own supervisory competence and skill set. The practice of supervision has been identified as one of the most noteworthy aspects in the training of professional counselors (Kindsvatter, Haag, Granello, & Duba, 2008; NASW & ASWB, 2013).

Leadership and Modeling

Gatekeepers (e.g., faculty and supervisors) have an important role in modeling ethical and professional behavior to students and supervisees. Bernard and Goodyear (2014) stated that "observing and modeling others is a powerful way to learn, and this extends to the learning of ethical behavior" (p. 278). Modeling leadership, professional conduct, ethical behavior, and the standards of behavior expected by the educational program or agency is an important supervisory activity. When gatekeepers act as role models, "the actions and advice of the supervisor are keenly observed by supervisees, and consequently, influence much of the supervisee's thinking and behavior" (NASW & ASWB, 2013, p. 14), often being emulated by supervisees in future professional practice.

Critical to leadership and modeling is the skill of providing *feedback*, defined by Bernard and Goodyear (2014) as "a process in which the supervisor verbally shares thoughts and assessment of the supervisee's progress, either explicitly or implicitly" (p. 233). To provide clear and helpful feedback to trainees, faculty and site-based supervisors need to have a clear understanding of the policies of the institution and profession they represent. Knowing about ethical and legal gatekeeping procedures such as documentation or consequential steps in remedying trainee behavior, as well as understanding their role in the evaluation process, are essential criteria for supervision and the tasks of gatekeeping (Bemak et al., 1999). By modeling a professional, nondefensive stance when addressing problematic behavior, supervisors and faculty teach supervisees professionalism through their actions (Behnke, 2008) and influence trainee responses and the potential for successful outcomes. This is especially important when instituting feedback and formal remediation procedures, as the purpose of both is to encourage successful change and positive development in the student or supervisee.

The supervisory role extends beyond leading and modeling. It is also intended to provide appropriate support and the opportunity for positive professional development while protecting the rights and vulnerable position of supervisees. Professional ethics codes charge faculty and supervisors with protecting trainees, using their influence respectfully and for good, facilitating the learning/clinical development process, evaluating trainee progress, and promoting ethical practice through supervisory and mentoring processes (American Association for Marriage and Family Therapy, 2015; National Association of School Psychologists, 2010; NASW, 2017). Supervisors and faculty members hold power inherent in their positions through knowledge, experience, and evaluative roles. Students and supervisees observe the ethical practices and legal compliance of those who are in positions of power, especially when they are in the early stages of training and professional development, and internalize these models of practice. As standard bearers for ethical and legal practices, interpersonal and intrapersonal behavior, and professional conduct, supervisors and educators cannot underestimate their influence—and their roles as gatekeepers.

Gatekeeping Activities

The remainder of this chapter focuses on the gatekeeping activities of faculty and supervisors as they pertain to the following seven areas: (a) providing support to trainees in their learning and development as clinicians; (b) preserving the safety and well-being of others, particularly the welfare of clients; (c) enlisting colleagues and coworkers to comply with policies and procedures; (d) providing students with opportunities to address concerns; (e) maintaining confidentiality; (f) intervening when injustices in the gatekeeping process are observed; and (g) managing liability risk.

Providing Support to Trainees in Their Learning and Development as Clinicians

A period of training and/or supervision culminates with the application of gatekeeping practices in determining whether a trainee is deemed ready to progress to the next level of training (e.g., from academic learning to clinical skills practice, to practicum, to internship, to graduation, to licensure). This progression requires the acknowledgment or endorsement of the faculty and supervisors responsible for overseeing the gatekeeping process as previously addressed.

Trainees, supervisees, faculty, and supervisors should have a clear understanding of the nature of the supervisory role in the gatekeeping process and how this role differs from other roles, such as counselor educator, therapist, or consultant (Behnke, 2005). This understanding is especially important for doctoral students, first-time faculty members, and practicing clinicians new to providing supervisory services. These groups are balancing both their new professional roles and responsibilities while simultaneously learning how to be effective gatekeepers. For example, new students and supervisees should be advised that faculty members and supervisors do not provide counseling services but are expected to address how the trainee's intrapersonal and interpersonal behaviors might impact clients, professional conduct, and interactions within the supervisory relationship (American Counseling Association [ACA], 2014a, p. 14). As previously mentioned, providing feedback to trainees is an important component of supervision and gatekeeping processes. It is recommended that feedback be (a) communicated regularly, (b) based on learning goals or competencies, (c) direct and clear, and (d) "balanced between support/reinforcement and challenge/criticism" (Bernard & Goodyear, 2014, p. 235). This allows educators and supervisors to support students in their developmental process as clinicians.

Inherent in the role of supervisor is the responsibility to provide educational and developmental support and opportunities to trainees while also monitoring trainees and supervisees for behaviors that indicate whether trainees may pose potential harm to future clients. Faculty and supervisors should advise trainees of the evaluative methods that will be utilized during the training program or supervisory period and the accompanying timeline. Trainee evaluation is discussed in detail in Chapter 9.

Supervisors and faculty must understand the range of problematic behaviors that might arise in trainee performance, such as difficulties with academic performance, interpersonal skills, clinical performance, professional conduct, or management of intrapersonal reactions and/or demonstrations of unethical behavior (Forrest, Elman, Gizara, & Vacha-Haase, 1999; K. W. Nelson, Oliver, Reeve, & McNichols, 2010). Being familiar with the various categories of problems and being able to notice concerns early allows faculty and supervisors to provide support for students and supervisees as they work to meet the challenges of learning and the personal and professional developmental process inherent in becoming clinicians. Problematic behaviors that occur with trainees could be the "result of competence never achieved, diminished functioning, or willful disregard" (K. W. Nelson et al., 2010, p. 3). Early intervention via conversations and feedback not only supports struggling students but can also differentiate the category of emerging problematic behavior so that educators and supervisors can provide the appropriate support.

Preserving the Safety and Well-Being of Others

Clinical educators, supervisors, and their institutions, whether based in an educational or agency setting, are responsible for the safety and well-being of others in relation to the actions of their trainees. This applies first and foremost to current or future clients of the trainees but also may pertain to the safety and well-being of other students or supervisees who may be negatively affected by a problematic supervisee. Faculty and supervisors "may be held liable if they endorse students to work with clients if they believe a student's personal limitations may cause harm" (Jackson-Cherry, 2006, p. 157). Polychronis and Brown (2016) concurred that supervision is on a short list of high-risk areas of clinical practice not only concerning the therapeutic services of supervisees but also because "by definition, strict liability regards supervisors as responsible for supervisees' conduct in the professional realm, including such egregious supervisee misconduct as deliberately concealed sexual involvement with a client" (p. 140).

Preserving the safety and well-being of clients is of vital importance, and trainees must understand the seriousness of adhering to the legal and ethical standards of the profession. Facilitating this awareness in trainees is the responsibility of educators and supervisors who must also inform students and supervisees about their obligations to take action as respondeat superiors when problematic and unethical behaviors are demonstrated (Baldo, Softas-Nall, & Shaw, 1997; Henderson & Dufrene, 2011). Mental health counseling and other clinical professional associations address the role of supervisors in preventing harm to clients in their ethics codes. Harm to clients can occur as a result of a lack of academic knowledge and judgment, inept clinical skill, and/or unprofessional conduct, areas of performance that fall within the responsibilities of gatekeepers.

Knapp, Younggren, VandeCreek, Harris, and Martin (2013) suggested that "as supervisors, psychologists assume full responsibility for the work product of their supervisees. They should undertake supervision with the expectation that they will take full legal responsibility for the services delivered" (p. 200) through direct or vicarious liability. *Direct liability* refers to a supervisor's own negligence, such as negligent supervision wherein his or her actions or misdirection as a supervisor cause harm to a client or supervisee (Welfel, 2006). *Vicarious liability* refers to a supervisor (or employer) being "held liable for actions of the supervisee regardless of any fault on the part of the supervisor" (Saccuzzo, 1997, p. 122). A supervisor is responsible for the actions of his or her supervisees by virtue of being the responsible or respondeat superior (Bernard & Goodyear, 2014; Disney & Stephens, 1994; Wheeler & Bertram, 2015).

Clinical educators and supervisors have an important obligation to ensure that students do not receive a degree and that supervisees are not licensed if they pose a risk to the welfare of future clients (Gaubatz & Vera, 2002; Hutchens, Block, & Young, 2013). As discussed throughout this book, establishing gatekeeping procedures and policies to monitor and evaluate the conduct of graduate students and supervisees throughout their training sequence is an important and necessary aspect of the clinical professions (Baldo et al., 1997). The *ACA Code of Ethics* (ACA, 2014a) states that supervisors are to "assist supervisees in securing remedial assistance" and recommend dismissal from training programs or counseling settings when supervisees are "unable to demonstrate that they can provide competent professional services to a range of diverse clients" (Standard F.6.b.). The goal of gatekeeping efforts is to protect future clients as well as others who are affected by a trainee's behavior.

Protecting Trainees and the Learning Environment

In addition to safeguarding clients, program faculty and agency supervisors have a responsibility to protect the welfare of colleagues in the related settings of the trainee. This may include, for example, student peers, professional and nonprofessional staff, other faculty members, future supervisors, and others engaged in the educational and work setting. These individuals may, under atypical circumstances, be subjected to distress or harassment by a trainee who displays problematic professional, interpersonal, and intrapersonal behaviors affecting the work performance of colleagues. Students displaying performance problems can disrupt the overall learning environment in an educational setting (Brown-Rice & Furr, 2013). According to surveys of students (Bemak et al., 1999; Brown-Rice & Furr, 2013), problematic behaviors that affect attention to learning include the following:

- Interrupting classroom dynamics with immature behavior
- Excessive interruptions and questioning due to personal anxiety about a topic that the student has difficulty comprehending
- Lack of ability to notice the social cues of others in an interactional setting
- Absence of personal insight
- Psychological problems that interfere with group dynamics and interpersonal interactions
- Overestimating one's clinical abilities
- Reluctance to take risks
- Failure to attend to client needs
- Moral character issues that result in poor judgment or unethical behavior

Even more disturbing to 85% of peer students was the incompletion of activities or assignments that required the participation of multiple students and that subsequently affected the grades of all involved in the team effort. Disruptive interpersonal behaviors can negatively affect or sabotage classroom demonstration projects such as cofacilitation of a group session or interactional processes when students are attempting to demonstrate clinical skills in a simulation.

Brown-Rice and Furr (2013) found that the top five problematic behaviors of students that most affected other learners were "difficulty regulating emotions (19%), inadequate academic skills (15%), psychological unsuitability (15%), inadequate clinical skills (13%), and unprofessional behavior (10%)" (p. 227). Conduct problems (e.g., chronic tardiness, excessive absences, and aggressive outbursts in class) also disrupt learning (Koppel Mitnick, 2001) by creating an unsafe learning environment and anxiety in other students.

In the clinical setting, unprofessional behaviors may include exhibiting extreme transference/countertransference responses to clients or supervisors, engaging in inappropriate self-disclosure or failing to listen to clients, undermining the goals of the supervisor or agency, treating staff disrespectfully, responding to clinical supervision defensively, demonstrating a reluctance to respond to feedback, or "engaging in undue conflict or withdrawal" with a supervisor (Bemak et al., 1999, pp. 26–27). Brown-Rice and Furr (2013) reported that although educators believed that only 3% of problematic students gateslipped through their training programs, students estimated the percentage of peers gateslipping at closer to 18%. In addition, 78% of students were concerned about the effect on the counseling profession when a problematic classmate was permitted to graduate and move on to the profession.

Across settings, unprofessional conduct, lack of judgment, interpersonal conflict, and emotional reactivity are disturbing to coworkers, peers, and others who have to witness the problematic behavior. Not only do these behaviors, when left unchecked, require the involvement of faculty and supervisors as gatekeepers, but they also put those in a nonsupervisory capacity in a bind. Students may prefer not to be in the position of reporting the problematic behavior of peers to faculty, and supervisees may avoid being held responsible for reporting other trainees to supervisors, as they may fear being labeled as complainers. They may also be reluctant to face potential retribution from the problematic individual who is causing the disruption or engaging in unethical behavior. Even though peer trainees may sometimes have the opportunity to observe actions that would not occur in front of a respondeat superior, they may have concerns that speaking up will have a negative effect on them.

Enlisting Colleague and Coworker Compliance During Gatekeeping

For gatekeeping processes and procedures to be effective in a training program or agency setting, all constituencies and appropriate shareholders need to work in concert to respond consistently to problematic situations encountered by trainees, a topic that is addressed in greater detail in Chapter 6 on gatekeeper collaboration. Professional colleagues and coworkers, including core faculty, adjunct and visiting faculty, field site supervisors, doctoral student supervisors-in-training, and even institutional administrators and risk management coordinators, must ally in their gatekeeping efforts. It is critical that all stakeholders have a common understanding of and agree with published standards for personal and professional conduct, evaluation and feedback procedures, and the remediation and dismissal policies of the educational or agency unit in order for gatekeeping practices to be successful. Because gatekeeping sometimes involves difficult interactions that include conflict and discipline, or potential liability, some individuals may be reluctant to carry out their gatekeeping role of addressing problematic supervisees. These colleagues require guidance and support in understanding the importance of gatekeeping processes and becoming active participants in the gatekeeping process to create uniform enforcement of the expected standards and consistent response to problematic students. This is important for both the inner working dynamics of the institution as well as management of liability risk.

There may be several logistical reasons why gatekeepers avoid addressing problems with students and supervisees. One of the main reasons has to do with a lack of established formal gatekeeping policies and procedures. If only informal policies and procedures exist, educators and supervisors will have difficulty differentiating objective data (e.g., the completion of documentation or timely attendance at appointments or client sessions) from subjective data (e.g., inconsistent moods that interfere with professional behavior, or awkward interpersonal skills that may be difficult to convey to the student; Bemak et al., 1999). In addition, clinical supervisors may have trouble evaluating the appropriate developmental level of clinical skill achievement and professional conduct demonstrated by supervisees in a practicum, internship, or postgraduation internship (Bemak et al., 1999). A lack of access to consultation or guidance pertaining to recommended procedures for addressing gatekeeping concerns throughout the various levels of graduate study may also deter faculty and supervisors from fulfilling their gatekeeping roles (Bodner, 2012; Homrich, DeLorenzi, Bloom, & Godbee, 2014).

Differences of opinion about an institution's commitment to gatekeeping practices, especially after a problematic situation has been encountered, can result in discouraged faculty or supervisors reluctant to initiate gatekeeping practices in the future, confusion among students and supervisees about professional expectations, and increased liability. Collaborative relationships with open communication help to ensure future productive collaboration among colleagues within and outside the program unit. (See Notes From the Field 5.1.)

Other factors that may influence engagement in gatekeeping processes include reluctant gatekeepers who may struggle with providing negative evaluations of students who have high grades but who are deficient in the areas of interpersonal, intrapersonal, and/or professional behavior. This may be because of concerns about the amount of personal time, effort, and financial resources students have invested in pursuing their

Notes From the Field 5.1

Gatekeeping procedures are challenging to trainees, and they can also be difficult for those who oversee the training process. Gatekeeping experiences are both emotionally and cognitively challenging for faculty members and supervisors. In a recent qualitative study about faculty experiences with and perspectives on gatekeeping, Chang (2017) found that faculty striving to be effective gatekeepers depended on the strengths and interactions inherent in four supporting processes.

The first was the internal processes of *integrating identities* and *balancing responsibilities* that emerge during the gatekeeping process. Chang (2017) found that faculty sometimes struggled to "balance their positive and supportive feelings towards students with the duties that arose when those students began to exhibit problems of professional competence" (p. 31). In encountering gatekeeping experiences, study participants admitted to needing to learn how to balance a range of expectations, functional tasks that consumed time and energy, and shifting roles that ranged from supporting to challenging to judging the outcome of a student's career path. Chang found that in faculty striving to be effective gatekeepers, learning how to successfully integrate various identities and balance responsibilities contributed to enacting effective gatekeeping responsibilities.

Practicing discernment, the "internal process of continuously enacting introspection and self-awareness in order to accurately appraise, evaluate, remediate and monitor" (Chang, 2017, p. 33) with problematic students, was the second experience of gatekeepers in their path to effectiveness. Because self-awareness combined with clinical skills and judgment is an important component of the process, those striving to gatekeep effectively consciously practiced discernment, which increased their self-perceived capability and effectiveness as gatekeepers.

The third component of faculty experiences of striving to be competent gatekeepers was the internal process of *managing challenging emotions*, particularly anxiety. "Because of the serious consequences of gatekeeping, their desires to be helpful and positive towards students and perhaps due to the investment made with students, participants experienced a wide range of difficult emotions involving the student with [problematic professional competence]" (Chang, 2017, p. 35). As Chang (2017) described in his study, faculty had to pay close attention to managing strong emotional reactions to the presenting situation, the student, colleagues, and even themselves in some circumstances. They found the difficult emotional reactions they experienced to be particularly burdensome. The range of emotional experiences included anger, disappointment, self-doubt, dread, worry, frustration, guilt, and sadness, as well as empathy for the student going through remediation or other gatekeeping processes. Often, their emotional struggle was most challenging to manage when they perceived themselves as doing something damaging or hurtful to a student. Chang determined that if participants manage the emotionally challenging aspects of gatekeeping, it helps them to sustain themselves as gatekeepers and counselor educators and leads to higher striving to be an effective gatekeeper. Conversely, if they have difficulty managing these challenging emotions,

(Continued)

Notes From the Field 5.1 *(Continued)*

it negatively impacts their striving to be an effective gatekeeper, especially over time.

The fourth aspect of internal experiences that influenced faculty engagement in gatekeeping processes was associated with the qualities of *cohesion and capability faculty perceived in their colleagues.* Chang (2017) found these qualities to include the sense of trust, mutual respect, support, and shared motivation or investment participants witnessed and experienced in their faculty colleagues. The task of gatekeeping is challenging intellectually as well as emotionally. Most faculty and supervisors would rather avoid the obligation of gatekeeping because of the internal and interpersonal factors involved in the process, and unfortunately some do. However, as dedicated faculty and supervisors strive to do their best work as gatekeepers, understanding the internal experiences of gatekeeping is valuable in creating support for the individuals involved in the process and one another.

graduate studies and future career (Bemak et al., 1999). Faculty and supervisors may personally be conflict avoidant and have difficulty dealing with stressful situations such as confronting others. They might also be unsure of their exact role in the gatekeeping process and thus hesitant to engage with supervisees who may prove to be unwilling to respond appropriately to the feedback identifying problematic concerns. The time demands and the documentation required to address problems of professional competence are other deterrents for gatekeepers, especially when documentation may lead to more time- and energy-sapping involvement required by formal remediation procedures, dismissal from a graduate program, or potential future litigation.

Individuals in gatekeeping positions are encouraged to develop and operationalize an ethical protocol to support students who encounter problematic peers and take action in accordance with the ethics codes of their profession to manage unprofessional or impaired colleagues (Brown-Rice & Furr, 2013). Professionals need to know how to manage or address misconduct or clinical deficiencies in their colleagues, an unsavory task for any clinical professional. Bemak et al. (1999) proposed a five-step process model of addressing both academic and personal/professional development to assist gatekeepers in their roles when monitoring clinicians-in-training:

- Clarify and communicate expectations to gatekeeper colleagues as well as trainees.
- Obtain consensual agreement on policies and procedures.
- Identify concerns of students and supervisees.
- Develop a process for providing feedback and recommendations to trainees.
- Monitor and evaluate trainee progress.

All gatekeepers (faculty and supervisors) should agree and collaborate on the enactment of the steps suggested by these authors. Ideally, this discussion and consensus would occur with all affected colleagues in advance of engaging in gatekeeping processes.

It is important that standards of conduct in clinical training be established and understood by everyone at every level involved in the gatekeeping process: from faculty to students, faculty to field site supervisors, field site supervisors to supervisees, and postdegree supervisors to prelicensure supervisees. Understanding should also be extended to administrators or people in other institutional positions who might be responsible in the event of litigation due to a gatekeeping situation. Because supervision is a necessary step toward achieving licensure, clinical supervisors, whether pre- or postdegree, need to be especially comfortable with and well versed in gatekeeping requirements, as most licensure laws require supervisors to formally attest to or endorse the fact that a supervisee is ready to enter the profession (Homrich et al., 2014).

Additional concerns of faculty and supervisors that can deter the initiation of gatekeeping procedures are fears that gatekeeping activities will impose negative career consequences, that institutional affiliations will not support gatekeeping recommendations, and/or that students who have been dismissed from programs or supervisees who have been denied endorsement will initiate legal retaliation (Bodner, 2012). Thus, the cooperative team approach described previously is both essential and beneficial in enlisting the support and participation of colleagues and coworkers in the gatekeeping process. Specifically, crucial actions include increasing interactions and communication among faculty, supervisors, and advisors when problematic student issues arise; ensuring timely and helpful feedback from the supervisory/faculty team to the trainee; and advocating for the protection of students' rights, such as due process, while also supporting colleagues personally and professionally when engaged in difficult actions or decisions (Bemak et al., 1999).

In addition to a common understanding and supportive position among all constituents who value gatekeeping, continued analysis and self-education is important at the respondeat supervisory level. Faculty and supervisors should not just proactively review gatekeeping practices; they should also spend time deconstructing cases in which they or others engaged in gatekeeping efforts. Some authors have suggested that ethical and legal issues in the practice of gatekeeping be discussed as they emerge in the contemporary literature across clinical professions (Jackson-Cherry, 2006; Lumadue & Duffey, 1999). For example, in the case of the student dismissal and resulting litigation that occurred at The College of William and Mary (*Plaintiff v. Rector and Board of Visitors of The College of William and Mary*) in 2005, the faculty involved shared their learning experiences in the professional literature (V. A. Foster & McAdams, 2009; McAdams &

Foster, 2007; McAdams, Foster, & Ward, 2007). In a case at Eastern Michigan University that involved ethical issues conflicting with the profession (*Ward v. Wilbanks*, 2010) both faculty and stakeholders of the profession provided context, decision-making strategies, and overarching considerations for gatekeepers who might find themselves in related situations (Burkholder & Hall, 2014; Dugger & Francis, 2014; Herlihy, Hermann, & Greden, 2014; Kaplan, 2014). The cases of others not only are educational from a procedural viewpoint but also contain excellent preventive information for faculty and supervisors and discuss the importance of enlisting the collaborative participation of other stakeholders.

Frequent review of standards and expectations of trainee behavior and conduct (which should be published for all to understand) is essential with doctoral students who are teaching or supervising, new faculty, adjunct faculty, field site supervisors new to supervisory practice, or partners with the educational institution that oversee field site placement. These individuals may not be familiar with the gatekeeping culture or expectations of the profession. These efforts would include providing one-on-one or small-group education about the detailed policies and procedures for addressing trainee professional conduct and interpersonal behavior required by the graduate program (Jackson-Cherry, 2006). It is also important for educational units to understand the expectations and gatekeeping practices of field sites affected by policies and human resources mandates because most interns are now treated as ex officio employees in relation to agency standards. Standards for the expected conduct of supervisees, evaluation policies, feedback procedures, and remediation and endorsement practices should be developed in concert with and conveyed to those affected. A discussion of how field sites and education faculty will communicate and collaborate is also important as a preventive measure. Difficulty arises when there is a lack of understanding of or commitment to the established policies and resulting application of procedural actions within or across training programs. Common understanding and commitment to gatekeeping reduces splitting or divisiveness by unhappy students, supervisees, and faculty or supervisors who are not in agreement on how to address a specific problematic situation. Lack of consistency can be destructive in the gatekeeping enforcement process.

Providing Students With Opportunities to Be Heard

Student evaluation by faculty is an ongoing process throughout the entire academic program. Policies and procedures pertaining to the expectations of students and supervisees should be provided to students when they begin their graduate studies and published on the college or university's website. It is recommended that a formal statement or informed consent be signed by students to confirm awareness and understanding of the program's policies and procedures, a procedure discussed in detail in Chapters 6 and 7. By verifying their agreement with the institutional policies, students acknowledge their understanding of and willingness to abide by such policies. A signed policy verification statement can be filed in the student's academic record (Jackson-Cherry, 2006) in the event that there is any future denial of awareness or understanding of program expectations for student conduct.

While learning about organizational and professional expectations, students and supervisees should be provided with the opportunity to inquire about any expectations, policies, or procedures that might need further clarification. When policies and procedures that address student performance and guidelines are introduced before or at the start of a program, faculty, supervisors, students, and supervisees will be better prepared to address and respond if areas of concern should arise.

Opportunities for students to be heard in regard to their progress in the program or pertaining to any trepidation expressed by faculty, supervisors, or peers should occur at the time the concern emerges. These can occur during individual meetings with faculty or supervisors in regard to coursework, clinical work, and/or specific performance considerations. They can also be scheduled during routine meetings with an assigned faculty advisor, especially after a regular progress review or evaluation period conducted for all students. Mandatory meetings with a faculty advisor are recommended during the first year of a training program to establish a nonclassroom relationship with a professional who can serve as a consultant. Students should be encouraged to meet with other faculty as needed when problems arise and/or to discuss challenges with a faculty member with whom they feel connected or comfortable. Student mentors who are further along in their program of study can also be assigned to entering students to provide guidance and support. This same structure can occur in a supervisory setting, allowing for multiple opportunities for supervisees to clarify expectations, consult about struggles, and/or address problems of professional performance.

Opportunities for cohort meetings may also be beneficial to students. First-year graduate students can participate in a mandated end-of-the-first-semester debriefing meeting in which all first-year students can meet and speak with faculty members about their experiences thus far in the program and receive guidance regarding their future program of study. Students who are experiencing difficulties can share their concerns in this cohort meeting or privately with their faculty advisor, other faculty educators, or student mentors—all of whom may be able to offer guidance to successfully address any concerns or challenges. Multiple cohort meetings throughout the duration of a graduate program should be considered, as they provide additional opportunities for students to share their experiences, ask questions, or express concerns. Examples of cohort meetings include new student orientation, clinical placement orientation, practicum/internship placement workshop, clinical orientation to practicum and internship, and Preparing to Launch (a final semester workshop that reviews preparation for postgraduation employment and licensure requirements; Rollins College, 2017b).

Students should be encouraged to address any academic concerns in a timely manner and directly with course instructors throughout their program of study. Because faculty members evaluate each student's progress, students should also be provided with opportunities to self-evaluate their progress. Examples include annual or biannual student self-evaluations as well as anonymous evaluative surveys or written forums for students to evaluate individual courses and their faculty at the conclusion of each semester.

As detailed elsewhere in this book, *due process* procedures are constitutional rights intended to protect trainees "from unfair or arbitrary actions by supervisors or other training program officials, and to protect those officials and programs from legal liability" (Koppel Mitnick, 2001, p. 25). Preventive actions to avoid charges of denying due process include providing expectations in writing for students when they begin their training program, communicating these procedures to trainees, making sure that the procedures are understood, and applying the procedures in a timely manner and uniformly when "serious performance, conduct, and ethical problems" occur (p. 25). This would also include allowing trainees to respond verbally and in writing to any concerns or charges that may hamper their progression through professional training. During practicum and internship, faculty supervisors must maintain open and frequent communication with site supervisors to convey any concerns that indicate the potential for harm to a client or clients based on the actions of the trainee. Faculty and supervisors must also document that the site supervisor has communicated these concerns, and requisite actions for remedying the concerns, to the supervisee (Jackson-Cherry, 2006). When student concerns are brought to the attention of the core faculty, a formal departmental student review meeting should occur in a timely manner, during which these concerns can be discussed and faculty consultation with colleagues can occur. (See What Would You Do? 5.1.) Strategies for documenting communication and implementing individual gatekeeping procedures are discussed in Chapters 3, 9, and 11.

Maintaining Confidentiality and Respecting Privacy

Sharing information between faculty and site placement coordinators and supervisors about the placement of students in a supervisory setting is common practice. Discussions often include observations of the student's performance in the academic setting. A recommended proactive risk management strategy is to explain in student handbooks and supervision contracts that student information is shared among faculty and with supervisors for the purposes of evaluation and to enhance both the department's and site agency's focus on trainee development and protecting client welfare.

What Would You Do? 5.1

Benny is a doctoral student in a highly regarded counseling psychology program. As part of his doctoral responsibilities, he supervises three master's-level counseling students in the program's in-department community mental health clinic. One of his supervisees is Santiago, who is in his initial practicum experience. Santiago attends supervision regularly but, from Benny's perspective, appears that he thinks he knows all that is necessary to be counseling clients. Benny has noticed two areas of concern: (a) Santiago is behind on his case documentation, although Santiago does not believe this is the problem that Benny perceives it to be; and (b) Santiago is documenting completion of experience hours that are incongruent with the clinic records; when asked about the discrepancy, Santiago blames the mistakes on other students running the clinic.

Benny has discussed his concerns about Santiago's professional behavior with his supervisor, Dr. Frost, who is also the department chair and oversees all supervision activities. Dr. Frost does not seem to want to engage with Benny on addressing Santiago and minimizes the problems as passing mistakes. Benny's concerns grow when an alarming incident occurs: Other practicum students inform him that Santiago has referred clinic clients to his own private practice where they are being seen by Santiago, unsupervised. When Benny asks Santiago about this, Santiago says no such thing has ever happened. Benny then confirms that Santiago is not being truthful and is seeing clients independently without a license.

Benny immediately goes to his supervisor and presents the information. Again, Dr. Frost minimizes the events and clearly avoids pursuing an investigation or engaging Santiago in disciplinary actions, much to Benny's frustration. Benny is conflicted about what steps to take next. He believes that there is an ethical responsibility to stop Santiago's actions and is concerned about clients being seen in illegal practice conditions. Benny does not believe Santiago should be allowed to graduate from the master's program. He is also concerned about going against his supervisor, Dr. Frost (who is also on his dissertation committee), as well as other faculty members who seem to want to avoid dealing with a highly problematic student.

What would you do?

If you were unable to gain support from your superiors to engage in gatekeeping procedures to stop unethical and illegal behavior on the part of a trainee, what avenues would you pursue on your own?

What could you do to stop the private practice of this trainee?

What else could you do to stop the progression of the trainee in the master's program?

How would you explain your actions to your supervisor/department chair, who wants to ignore the problem until it goes away?

Policies and regulations regarding student or intern/employee confidentiality in program, university, institutional, and agency settings can be multifaceted and may influence consultation inherent in the gatekeeping process when discussing trainees who have exhibited problematic behaviors in their clinical work. Kaslow et al. (2009) recommended a multisystemic and structured approach to addressing confidentiality concerns by establishing communication boundaries whereby supervisors and supervisees understand how concerns about student performance will be shared among educators, supervisors, other students (Forrest, Shen-Miller, & Elman, 2008) and when consultation regarding student problems will need to be addressed and shared with other professionals, such as those working in partnering site agencies or in university or agency administration. When addressing issues of confidentiality, clinical educators and supervisors need to be aware of the limitations to individuals' rights to privacy and confidentiality pertaining to ethical, legal, and regulatory standards that require students to disclose information that is personal (Kaslow et al., 2007). *Privacy* refers to "the right of an individual to keep oneself and one's personal information free from unauthorized disclosure" (ACA, 2014a, p. 20).

A primary example of the privacy rights of students is the Family Educational Rights and Privacy Act (FERPA), which regulates disclosure of students' education records. The purpose of this federal legislation is to provide students (or parents in the case of minor students) with privacy rights over access to their written records. It applies to all institutions that receive funds from the U.S. Department of Education. FERPA governs recorded information that is (a) directly related to a student and (b) maintained by an educational agency or institution or by a party acting for the agency or institution. Students' medical and counseling treatment records are also covered by FERPA guidelines (U.S. Department of Education, 2015).

An exception to FERPA is that institutions can "release information without consent to school officials with legitimate educational interests" (Kaslow et al., 2007, p. 487). This specific clause was later clarified in the 2008 *Federal Register* to extend to those contractors performing services for the educational institutions, such as joint degree programs, and those overseeing practicum and fieldwork students, including unpaid interns. At the discretion of individuals representing the educational institution, such as faculty, pertinent student information that has been recorded in student records may be disclosed to placement sites based on a legitimate educational interest, as long as reasonable methods are applied to limit disclosure and restrict access to the information ("Family Educational Rights and Privacy," 2008). Partner sites may only use the information for the purposes for which it was disclosed and must also protect the information from further distribution. In other words, site supervisors may be regarded as partners of the educational institutions under FERPA when appropriate documentation is in place at the institution ("Family Educational Rights and Privacy," 2008; Springer, 2009; U.S. Department of Education, 2015).

In any circumstance involving legal issues, best practice measures call for consulting with institutional leadership and/or legal counsel to verify compliance. Graduate students should be informed about what information in their record is being shared, with whom, and why, even when their consent is not necessary. Being respectful of sharing students' information on a need-to-know basis and obtaining informed consent from trainees in advance of exchanging information are also recommended as best practice (Springer, 2009).

Educators and supervisors should consult their jurisdictional licensure requirements and the ethics codes of their professional associations to determine requirements regarding confidentiality. For example, *Ethical Principles of Psychologists and Code of Conduct* of the American Psychological Association (2017c) addresses student disclosure of personal information, stating that

> Psychologists do not require students or supervisees to disclose personal information in course- or program-related activities . . . [unless] (1) the program or training facility has clearly identified this requirement in its admissions and program materials or (2) the information is necessary to evaluate or obtain assistance for students whose personal problems could reasonably be judged to be preventing them from performing their training- or professionally related activities in a competent manner or posing a threat to the students or others. (Standard 7.04)

In terms of maintaining the confidentiality of trainees, marriage and family therapists are advised by their ethics codes that they

> do not disclose supervisee confidences except by written authorization or waiver, or when mandated or permitted by law. In educational or training settings where there are multiple supervisors, disclosures are permitted only to other professional colleagues, administrators, or employers who share responsibility for training of the supervisee. Verbal authorization will not be sufficient except in emergency situations, unless prohibited by law. (American Association for Marriage and Family Therapy, 2015, Standard 4.7)

Even when justified, revealing private information about supervisees and students should be limited to a need-to-know basis, especially with individuals outside of the faculty or supervisory circles. However, the "appropriate use of confidentiality should not interfere with assessment of or intervention with those who have competence problems" (Kaslow et al., 2007, p. 486).

It is important that trainees be informed of the limits to privacy or confidentiality across educational and supervisory settings at the beginning of their enrollment in a training program. It is also prudent for programs to obtain a three-way informed consent form signed by faculty supervisors, site supervisors, and trainees during the field placement process. Such an action allows for the exchange of information on an as needed or need-to-know basis for the purposes of faculty and supervisor evaluation and consultation. It is also important in order to take the necessary steps to support a problematic trainee if remedial intervention is needed and, primarily, when information is required to make decisions about client protection. Such a statement can be included in the three-way trainee placement agreement among the graduate program, the site agency, and the student or constructed as a separate informed consent or release of information document that is signed by all parties involved. Proposed phrasing may be as follows:

> The student supervisee, faculty supervisor, and agency supervisor agree that client protection supersedes all training experiences and educational or other goals of the trainee, agency site, and educational institution. The student trainee acknowledges that faculty supervisors and site supervisors may exchange information about the student trainee's performance in the form of reports or evaluations and in consultation with other training-related professionals (e.g., faculty, clinical staff, institutional administrators) when directly related to any concerns or incidents on a need-to-know basis. The purpose of discussing student performance will be to (a) protect client welfare, (b) support the process of student development and remediation, and (c) permit the initiation of gatekeeping procedures and processes when needed. Student privacy will be protected to the extent possible, but confidentiality and privacy across institutions is not guaranteed.

Graduate programs and agency sites may adapt this statement and determine appropriate placement in their procedures for informing students, such as a clinical placement handbook or placement agreement with sites. It is recommended that both informed consent from trainees to verify that they understand and agree to this policy and a release of information to and from clinical respondeat superiors (faculty and site supervisors) be obtained from trainees. As with all documentation in the gatekeeping process, obtaining signatures from all involved affirming understanding and agreement is essential.

Intervening When Injustices Occur

Injustices in the gatekeeping process happen. They can occur when there is a misunderstanding, overzealousness, or avoidance of a particular policy or procedure and when action is taken without hearing the trainee's perspective on the situation in question. Personal reactions, such as the countertransference of a supervisor toward a supervisee, can also be unknowingly activated, setting off an undeserved chain of events. *Countertransference* refers to a triggering event that "can be related to the supervisee's skills . . . or . . . to issues related to his or her personhood" (Bernard & Goodyear, 2014, p. 39). Countertransference can result in failure to apply due process procedures, inconsistent enforcement of published standards for interpersonal and intrapersonal behavior, and erratic application of expectations for professional conduct. These missteps can lead to inconsistent disciplinary actions that not only are unmerited but also may fall within the legal definition of arbitrary and capricious. Undeserved or overly harsh actions on the part of a faculty member or supervisor may destroy a trainee's career and lead to significant financial and psychological harm.

Injustice can also occur when faculty and supervisors who are not directly involved in a specific situation observe unfair actions but fail to object to inappropriate or professionally unacceptable treatment of trainees, allowing the harm to continue. When injustices are observed, professionals should intervene with colleagues as directed by ethics codes and professional standards and raise awareness among the rest of the faculty or supervisory unit of appropriate practices concerning evaluation, remediation, due process, and gatekeeping for clinical trainees.

Intervening when injustices appear to be occurring is important to reduce the risk of liability regarding selective enforcement of standards, incidents in which trainees may be ganged up on while others are favored, and potential violations of procedural or substantive due process. *Arbitrary* and *capricious* describes punitive actions that are considered an unreasonable or unjust exercise of power by an institution or individual, without cause, indiscriminately applied, or with inadequate consideration for the circumstances.

Recommendations to guard against the violation of substantive due process include having programs treat "similar student problems consistently between and among students" and linking "evaluations, warnings, and decisions about problematic actions to training goals" (Gilfoyle, 2008, p. 204). Institutions can reduce the risk of liability by openly addressing identified problematic concerns, providing both written notice to students and opportunities for students to respond, and maintaining documentation of actions taken (Gilfoyle, 2008).

It is incumbent on faculty and supervisors to maintain their professional roles consistently and appropriately while also maintaining standards, supporting colleagues, and initiating consultation meetings while not undercutting colleagues, students, or supervisees. It is advised that a team or unit approach be utilized once a gatekeeping case becomes about more than providing simple feedback. Involving colleagues, especially in the case of multiple supervisors, is a prudent way to avoid unchecked countertransference and cross-check one another to avoid favoritism or unfair punitive actions that may lead to charges of arbitrary and capricious treatment of a supervisee or student. When formal procedures are called for in the gatekeeping process, no single faculty member or staff supervisor involved in overseeing a trainee should go it alone in pursuing a problematic situation.

In addition, there will be times when faculty should not act alone, even when providing informal feedback to students based on the presenting problem, such as issues pertaining to gender or culture. It is better to initiate a team or committee approach before procedures addressing a problematic situation become too complex.

Consultation is one of the most important actions that faculty members and supervisors can engage in as part of the gatekeeping process. Detailed documentation across all gatekeeping efforts substantiating the involvement of multiple supervisory or training team members and/or consultation with appropriate decision makers can also help to reduce the liability risk. Overall, programs and agencies should follow and consistently apply their previously established and published program objectives and policies.

Managing Liability Risk in Gatekeeping

As respondeat superiors, supervisors are responsible for their supervisees' clinical actions and thus assume legal and professional risk. (See What Would You Do? 5.2.) Supervisors are ethically and legally mandated to ensure that gatekeeping policies and procedures are implemented

What Would You Do? 5.2

As a supervisor of postdegree interns, you strictly adhere to your state's supervision requirement of meeting a minimum of every 2 weeks with the registered interns who are accruing clinical experience to fulfill licensure requirements. One of the interns you supervise, Jenna, mentions activities such as meeting with clients in their homes or at coffee shops rather than her office because "it helps to make the clients feel more comfortable." You immediately initiate a discussion with Jenna about boundaries and include a review of ethical standards and the laws and rules of your state (information with which Jenna is familiar). You review the obligation to clients to provide confidentiality and create a therapeutic space that is different from that of other relationships. You also discuss the boundaries between personal and therapeutic relationships and the risk of client confusion. Jenna expresses understanding and appreciation for your guidance.

You begin to notice that Jenna starts to omit information about where she meets her clients, although she has a very nice office space that is accessible at all times. As your supervisory meetings continue, Jenna becomes increasingly vague and avoidant about specifying details about her work with clients, to the point that you are realizing you do not have the information necessary to fully understand the standard of care clients are receiving. Jenna then begins to miss scheduled supervision appointments and fails to respond to your requests to reschedule the meetings.

What do you do?

What are your immediate concerns about Jenna's performance?

How do you address these concerns with her?

If Jenna fails to respond to your requests to meet, what are your responsibilities as a supervisor?

and followed at their institutions and to intervene when unfair treatment occurs in the gatekeeping process. It is of vital importance for supervisors to manage liability risk while also fulfilling their supervisory responsibilities. Avoiding the role of gatekeeping leads to gateslipping of problematic trainees, which risks the licensure of incompetent clinicians. As W. B. Johnson et al. (2008) described, faculty and supervisors engaged in the clinical training process

> bear a weighty ethical and professional burden to guard entry into the profession and ensure that those who graduate have sufficient character, psychological fitness, and competence to function autonomously. However, it is often quite difficult to actively foster growth and development, to be compassionate and supportive, and to engage students as a mentor while simultaneously rendering objective and accurate summative evaluations. (p. 591)

This statement describes the dilemma that clinical supervisors and faculty members encounter in fulfilling their various obligations and roles while also ensuring the professional competence of the supervisees whom they supervise (Bernard & Goodyear, 2014). Failure to strike a balance can potentially result in unjust consequences for clients and/or trainees.

Risk management, the action of minimizing exposure to legal risk, is an important consideration of the gatekeeping process (Behnke, 2008), although it should not prompt avoidance of gatekeeping obligations. Faculty and supervisors need to be aware of the legal concerns relevant to their oversight of supervisees and find ways to minimize their risk while still fulfilling their roles as just and fair gatekeepers for the professions they represent. Statutes are instituted by legislative bodies or regulatory boards that have been given authority to protect the rights of individuals—including clients, students, and supervisees. The same is true about the development and enforcement of ethics codes, which are designed to protect the profession, clients, and others with whom the professional interacts. Ethics codes may be cited as best practice standards in a legal proceeding. Welfel (2006) suggested that "the most important legal issue in supervision relates to the degree of liability a supervisor bears for the actions of supervisees" (p. 308). Strategies to reduce the likelihood of liability risk include the following (Bernard & Goodyear, 2014; Wheeler & Bertram, 2015):

- Maintaining a trusting supervisor–supervisee relationship
- Reviewing every client case for which a supervisee is providing services
- Viewing raw data (video or audio recordings of sessions, case files)
- Maintaining current knowledge about legal issues that affect the clinical training profession
- Consulting with colleagues when the outcome of decisions is not clear or in high-risk situations

- Obtaining legal services when needed
- Establishing record-keeping procedures
- Documenting specific directives for supervisees
- Requiring that both the student or supervisee and supervisor maintain and provide proof of liability insurance

Consultation is an especially important component of risk management. Seeking the guidance and counsel of professional colleagues, such as others involved in training clinicians, is strongly recommended in all cases involving high-risk students or supervisees. Supervisors can also consult with experts in their professional groups, other faculty members, and legal consultants (Jackson-Cherry, 2006). In the event of highly problematic situations that cross multiple legal and ethical concerns, faculty and agency supervisors should not hesitate to consult with their professional association or institution's attorneys if legal counsel is needed. Professional advice from a lawyer versed in educational law and/or health law, ideally with experience in legal issues affecting the clinical mental health professions, might be invaluable in some situations.

The laws pertaining to the requirements of postdegree, prelicensure supervision vary from state to state and across the clinical professions (e.g., psychology, mental health counseling, clinical social work, or marriage and family therapy). The requirements for qualified or approved supervisors for postdegree interns vary; thus, it is important that prior to providing postdegree supervision, supervisors are fully aware of their legal obligations and the penalties that could occur as a result of violations of practice. When laws and rules are not followed, licensure boards that regulate and discipline licensed clinicians can take disciplinary action against postdegree supervisors who do not fulfill eligibility requirements or their obligations as supervisors.

Conclusion

In conclusion, faculty and supervisors have an obligation to the counseling profession in their role as gatekeepers. The reputation of the clinical profession is diminished in the eyes of the public, other behavioral and medical health groups, and policymakers when a problematic student is graduated or a problematic supervisee is endorsed for licensure. In addition, the care of future clients is jeopardized.

One of the most influential factors in the training of clinicians is the education and supervision that occurs during graduate school and after graduation while interns are accumulating clinical experience toward licensure (Kindsvatter et al., 2008). Clinical supervision is a high-risk endeavor that can place the credentials of supervisors at considerable threat, which suggests that "careful consideration should be given to risk management in the practice of clinical supervision" (Polychronis & Brown, 2016, p. 145). Faculty and supervisors should be well versed in gatekeeping procedures as they pertain to the seven areas discussed in this chapter. Behnke (2005) stated that faculty and supervisors in their gatekeeping role need to understand the consequences when appropriate gatekeeping practices are not followed to avoid the "*promoveatur ut amoveatur* principle, loosely translated from Latin as, 'Let us move this supervisee along in order to have the supervisee gone from our placement'" (p. 91). As the respondeat superiors in the clinical supervision process, faculty and supervisors are responsible for the ethical and legal expectations of addressing problematic trainees and gatekeeping for the profession and the consumers of clinical services. (See What Would You Do? 5.3.)

Key Points and Best Practices

- Faculty members and faculty and site supervisors are the first line of gatekeepers in the clinical field. Clinical professionals outside of the academic arena who supervise postgraduation, prelicensure supervisees under the mandate of their state's licensure law requirements are the secondary line of gatekeepers critical to ensuring the quality of the profession.
- In clinical education, faculty members overseeing clinical activities and (pre- or postdegree) field supervisors are considered the respondeat superiors of supervisees. This legal term identifies supervisors as having responsibility and vicarious liability for the actions of their trainees.
- Ethical definitions of standards for supervision and practice differ across the clinical professions, and legal requirements vary from state to state as defined by regulatory boards. Those supervising pre- or postdegree trainees, whether faculty or agency based, need to be familiar with the ethical and legal mandates under which they practice supervisory oversight.
- *Endorsement*, a critical aspect of gatekeeping, is the formal pledge by a supervisor or faculty member that a trainee is ready to advance in the training or professional practice process (e.g., candidacy, practicum, internship, graduation, licensure, or certification in the case of a specialty area).
- *Feedback* is a skill that is critical to effective gatekeeping. Feedback to students and supervisees should (a) be communicated regularly, (b) be based on learning goals or competencies, (c) be direct and clear, and (d) strike a balance between supporting and reinforcing a student or supervisee while also being able to challenge or offer constructive criticism for the purpose of professional development.
- Faculty and supervisors should have a clear understanding of how their gatekeeping responsibilities interface with their other roles and responsibilities with trainees.

- Inherent in the role of educator or supervisor is the responsibility to provide educational and developmental support and opportunities to trainees while also monitoring for behaviors that may signal that a trainee might pose potential harm to current or future clients.
- When inappropriate or professionally unacceptable treatment of trainees is observed in the gatekeeping process, clinical professionals should intervene with their peer colleagues as directed by ethics codes and professional standards and raise awareness among the rest of the faculty or supervisory unit of appropriate practices concerning evaluation, remediation, due process, and gatekeeping for clinical trainees.
- *Risk management*, the action of minimizing exposure to legal risk, is an important consideration of the gatekeeping process. Strategies to reduce the likelihood of liability risk include the following:

    –Maintaining a trusting supervisor–supervisee relationship
    –Reviewing every client case for which a supervisee is providing services
    –Viewing raw data (video or audio recordings of sessions, case files)
    –Maintaining open communication with training partners, such as university program faculty and supervisors, agency site supervisors, or clinical colleagues working with the same trainee
    –Maintaining current knowledge of legal issues that affect the clinical training profession
    –Consulting with colleagues when the outcome of decisions is not clear or in high-risk situations
    –Obtaining legal services when needed
    –Establishing record-keeping procedures
    –Documenting specific directives for supervisees
    –Requiring that both the student or supervisee and supervisor maintain and provide proof of liability insurance

What Would You Do? 5.3

You are the training coordinator of a graduate social work program. A student in your program, Aasma, is in her final semester as a social work intern. She had a tragic loss about 3 years ago when her teenage son died of a drug overdose. Throughout the program, Aasma seemed to do well while also acknowledging that she was grieving the loss of her son. You receive a call from Aasma's faculty supervisor that Aasma called her to say that she had been dismissed from her internship site. The last time the faculty supervisor had checked with the site supervisor, everything had been going very well. The student states that she does not understand why she was dismissed. You call the site supervisor, whom you know well from working with him regarding past student placements and site visits, to ask him what happened. He declines to tell you because he says he is protecting Aasma's confidentiality. You assure the site supervisor that there is no obligation of confidentiality and, in fact, you have an obligation as the training coordinator to be aware of student problems for gatekeeping purposes. After some convincing, the site supervisor explains that he realized that Aasma had been arriving at her site under the influence of alcohol. He believed it was his duty to protect clients from harm, so he dismissed Aasma immediately.

What would you do?

Do you agree with the site's decisions to dismiss Aasma after they realized a pattern of using alcohol while seeing clients?

What is your opinion of the site supervisor's understanding of confidentiality in relation to interns?

What would you do in the future to inform sites and create working alliances that would prevent an abrupt dismissal such as this and allow for a student to have the opportunity to change?

Chapter 6

Collaboration During Gatekeeping

Roxane L. Dufrene

Faculty and supervisors are not alone when encountering a trainee who is experiencing challenges. Gatekeeping actions affect and are affected by organizational administrators and policies, professional standards, jurisdictional legal mandates, societal and client trends, and all of the related colleagues inherent in these various institutions. Adopting a systemic and holistic approach to gatekeeping that attends to trainee problems offers substantial educational and training benefits for participants at all levels, including trainees. For the purposes of this chapter, the term *stakeholder* is defined as all individuals, departments, agencies, and institutions that are involved with and/or invested in the system of developing trainees to become effective clinical practitioners ("Stakeholder," 2014). There are many benefits to embracing a systemic approach to training and the gatekeeping processes. For example, program leaders who involve all stakeholders in developing programmatic gatekeeping policies based on professional ethical principles and accreditation standards reduce legal risks (Gilfoyle, 2008). An emphasis on and inclusion of various systemic stakeholders' perspectives enhance training quality, trainees' standing in a program (Behnke, 2008), and the reputations of the clinical professions and training institutions while also ensuring increased success of gatekeeping outcomes and the ultimate protection of client welfare.

Faculty/Supervisor Leadership

Leadership in clinical and educational settings, and the culture in which it occurs, is important to the gatekeeping process. The conceptualization of leadership can be viewed from a standpoint akin to Bronfenbrenner's (1979) ecological systems perspective, which depicts all stakeholders at different levels in a systemic framework (Forrest, Shen-Miller, & Elman, 2008; J. Miller & Koerin, 2002; Wester, Christianson, Fouad, & Santiago-Rivera, 2008). At the *macro* level are the institutional and contextual factors of the framework. At the *meso* level are the leaders or policy setters themselves (e.g., faculty, staff, and administrators) who design and/or decide on gatekeeping practices. The *exo* level contains the outside groups (e.g., legal system, ethical standards, accreditation bodies, licensing boards, and clinical professional associations) that influence the practice of gatekeeping. At the *mezzo* level the supervisors, staff, and professionals in field practice settings who are in nonleadership roles appear; this level may also include others who are not in decision-making roles, such as adjunct faculty, who are responsible for policy implementation, or clients who receive the services provided by trainees. All levels influence trainees represented at the *micro* level. In both educational and clinical practice, the macro level should be considered and understood as holding the overarching concern of accountability in gatekeeping across all of the other ecological levels (see Figure 6.1).

Gatekeeping in a training program provides an important element of professional leadership and cross-discipline relationships that serve as a means of exercising each of the stakeholders' responsibilities. Viewed from the ecological approach, transparency in the leadership culture is important because it can prevent problems that occur at all levels of the ecological system (West, Bubenzer, Osborn, Paez, & Desmond, 2006). Urwin, Van Soest, and Kretzschmar (2006) believed that the different viewpoints of all stakeholders, including clinical program directors and faculty, department chairs, deans, administrators (both university and site), supervisors (both university and site), accreditation organizations, other students or colleagues, attorneys, staff (both university and site), site professionals (nurses, doctors, etc.), state

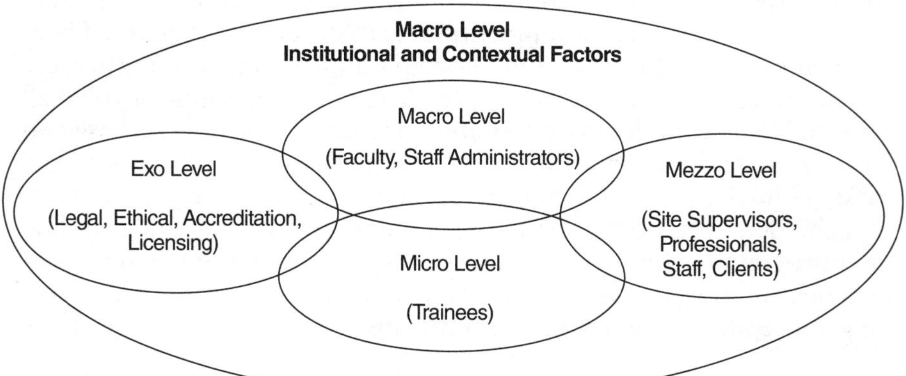

Figure 6.1 • Ecological Collaborative Gatekeeping Approach

licensing boards, professional associations, clients or consumers, and the other various constituencies they represent, should be represented when developing standards and procedures for gatekeeping.

Forrest et al. (2008) suggested using the ecological framework to conceptualize gatekeeping collaboration among all involved in policy setting because it can identify multiple stakeholders and processes in and among a programmatic gatekeeping effort. Considering a trainee problem from the multiple levels of an ecological framework and the influence that those levels have on a trainee can assist in understanding a problem situation. Also, worthy of consideration in the system of gatekeeping, though not necessarily as a policy-setting entity, are others affected by a student's or supervisee's problematic behavior, such as other students, site colleagues, and, most important, current and future clients. An ecological framework provides a holistic perspective, rather than a linear perspective, and that approach frames mutual collaboration across all levels and attends to the individuals at each level. All stakeholders in each level should be identified and included in the collaborative effort. J. Miller and Koerin (2002) stated that specific challenges and liabilities for all stakeholders are best managed with open communication that includes information about the criteria for gatekeeping and how they relate to the roles of each stakeholder.

Several professionals have proposed many useful implications utilizing the ecological approach in training programs (Forrest et al., 2008; J. Miller & Koerin, 2002; Wester et al., 2008). For example, when gatekeeping or remediation is not implemented consistently at the program (meso) level, poor faculty cohesion and lack of collaboration between faculty and administrators can result. Perspectives and programmatic or institutional priorities can differ between the faculty or clinical field supervisor level and administrators regarding the nature and importance of enforcing gatekeeping or remediation practices. Such differences and inconsistencies can impact other stakeholders and will likely also trickle down to the trainee (micro) level, leading to confusion. The lack of cohesive leadership at the meso level (faculty, staff, administrators) can also influence an individual trainee's academic achievements and clinical performance as well as trainee peer interactions at the micro level (Forrest et al., 2008). For example, when collaboration does not occur between the meso level (clinical faculty supervisors representing program policy and learning requirements) and mezzo level (site supervisors representing agency policy), trainees may align with site supervisors and improperly convey documentation or supervision requirements from the program and accreditation perspective, creating inconsistency in the enforcement of trainee competency standards. Also, because professional training initially consists of didactic classes that are typically followed by practicum and internship placement in the clinical field community (mezzo) where clients are provided services, conflict between the theoretical application of state, legal, and ethical situations (exo) can occur when real-life application of theory to actual clients comes into play. Thus, consistent leadership is needed at the meso level and in collaboration with the mezzo and micro levels to avoid inconsistency and resulting gatekeeping dilemmas. For example, a participant from West et al.'s (2006) study used the term "lone ranger" (p. 12) to describe faculty who make quick decisions and choose to work alone when engaging in gatekeeping or remediation. This lack of consultation can result in inconsistent application of program gatekeeping practices, which could lead to charges of arbitrary enforcement. Behnke (2008) stated the importance of leadership, as a cohesive entity, to provide a perspective that reflects the program's written policies and procedures to inform stakeholders and trainees, not just individual faculty members.

Using an ecologically collaborative gatekeeping approach, professionals can assume complementary roles, work together, and share responsibilities by making decisions that work toward solutions to problems. This works best if it occurs in a proactive environment (Crawford & Gilroy, 2012), avoiding the breakdown of training relationships and preventable problems at the meso, exo, and mezzo levels. For example, when field site supervisors are provided collaborative training by program faculty about learning goals and accreditation standards in advance of internship placement, such as documentation requirements, triangulation among site supervisors, faculty supervisors, and trainees is less likely to occur and field site supervisors can align with and receive support from faculty supervisors to provide more effective and consistent learning opportunities across sites.

From a leadership perspective, as suggested by Gilfoyle (2008) and Forrest et al. (2008), the shift from an individual linear perspective to a holistic collaborative framework places risk management principles in the broad context of multiple levels of responsibility of all stakeholders. A collaborative leadership framework focuses on principles that value the priorities of all stakeholders and simultaneously benefits training programs in terms of consistency, quality, and effectiveness. (See Notes From the Field 6.1.) Best practices for risk management from a program perspective should involve

> comparisons to other external influences on training programs (e.g., accreditation standards and ethical principles). . . . [that] can be integrated into a partnership role as a valuable participant in the training exosystem, with good results for all those who have a part in that system. (Gilfoyle, 2008, p. 209)

Notes From the Field 6.1

A student shows up at a dean's office with a local news crew alleging mistreatment by the counseling program faculty during his remediation. The dean was not aware of any problems with the student or that the student was on a remediation plan.

Stakeholders who demonstrate collaborative working relationships tend to adhere to best practices adapted to meet the needs of their training programs (Kerl, Garcia, McCullough, & Maxwell, 2002; Lamb et al., 1987; McAdams & Foster, 2007; McAdams, Foster, & Ward, 2007). Positive working relationships among stakeholders who understand and value interprofessional roles and agreements regarding gatekeeping policies and enforcement encourage consensual collaboration that recognizes the broader aspects reflected in each participant's guiding policies. Examples include university policies related to the Family Educational Rights and Privacy Act of 1974 (FERPA; U.S. Department of Education, 2015), site policies regarding the Health Insurance Portability and Accountability Act of 1996 (HIPAA; U.S. Department of Health and Human Services, 2013), professional ethical standards, training program accreditation guidelines (such as those from the Council for Accreditation of Counseling and Related Educational Programs, Commission on Accreditation for Marriage and Family Therapy Education, American Psychological Association, Council on Social Work Education), mandates of licensure legislation, and overall best practice standards of the clinical professions intended to protect clients.

Collaborative Commitment

Collaboration is a decision-making process that is implemented among an interactive group of faculty or professionals rather than a chain of activities in which one faculty member consults with another faculty and so on to make decisions. Collaboration includes individual consultation but also involves a more complex skill set (Wester et al., 2008). Collaboration draws on the following skills:

- Using engagement practices to create collegial working relationships among stakeholders to enhance understanding of and communication during problem-solving processes
- Applying the collective experiences and knowledge bases of all stakeholders
- Reducing stress or distributing stress across all stakeholders
- Using collaborative team approaches to increase faculty's involvement
- Increasing available resources when problems occur
- Encouraging stakeholders to fulfill the gatekeeper role
- Enhancing protection of faculty, professionals, trainees, and clients

Involving all stakeholders and recognizing differences can be one of the most difficult factors to manage in any training program, especially because the gatekeeping process can be conflictual. Collaboration in a program is considered a comprehensive method of addressing trainee issues, from admission into the program, through all trainee experiences, to successful completion of a program (Crawford & Gilroy, 2012).

Stakeholders' collaborative communication in a training program necessitates knowledge of organizational and systemic perspectives that include behaviors, policies, laws, theories, standards, data, and clinical practice (Arredondo, Shealy, Neale, & Winfrey, 2004). A faculty member's ability to recognize the need for collaboration with other professionals, along with the ability to seek out and engage other professionals in the principles and actions of the gatekeeping process, creates the basis for collaboration, resulting in effective systemic alliances across all levels of the ecological collaborative gatekeeping approach. These alliances can promote best practices and extend to various combinations of relationships, including those with university personnel, supervisors, professionals at sites, and professionals in organizations such as the American Counseling Association, American Psychological Association, National Association of Social Workers, and others (Crawford & Gilroy, 2012). Faculty who act collaboratively in their programs tend to work with shared goals. When taking a collaborative approach, faculty are committing to the best interest and benefit of the trainee during the gatekeeping process.

Evidence of the benefits of collaboration among faculty and administrators can be found in a court case regarding the remediation of a trainee, *Plaintiff v. Rector and Board of Visitors of The College of William and Mary* (McAdams & Foster, 2007). McAdams et al. (2007) stated that "consensus among all stakeholders," which included the full program faculty, associate dean, dean of the college, and school administration, was "the greatest strength" (p. 222) in the dismissal decision that initiated the court case. Consultation with administrators prior to all faculty gatekeeping decisions and endorsement from both school and university administrators as the processes of remediation and dismissal unfolded are examples of faculty collaborative efforts that resulted in a positive outcome for all invested constituencies.

Balancing the differences among the priorities and perspectives of all stakeholders is one of the most challenging aspects of collaboration. (See Notes From the Field 6.2.) To prevent problems in communication, Lamb (1999) suggested that faculty clarify the criteria for gatekeeping policies and procedures, framing the importance of trainee evaluation

Notes From the Field 6.2

An instructor allows one student to earn practicum hours over a semester break at a site (or ignores the fact that the student is doing so), which is outside of the licensing board policies and Council for Accreditation of Counseling and Related Educational Programs policy, whereas another instructor upholds the policy by not allowing two students to collect practicum hours at their site during the semester break. Student unrest starts with the two students who are not allowed to collect hours over the semester break. They complain to the site supervisors and faculty.

from a program and site perspective, using a collaborative process with all stakeholders. Each stakeholder has different roles and responsibilities based in the mission and priorities of his or her professional standpoint, and those must be clarified for collaboration to occur effectively. For example, faculty's role is to know, understand, endorse, and apply due process procedures consistently across students and supervisees in the educational context (American Counseling Association, 2014a; Bemak, Epp, & Keys, 1999; Wilkerson, 2006; Ziomek-Daigle & Christensen, 2010), which typically is not a role or responsibility for site stakeholders who are also following agency policies guided by other systems with which they interface (such as Medicare or Medicaid requirements).

Faculty Role and FERPA Implications

Another systemic point of view involving faculty responsibilities can be illustrated in relation to policies at the university level. Jasonson et al. (2008) pointed to the progress made in understanding and implementing FERPA guidelines regarding privacy and record keeping of students, which faculty can and should embrace in training programs when engaged in collaborative gatekeeping practices. Understanding FERPA helps faculty prepare and enact program policies and procedures that align with FERPA requirements. Using a collaborative approach to understand and implement policy obligations across various systemic levels can enable educators, staff, and administrators in colleges and universities to create practical strategies for evaluating and discussing trainee competencies with site supervisors when a supervisee is placed at a site. This collaborative approach creates strategies that are consistent, are integrative, and account for problem behaviors while at the same time adhering to FERPA guidelines.

Although the obligations of stakeholders or other considerations affecting various levels of operation in universities or clinical field sites can hamper collaboration between programs and across disciplines, faculty can use the collaborative process to establish training program policies and procedures that adhere to FERPA and HIPAA guidelines when constructing their program requirements. For instance, when trainees reach practicum or internship, trainee information, such as remedial plans, may not be fully disclosable to individuals not affiliated with the campus system (Elman, Forrest, Vacha-Haase, & Gizara, 1999). This can become a concern because sites are responsible for the impact of trainee problems on clients and may need information about the student from the educational institution to oversee client protection. Or doctoral trainees may be involved in supervising master's-level trainees with behavioral issues, potentially crossing the boundaries of students knowing private information about other students. Thus, it is important to have policies regarding communication within training programs and between sites based on a need-to-know approach that aligns with FERPA requirements. For example, before problems occur, informed consent documents should be provided to trainees that explain how their information is protected and when it may be conveyed (such as when they apply for practicum and internship field site placement) or shared in cross-supervision scenarios. Also, throughout their training process, students and supervisees should be updated about changes in gatekeeping and remediation policies (Frame & Stevens-Smith, 1995; W. B. Johnson et al., 2008; Kerl et al., 2002; Lamb et al., 1987; McAdams & Foster, 2007; McAdams et al., 2007) and given the opportunity to provide signed informed consent demonstrating their understanding and acceptance of the implications of such changes. In addition, clinical field sites should be informed of the limitations involving FERPA laws that affect supervisees when they are placed in off-campus training settings. Similarly, programs and sites should have jointly constructed and/or agreed-on policies regarding communication about clients and trainee responsibilities that are consistent with HIPAA requirements. Sharing information with stakeholders about changes in established policies and obtaining consent or agreement from those at other levels in the ecological gatekeeping system allows for potentially conflicting issues to be addressed proactively and also strengthens the working relationship and trust developed among collaborators at all levels.

Collaboration During Graduate Clinical Fieldwork

Vacha-Haase, Davenport, and Kerewsky (2004) advised that collegial collaboration is especially necessary when developing remedial interventions for supervisees engaged in the clinical aspect of their training program. It is critical that the educational unit and all individual faculty members involved in the training process understand and are consistent in their approach to evaluating trainees and implementing standardized gatekeeping policies before they can effectively collaborate with outside stakeholders, such as administrators and field site supervisors. Faculty units that struggle with agreement about their own roles and/or a common understanding of gatekeeping will complicate collaborative efforts at times when proactive working alliances are critical (Dufrene & Henderson, 2009; Forrest, Elman, Gizara, & Vacha-Haase, 1999). Consensus among faculty is needed to prevent conflicting expectations of trainees, minimize inconsistent enforcement of standards, and eliminate disagreement between faculty in order to create a culture of respect for stakeholders and current and incoming trainees.

Clear discourse about policies and procedures also acknowledges the importance of professional ethics and best practice standards. These efforts create a positive and professional learning environment for trainees and a culture for professional practice modeling to trainees that remediation or dismissal is based on the collaborative judgment of the entire faculty, not one person (Dufrene & Henderson, 2009; Homrich,

2009). Trimble, Stroebel, Krieg, and Rubenstein (2012) reported that survey respondents in their study suggested that frequent communication, transparency, and shared responsibility between faculty encourage a collaborative environment and decreased problems in a training program.

Such alliances are important not only among faculty in a program but also in maintaining a positive working relationship between faculty from the educational unit and the clinical field site systems once educational program policies are established. Ongoing communication and collaboration are encouraged between field sites and academic programs in order to develop clarity of criteria and congruent strategies for the evaluation of trainees across settings. For example, accreditation standards and ethics codes are considered excellent resources for identifying trainee competencies and serve as the foundation from which to infer insufficient supervisee performance from the perspective of clinical faculty and site supervisors who hold professional licenses (Forrest et al., 1999; Henderson & Dufrene, 2011). However, although these resources may inform clinicians, they may not influence the priorities or actions of administrators at higher levels of both related institutions (agencies and universities). Collaboration also involves educating participant partners who have disparate interests about foundational principles such as professional association ethics, legal mandates, and the doctrine of procedural due process that allows the trainee the opportunity to respond to a decision to take corrective action (Dufrene & Henderson, 2009; Frame & Stevens-Smith, 1995; Jackson-Cherry, 2006; Kerl et al., 2002; Lamb et al., 1987; McAdams & Foster, 2007; McAdams et al., 2007). Thus, inherent in the ecological collaborative gatekeeping approach is the need to establish within-group collaboration (in a faculty group or among the representatives of the clinical professions at both universities and field sites) as well as develop alliances across group constituencies at the meso, exo, and mezzo levels. As suggested by Lysaght and Altschuld (2000), maintenance of competency issues goes beyond training programs and extends to professional practice and all stakeholders at that level. Professional organizations, licensure boards, and individual professionals are groups that should address competency issues as an ongoing responsibility to the standards of the profession.

Collaboratively Maintaining Gatekeeping Systems and Procedures

Although gatekeeping policies and procedures in training programs are important, it is also essential to maintain such policies and procedures in a way that supports collaboration. Just as faculty in programs may discuss the necessity of gatekeeping, site supervisors and professionals in the field are also concerned about gatekeeping but may not engage in advanced prevention-based discussion or policy setting. In

Gillis and Lewis's (2004) study, site supervisors' concerns included the need for communication and closer collaboration between the site and the training program, increased training for sites, ways to discuss trainee problems with faculty early in trainee placements as well as when problems develop across the placement period, procedures for how problems are identified and remediated, support from training programs for solutions to problems, and clarification of the roles of everyone involved. Between field sites and educational institutions, faculty are the primary holders of information and procedure setting and should provide leadership about gatekeeping practices when problematic trainee situations arise, collaborating with sites around the individual situation.

Formal Policy Reviews

Periodic reviews of existing policies and procedures in concert with field sites allow for policy updates, revisions, and recognition of changing collaborative interests and efforts and should be instituted as a continual process in training programs (Vacha-Haase et al., 2004). To prevent conflicting policies, the benefits of a periodic review should include the identification of policies that are out of compliance or that conflict with current accreditation standards, ethical standards, licensure requirements, site policies, and university policies. Faculty should reach out to all stakeholders when reevaluating or updating their gatekeeping policies and are strongly encouraged to collaborate with the various stakeholders to compare policies and discuss what has been revised or what will be revised in their program as well as in various field site settings (Gilfoyle, 2008; Urwin et al., 2006; Vacha-Haase et al., 2004). In other words, the development of gatekeeping policies and procedures should not be limited to the meso level of a faculty department.

Lamb, Cochran, and Jackson (1991) stated that interaction with sites should occur on an ongoing basis and possibly at prescribed formal intervals, such as at annual or biennial joint meetings. Collaboration between sites and training programs regarding the communication, refinement, and maintenance of gatekeeping policies and procedures can enhance the relationships between site supervisors and faculty (Gonsalvez & Freestone, 2007) by strengthening the partnership toward the common goal of preparing ethical and effective future clinicians. Having relevant stakeholders present at meetings enables collaboration around what is expected and/or required of trainees. Also, collaboration should involve notifying trainees of program requirements and alerting collaborative partners when trainees are not meeting those requirements, such as when a supervisee is placed on remediation. A study by Brown (2013) found that 17 out of 47 programs used a collaborative approach with trainees when notifying them of remediation.

When collaboration between the educational unit and site occurs, it reduces the likelihood that a trainee will blame one individual (i.e., faculty, stakeholder) or twist information for the actions taken regarding remediation (Lamb et al., 1991).

Specific to the evaluation of trainees with behavior problems, Forrest et al. (2008) stated that gatekeeping policies or trainee problems should be periodically reviewed by stakeholders who are involved in evaluations of trainees (e.g., site professionals, faculty) and/or may be drawn in to the more complicated cases of remediation and gatekeeping with highly difficult trainees (e.g., deans, administrators, attorneys). Ideally, these stakeholders should be assessed for their willingness to conform to and support trainee evaluation and disciplinary procedures in advance of their involvement in a specific case (Bemak et al., 1999; Frame & Stevens-Smith, 1995). Maintaining clear communication among all stakeholders (e.g., faculty, supervisors, department chairs, deans) both in and outside the training program is essential and creates support across all involved in trainee evaluations. Prior to engaging with trainees and depending on the gatekeeping scenario, stakeholders involved in the situation should be provided with program forms and rubrics required for evaluation and understand their responsibilities in the evaluation process. For example, gatekeeping and/or remediation evaluation scales and procedural policies should be provided to site supervisors when trainees experiencing problems are placed at a site along with additional points of expectations or behaviors that are part of the specific remediation plan for a given trainee.

Challenges and Transparency

According to Lysaght and Altschuld (2000), factors working against successful maintenance of competency issues are "the costs of continuing education, increasing workload, and trends towards restricted institutional support for professional development" (p. 103). Also, "there will be factions in any professional group who do not actively pursue competency maintenance" (p. 102). V. A. Foster and McAdams (2009) stated that to proactively maintain policies that address competency issues, faculty should ensure that policies include transparent, formalized methods of professional performance expectations. They believed that transparency occurs in a nonpunitive environment in which all stakeholders are respected during the learning process. Maintaining policies whose expectations are fair and informing all trainees about such policies should start when trainees apply to a program and continue until they graduate or are dismissed from they program (V. A. Foster & McAdams, 2009; Vacha-Haase et al., 2004). Foster and McAdams suggested that maintaining policies in a positive environment ensures that trainees will believe that they are valued as part of the program requirements and expectations that are consistently represented by all stakeholders.

Part of maintaining a gatekeeping system, as suggested by Urwin et al. (2006), is to document and communicate positive gatekeeping and remediation outcomes to all program faculty as part of an ongoing effort to encourage participation in gatekeeping and remediation with all stakeholders. In general, there are more positive responses by trainees to gatekeeping efforts than negative, yet good outcomes or problem resolutions are often overlooked and not shared as success stories. Also, trainees could be informed of some of the positive results (without identifying information) to communicate transparency in the program and to promote gatekeeping and remediation as nonpunitive and proactive steps in supporting the success of trainees. Examples provided by Urwin et al. included the following six outcomes:

1. Less time spent by administrators on trainee complaints
2. Reduced overturned decisions regarding remediation by administration
3. Remediation success for the majority of trainees with problems
4. Faculty and administrators feel supported with the team effort
5. Less legal liability for the training program
6. Satisfaction among faculty because problems were addressed effectively

Homrich (2009) suggested that training programs could offer a workshop for site supervisors and other site professionals on how to supervise trainees with problem behaviors, develop evaluation methods that are behaviorally specific, collaborate with trainees to improve behaviors, and work closely with faculty supervisors to avoid triangulation and support maximal supervisee development. Sample evaluation rubrics, remediation plans, and remediation assessment forms could be provided at the workshop for site supervisor participants to practice conceptualization skills and strategies on how to address trainee behaviors that need to be addressed at the field site level.

Consistent Monitoring or Gatewatching

It is important that all stakeholders agree to consistent monitoring or gatewatching of trainees that includes adherence to the following:

1. Accreditation standards and ethical principles
2. Legal mandates expected of future licensees
3. Procedures for how, what, and when to inform sites about identified problems
4. Procedures for how and at what point sites should inform training programs about problematic situations with trainees
5. Requirements for accurate and complete communication about and documentation of problems, responses to feedback and interventions, and changes in problem behaviors

6. Written suggestions detailing appropriate interventions to use and timeline expectations to apply during the evaluation process
7. Expectations for providing trainees with the opportunity for due process
8. Delineation of the roles and responsibilities of all stakeholders during the monitoring process

Homrich (2009) suggested that training programs should consider strategies for dividing up the potential roles of each faculty member in the gatekeeping process—as mentors, advisors, instructors, and evaluators of the student or supervisee—to balance the trainee's perceptions that faculty may be ganging up on him or her. For example, one faculty member can give corrective feedback, whereas another faculty member can be a mentor who provides space for debriefing. The same can occur across faculty and field site supervisors when appropriate. Consistent monitoring using this method includes transparency about each participant's roles and the requirement to inform the other stakeholders, including the trainee, about the trainee's progress or lack of improvement regarding the concerns to avoid the development of conflicting perspectives and conceptualizations of problem issues.

Shen-Miller et al. (2011) found that norms in a program environment can prevent problems from worsening if they are supportive of and collaborative with stakeholders, which can have positive impacts on trainees. In a supportive environment, regular checkups, reviews of evaluation reports, and discussions regarding trainee problems occur. These actions should also include following up on reports of problems with trainees or individual remediation plans to ensure that improvements in problem behaviors are being seen and documented by all affected.

Agreement Among Gatekeepers

Collaboration and a sense of teamwork that facilitates faculty buy-in to gatekeeping policies and procedures create a program environment that results in agreement among gatekeepers (Urwin et al., 2006, p. 176). In a program that interfaces with various ecological levels, the ability of all professionals from all contexts and institutions to engage in sustained, respectful communication is critical to collegial consultation and collaboration. Ongoing communication among all relevant stakeholders strengthens commitment to both the training requirements and the site requirements. Support for norms that are framed in a collegial and respectful manner sends a consistent message to all professionals and trainees that is helpful to everyone and the training program (Shen-Miller et al., 2011).

Gizara and Forrest (2004) suggested that when program norms are not supported, faculty and/or supervisors can come to believe that they have to be careful about how they present their concerns because their perspective about a trainee may be the opposite of what a key faculty member thinks about a favorite student or supervisee. Such disagreement can often result in differences in perspectives about a trainee as well as how to approach problematic behavior. One faculty member may perceive a trainee as struggling with emotional issues like frustration, anger, manipulation, entitlement, or refusal to accept feedback, whereas another faculty member may not perceive the trainee as struggling with those emotions. This difference in perspectives can sometimes result in faculty struggling with similar emotions (Gillis & Lewis, 2004). Trimble et al. (2012) stated that a lack of collaboration in such circumstances creates disagreement and exacerbates problem situations in gatekeeping that can result in negative program dynamics. Delays in addressing trainee issues and recurring problems from unresolved concerns are often the result of not addressing differences in viewpoints about gatekeeping and/or specific student or supervisee situations when they first occur.

Another factor that can impact program norms is social loafing, in which an individual faculty member does not participate in faculty responsibilities or does not collaborate with others. Social loafing by a faculty member can contribute negatively to program norms and the resolution of specific problem situations (Karau & Williams, 1993). Other factors, like splitting or subgrouping among stakeholders, can be harmful to agencies, professional relationships, and the training program in general (Homrich, 2009; Trimble et al., 2012). For example, when professionals in different disciplines, such as social work, counselor education, or psychology, have specialized training, their training sometimes has the effect of narrowing their professional views and approaches to client services, which can create specific problems related to trainees. Okech and Geroski (2015) stated that many site supervisors are able to articulate concerns and issues related to clients but are slow to pick up on trainee issues. An example of this is when splitting occurs in the alignment of a site supervisor and a problem trainee in which the trainee and supervisor believe that the program is the source of a problem. Another example is when trainees are required to demonstrate certain abilities, such as utilizing a theory when working with clients; however, site supervisors do not assess or evaluate the trainee's abilities based on the theoretical framework. In both examples, splitting can occur between faculty and other stakeholders.

Conversely, many university administrators do not have a clear understanding of clinical requirements because they have no basis or need for understanding the unique expectations of professional conduct and interpersonal behavior in clinical training. (See What Would You Do? 6.1.) The conflict that can arise from differing perspectives, such as the university's need to increase enrollment, the training program's ethical and legal requirement for gatekeeping, or the site's mandate to protect its clients and the public, can negatively

What Would You Do? 6.1

Jason is a 30-year-old master's-level student enrolled in a practicum. His practicum site is in a school setting with a site supervisor who has been a school counselor for 20 years. His university group supervisor is a female doctoral trainee who is being supervised by a faculty member of the program. Throughout the semester, when listening to tapes from Jason's individual sessions with clients, Jason's group supervisor and faculty supervisor began to have concerns that Jason was having problems applying his chosen theory, acceptance and commitment theory, in his sessions. Based on several taped client sessions, Jason was given feedback by the doctoral student supervisor that he was not addressing clients' painful thoughts and feelings during sessions but instead focusing on solutions to their distress. When this concern was expressed during his group supervision, Jason reported that his site supervisor had said that Jason was doing great and, because they were in a school setting, Jason's approach needed to focus on solutions, as that was the theory that worked best in school settings. The solution-focused approach was his site supervisor's theoretical model. At midterm, Jason was given documented feedback from his group and faculty supervisor regarding theoretical concerns, poor ability to receive feedback, lack of implementation of feedback from supervisors, and externalization of personal responsibility that affected his clinical performance. Jason's site supervisor gave him all excellent scores on his evaluation.

What would you do?

What would you do about these inconsistent supervisee evaluations?

What types of collaborative efforts should be initiated?

Who should be a part of those collaborative efforts?

impact the working relationships among stakeholders and trainees if not attended to proactively.

Balancing all stakeholders' perspectives with the program's requirement can be a challenge. This context is further complicated by each system's hierarchy (Delunas & Rouse, 2014; Meyers, Hales, Young, Nesbitt, & Pomeroy, 2013). When one or more professionals in the different system hierarchies are undervalued, collaboration is negatively impacted. Okech and Geroski (2015) reported that it can be difficult for various professionals who are stakeholders in a clinical training program to acquire the skills needed for communicating and collaborating across disciplines when professionals become strongly acculturated to their own professional language and setting. For example, various professionals from different disciplines, like administrators or attorneys, may question the utility of exploring trainee problem behaviors, believing that trainees have a legal right to a degree. Universities and field site agencies typically place administrators at the top of the hierarchy, which makes interdisciplinary collaboration a challenge (Delunas & Rouse, 2014; Meyers et al., 2013) because constituents at these higher levels are least likely to understand the necessity for professional and interpersonal requirements of clinical trainees.

When splitting or subgrouping in the hierarchical systems occurs, disagreements among faculty or stakeholders can lay the foundation for conflicting perceptions and expectations in departments or agencies. Not trusting others, blaming, and being accusatory add to negative situations and relationships, resulting in the potential for splitting or triangulation among faculty and stakeholders in and between the exo, meso, mezzo, and micro levels. Faculty's and stakeholders' ability to discuss when splitting occurs contributes to positive program norms and increased trust among all participants in the ecological collaborative gatekeeping model. Consistent enforcement of standards by all stakeholders for all students and supervisees reduces confusion and creates success for the program and trainees. If stakeholders engage in respectful conflict, consistency in communication with others and trainees occurs. Follow-up communication from meetings that includes common points of agreement by faculty or stakeholders establishes healthy program norms that assist all stakeholders and the training program goals in general. These positive norms and consistent messages encompass a help-seeking approach with trainees in the gatekeeping process (Gizara & Forrest, 2004; Homrich, 2009; McCarthy, 2008; Trimble et al., 2012).

Consulting With Colleagues

Kaslow et al. (2007) stated that many clinical training programs lack the expertise or perspective of the various stakeholders and constituencies, so it is important that a training program have support and collaboration across the various levels of the ecological collaborative gatekeeping approach. Beyond the academic training and the field site units, representative participants may include administrators in higher education institutions, various ancillary university units (e.g., trainee affairs, disability services, the Title IX office, student conduct councils), attorneys in the legal department, human resources professionals, and medical professionals in related disciplines (e.g., physicians, nurses) affiliated with the core cooperating units. Common barriers to effective communication and collaboration during gatekeeping and remediation can include the multiple hierarchies involved in both university settings and health care settings. Communication failures can arise from vertical hierarchical differences, conflict and ambiguity in roles, and struggles with institutional and interpersonal power dynamics. In cases of hierarchical differences, communication is likely to be distorted or withheld. Communication failures occur, particularly when one person is concerned about the power difference and either does not want to offend others or perceives that others are not open to communication.

In hierarchical university environments, administrators are typically at the top of the hierarchy (Delunas & Rouse, 2014; Kaslow et al., 2007; Meyers et al., 2013). Consequently, although faculty may believe that their immediate environment is collaborative and that communication is open, administrators may have a different perspective of trainee requirements and needs. Hierarchy differences can diminish the collaborative interactions necessary to ensure that profession-specific program requirements, ethical guidelines, and/or accreditation standards are adhered to. When differences in viewpoint exist in a hierarchical structure, people on the lower end of the hierarchy who have "limited power" tend to be uncomfortable speaking up about problems or concerns (Lysaght & Altschuld, 2000, p. 102). Furthermore, intimidating behavior or the imposition of authoritarian power by individuals at the top of a hierarchy can hinder communication and give the impression that an individual is unapproachable. In a hierarchy, faculty, supervisors (both university and site), and trainee peers who witness the poor performance of a trainee with behavioral issues may be hesitant to speak up because they perceive that doing so will result in no action being taken or cause conflict. Reasons for this include intimidation, fear of being drawn into a confrontational discussion, lack of confidentiality, or concerns about retaliation. Many of these issues depend on individual personality and communication style as well as institutional or hierarchy reputation.

Inconsistent collaboration and gatekeeping practices in and across levels result in problems at and beyond the macro level of the ecological collaborative gatekeeping approach. Failure to gatekeep due to failed collaboration or consensus leads to gateslipping: allowing impaired or problematic trainees to move into professional practice, impacting the reputation of the clinical professions in general and, more critically, the potential health and welfare of future clients. For example, W. B. Johnson et al. (2008) stated that many mental health professionals who have worked in education or credentialing agencies believe that stakeholders in each professional area perceive little transparency or sense of shared responsibility with other professional areas regarding gatekeeping. They suggested that professionals working at clinical sites generally blame educators for not addressing problems with trainees, and professors sometimes believe that clinical sites ignore or take no responsibility for addressing supervisee issues of personal conduct and professional behavior. Licensing boards believe that the fault lies with both educational programs and clinical sites allowing incompetent trainees to graduate and pursue licensure in their respective clinical field of professional practice.

W. B. Johnson and Campbell (2004) stated that better working relationships should also be initiated between stakeholders in university settings like trainee affairs departments or outside the university with constituencies like the state licensing board. They provided an example of working relationships with the legal profession in Oregon, where the Board of Bar Examiners collaborates with each law school in Oregon annually to exchange information with university faculty and deans on the admission criteria for the bar. These scholars said that if licensing boards worked with training programs regarding requirements, training programs would be more likely to enforce gatekeeping during student admission and throughout training, thereby reducing the number of disciplinary problems that would occur after trainees have graduated, obtained their licenses, and are working in the field.

Programs should assess the prevalence, contextual influences, and impact that the actions and behaviors of individual stakeholders can have on a problem situation in an effort to identify potential opportunities for improvement in communication and collaboration. Support and educational funding for collaborative efforts that promote discussion and education about gatekeeping to outside constituencies is important and worthy of consideration. Clinical programs have a responsibility to educate partner constituencies and systems—that affect and are affected by the various contexts, institutions, professions, and hierarchical levels discussed here—about the obligation of gatekeeping in clinical training programs. One recommendation that Kaslow et al. (2007) made was to have an award that recognizes collaboration. Awards can encourage proactive working alliances in a program, and they can also encourage cooperative partnerships beyond an institutional program, such as with a site or supportive professional organization.

W. B. Johnson et al. (2008) stated that progress has been made conceptually and in policies regarding gatekeeping. First, specific professional organizations have addressed professional competencies issues by helping the public and professionals understand that addressing problems of professional competence is a responsibility of all stakeholders. This can be illustrated by the inclusion of gatekeeping practices, such as trainee oversight, evaluation, and remedial intervention, in professional ethics codes. Second, efforts to collaborate across systems (e.g., faculty, university administrators, site supervisors) have increased among professional levels. Third, progress has been made in understanding due process and legal issues, including laws such as FERPA and HIPAA, that help training programs to develop policies and procedures in collaboration with all stakeholders.

Conclusion

Leadership in a training program is important to the gatekeeping process. Conceptualizing leadership in a training program from an ecological viewpoint helps strengthen program perspectives from a variety of professionals and disciplines. Collaboration across the many varied disciplines and hierarchical structures that affect and are affected by gatekeeping practices involves decision-making processes that are implemented by an interactive group of professionals as opposed to one faculty member, a single supervisor, or a sole administrator making decisions or policies about or during the gatekeeping process. Collaboration includes consultation but involves more specific skills that engage proactive planning, problem solving, collegial agreement, collective knowledge, and the protection of all stakeholders.

Maintaining gatekeeping policies and procedures is as important as developing the policies. Consistency is one of the main skills for all stakeholders to use during communication, documentation, and implementation of policies. Consistency of communication complements problem solving and collegial agreement; the collective knowledge of all stakeholders; the reduction of problems and stress; increased fulfillment of the roles and obligations of gatekeeping; and protection of faculty, professionals, institutions, trainees, and clients. Once collaboration at all levels is established, the ecological collaborative gatekeeping approach should be used to monitor policies and conduct periodic reviews of individual trainee problems. Faculty should work collaboratively to prevent subgrouping or splitting in faculty and among all stakeholders. Programs that are not collaborative encourage norms that lack transparency, poor communication, punitive climates, a lack of trust, and accusatory attitudes. (See What Would You Do? 6.2.)

Key Points and Best Practices

- A systemic and holistic approach to gatekeeping that attends to trainee problems is important.
- Gatekeeping should include a collaborative commitment to decision making that is implemented in an interactive group that includes all faculty and professionals.
- Gatekeeping policies and procedures should be maintained in a way that supports collaboration through consultation, consistent formal policy reviews, and monitoring of gatekeeping.

What Would You Do? 6.2

Toni is a 35-year-old master's-level student. She completed her practicum and is now in her first internship. She is interning at a community mental health clinic where she has a male supervisor. Her university group and individual supervisors are both female doctoral trainees who are being supervised by a faculty member of the program. At the end of last semester, Toni's faculty supervisor for individual supervision at the university began to report concerns that Toni was having problems with timeliness in attending individual supervision. When the individual faculty supervisor met with Toni's site supervisor during the third week of her internship, he indicated that Toni was doing fine.

At midterm, Toni's group and individual supervisors documented that they had given Toni feedback regarding their concerns about her behaviors during individual and group supervision: lack of timeliness with assignment completion (documentation at the beginning of the semester, weekly recording transcripts and case work for a client session, weekly logs of hours, etc., were submitted past assigned due dates), lack of timeliness in attending supervision, poor ability to receive feedback, lack of implementation of feedback from supervisors, externalization of personal responsibility, poor decision making and balance in professional and personal lives that affected her clinical performance, and lack of insight regarding the causal link between personal behaviors and the consequences of her actions. The faculty decided to put Toni on a remediation plan designed to address these professional and interpersonal deficiencies. When Toni was informed that she would be placed on a remediation plan, she provided faculty with a form from the university's disability services office regarding her necessary accommodations, such as absences from class, allowances for lateness to class, and assistance with note taking.

What would you do?

What types of collaborative efforts should be initiated?

Who should be a part of those collaborative efforts?

What steps should be taken by faculty that allow for a student to have the opportunity to change?

Chapter 7

Informing Trainees About Gatekeeping Policies

Page L. Thanasiu

One of the biggest concerns of educators and supervisors engaged in gatekeeping practices is the fear of litigation resulting from the dismissal of a student. Across the helping professions, faculty have admitted to considering legal risks when contemplating gatekeeping options (Barlow & Coleman, 2003; McAdams, Foster, & Ward, 2007). Some consider the appraisal of students' professional suitability as a subjective process and are unsure whether they can include elements they consider to be nonacademic in dismissal decisions. In fact, authors in both the mental health and judiciary fields have maintained that interpersonal functioning, professional performance, and psychological fitness can be included in the academic domain when they are requisite competencies for the profession (Darr, Moore, & Snyder, 2003; Forrest, Elman, Giazara, & Vacha-Haaze, 1999; Kerl, Garcia, McCullough, & Maxwell, 2002; Olkin & Gaughen, 1991). Granted, there have been several cases in which students dismissed from mental health training programs have brought legal action against their universities claiming that the dismissals were arbitrary, prejudicial, capricious, and/or unrelated to academic performance. However, thus far, case law decisions have ultimately upheld universities' rights to evaluate and determine student performance and to dismiss trainees for reasons of interpersonal performance and/or psychological competence (e.g., *Keeton v. Anderson-Wiley*, 2010; *Plaintiff v. Rector and Board of Visitors of The College of William and Mary*, 2005; *Ward v. Wilbanks*, 2010).

In court, the critical task for the university becomes demonstrating that the department followed all necessary steps to ensure that the student was afforded due process (Dugger & Francis, 2014). Consequently, it is recommended that training programs create and publish a specific review and retention policy that clearly outlines procedures for due process (Baldo, Softas-Nall, & Shaw, 1997). To assist with this goal, the objectives of this chapter are as follows:

- To identify the progressive points of opportunity that programs and supervisors should utilize for informing clinical trainees of required standards and accompanying policies prior to and through to the end of the pre- and postdegree training process
- To introduce best practice strategies for communicating standards and policies to students and supervisees in a manner that supports the principles of informed consent, understanding and compliance, enforcement of gatekeeping, and due process

As discussed in detail in Chapter 3, *due process* is a legal term that refers to the rights to life, liberty, and property protected by the Fourteenth Amendment of the U.S. Constitution and "is applicable to the gatekeeping procedures of counselor educators and supervisors with regard to intrapersonal and interpersonal functioning of trainees" (Homrich, 2009, p. 4). A program that maintains sound due process is one in which standards are clearly defined, made widely available, and communicated to students or supervisees often. Furthermore, students/supervisees exhibiting problematic professional behaviors are notified in a timely manner when they are not meeting published expectations and are then given the opportunity to respond followed by sufficient time and support to remediate problematic behaviors. Homrich further emphasized that "due process requires that both the standards and procedures that govern counselor education programs be applied consistently and fairly to all students in the program" (p. 4). In order to best protect programs that may encounter litigation, "all faculty must understand due process procedures, actively endorse them, and learn to apply them consistently" (Crawford & Gilroy, 2012, p. 35).

Chapter 8 addresses how a graduate program or postgraduate supervisor should construct standards for the personal and professional behavior of trainees. Sometimes there are different and conflicting standards among the professional organizations (e.g., Commission on Accreditation for Marriage and Family Therapy Education, American Psychological Association Commission on Accreditation, Council on Social Work Education, Council for Accreditation of Counseling and Related Educational Programs), the ethics codes of the mental health professions, and the codes of conduct for students as determined by academic institutions and departments. This places responsibility on individual mental health training programs to weave together a cohesive set of standards to apply to their own students that reflect the professional, institutional, and programmatic constituencies that govern the major. (See On the Legal Side 7.1.)

Supervisors at the postdegree level must also consider not only the policies dictated by the organization for which they work and the ethical guidelines of their profession but also the statutory requirements within their particular jurisdiction (state) when composing written expectations for their supervisees expecting endorsement for licensure. Standards need to include specifically defined criteria that clearly communicate precisely what is expected of trainees in the domains of professional, interpersonal, and intrapersonal conduct. Furthermore, each supervisor or program is responsible for determining the evaluation strategies and intervention policies and procedures it will follow when students/supervisees are not meeting the predefined criteria. Once these criteria are solidly in place, the next important step is to establish a routine through which all students/supervisees are notified of required standards, policies, procedures, and processes at multiple points along their professional journey, beginning with their consideration of a graduate program through to endorsement for licensure (see Figure 7.1).

On the Legal Side 7.1

Once a training program or professional supervisor has developed written documentation of an agreement, event, or action, an important step prior to publishing the documentation or utilizing a supervision contract can be to seek counsel, whether it be legal or administrative (Wheeler & Bertram, 2015). Professionals may be able to obtain legal consultation from their associated professional organizations (e.g., American Counseling Association, American Psychological Association, National Association of Social Workers) or may seek personal legal counsel. Training programs can follow these same avenues; however, they should also have published documentation reviewed and approved by their institution's legal counsel, particularly graduate catalogs and graduate student handbooks that stipulate adherence to professional standards not typically addressed in the academic realm.

When colleagues have sought personal legal counsel while developing informed consent and other professional documents, there have at times been differing legal opinions (K. Henderson, personal communication, February 5, 2016). Therefore, it is recommended that professionals document the guidance and legal advice they have received in case a situation occurs whereby it becomes necessary to defend the rationale for future policies and procedures related to published professional documentation. Records may include the date of the legal consultation, the legal consultant's credentials and areas of expertise, what exactly was requested or presented for approval, the resulting advice or directive, and/or whether approval was ultimately ascertained.

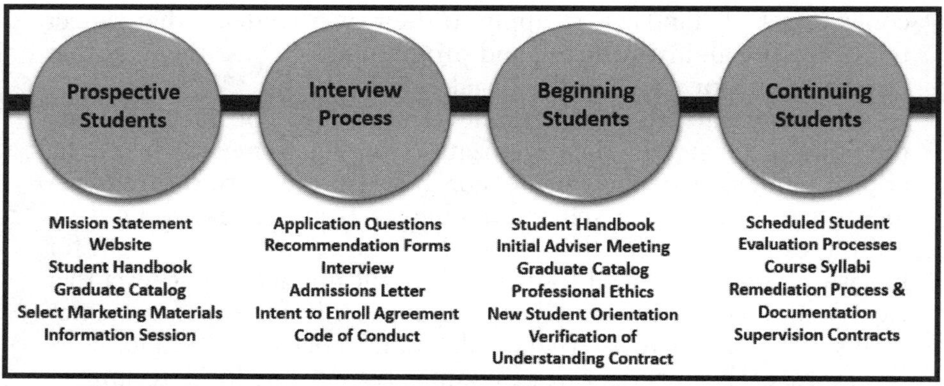

Figure 7.1 • Timeline for Informing Graduate Students of Program Standards and Policies

Informing Students of Program Expectations and Professional Standards

Informing Prospective Students

Prior to the application process, prospective students/supervisees should be informed of any standards and/or policies that will apply to them while enrolled in a training program during the consideration stage. Homrich (2009) suggested that programs address expectations for students throughout their marketing and recruiting efforts. A training program's standards and disciplinary policies should be published in multiple locations that are easily accessible to both current and prospective students. "This may be accomplished by including them within the program's student handbook, posting them to the department's website, and/or including them (or a link to them) within the letter of admission sent to new students" (Dugger & Francis, 2014, p. 139). A program's website should also include a link for prospective students to the graduate catalog, another source of critical standards and policies at the institutional level. Finally, a department's mission and values statements provide an additional avenue for including terminology that communicates program expectations. For instance, departments may choose to incorporate wording such as:

- learners who value personal and intellectual growth . . .
- self-reflective practitioners competent in serving diverse populations
- students who actively engage as self-reflexive practitioners . . .
- experiences that promote awareness of self and one's impact on others . . .
- practitioners who possess a deep awareness of themselves . . . (Homrich, 2009, p. 8)

As Homrich (2009) further observed, "Specification of academic expectations, including personal and professional competencies, accompanied by advance notification of remedial and disciplinary procedures and consequences if students do not fulfill standards, serves as informed consent for applicants" (p. 9).

Informing Applicants During the Admissions Process

Many training programs choose to conduct information sessions and individual and/or group interviews during the admissions process. These opportunities are valuable for enabling potential applicants to evaluate training and supervisory options during which transparency can minimize the risks of future charges of breach of contract (Homrich, 2009). For instance, at one department's mandatory information session, the American Counseling Association's (ACA's) position on value conflicts between counselors and clients (Kaplan, 2014) is presented and discussed with potential applicants as it relates to referral practices and the program's emphasis on valuing diversity. The program's goal is to assist applicants in deciding whether the professional values of the program will be compatible with their own personal values prior to application and enrollment. Additional areas to cover, at least briefly, during these face-to-face experiences could include the following:

- The departmental philosophy, mission, and values
- The ethical standards of the profession
- A select list of the most salient personal and professional competencies expected of students/supervisees
- The location of written standards and policies, specifically the student handbook, the graduate catalog, and the specific profession's code of ethics, for applicants to review prior to accepting a position in the training program

Although most training programs expect the application packet to provide valuable insight into the characteristics, goals, and qualifications of the applicant, elements of the application can also serve as an additional avenue for communicating program expectations. Responses to application questions or interview activities can be evaluated for appropriateness in terms of intrapersonal insight, interpersonal awareness, or the candidate's match with the values for the profession or program. For example, Homrich (2009) proposed the following structured essay question for possible inclusion in a training program application:

> This counseling program is known for valuing diversity and social justice for oppressed groups in terms of race, ethnicity, culture, class, gender, sexual orientation, gender identity, age, spiritual tradition, ability, etc. Graduate students are expected to self-evaluate and resolve any values that they hold that perpetuate discrimination and marginalization of oppressed or minority groups, as such values, rigidly and inflexibly held,

> can prevent students from performing the behaviors and competencies expected in our program and in the profession of counseling (Mintz & Bieschke, 2009). How will you begin the process of reflecting on and addressing any attitudes, beliefs, assumptions, or feelings that may negatively impact your ability to work with a client or a colleague holding an identity or social location different from your own? (p. 9)

Responses to this question can indicate a candidate's ability to self-reflect and problem-solve and/or his or her willingness to "respect the diversity of clients . . . and seek training in areas in which they are at risk of imposing their values onto clients, especially when the counselor's values are inconsistent with the client's goals or are discriminatory in nature" (ACA, 2014a) as described in Standard A.4.b. of the *ACA Code of Ethics*.

This same question could be modified and/or incorporated into a face-to-face interview for either a program applicant or a potential postdegree supervisee. In a similar manner, recommendation forms are another place wherein departments can inform others about programmatic expectations and assess suitability for the profession during the admissions stage—the first gate of the gatekeeping process. Homrich (2009) discussed another example in which

> Portland State University prints four aspects of the graduate school of education's conceptual framework directly on their recommendation forms (http://www.pdx.edu/coun/admissions-and-registration). The items are succinct and include one or two bulleted outcome statements for their graduates, such as the expectation "to work in diverse settings" and "to promote inclusiveness and therapeutic environments." (p. 10)

Once applicants are extended an offer of admission, they are often asked to respond with a signed intent to enroll agreement accompanied by a monetary deposit securing a place in the next class. This form, which requires a signature, provides an additional opportunity to indicate the parameters of matriculation reflecting standards and expectations of the program.

Informing Beginning Students

Once enrolled, entering students typically participate in a mandatory new student orientation meeting. This meeting, when the new cohort is together, is an excellent time to emphasize the philosophical intent of professional standards, the program's commitment to maintaining professional standards, and the legal and ethical obligation of the program faculty and supervisors to enact the gatekeeping process in an effort to support student development. Some programs may choose to go into detail about specific standards; yet at this first official meeting, new students have found specific details to be overwhelming and anxiety provoking. Research has indicated that new students do not retain the specifics discussed at orientations related to gatekeeping policies (J. M. Foster, Leppma, & Hutchinson, 2014; Parker et al., 2014). Thus, a general overview of professional standards is suggested with specific opportunities to continue the discussion in the introductory course during the first semester.

As a way to inculcate new students to the expectations and standards of their graduate program and the counseling profession, one counselor education program asks students to take a professional pledge at the new student orientation meeting that affirms their understanding of the commitment that will require their engagement as a student and a professional. The purpose of this activity is twofold: (a) to introduce new students to the seriousness of the program's standards and regard for the professional responsibility they are about to undertake by entering the mental health field, and (b) to instill a sense of unity among the cohort as a team of people engaging in this endeavor together. The pledge, with multiple signature lines, is printed on a large piece of paper and is laid out on a table in the front of the room. At the conclusion of the new student orientation, the department chair introduces the ceremony; asks students to step forward, announce their name to their new peer colleagues, and sign the pledge; and asks the group to applaud their commitment. The professional pledge with signatures is then framed and hung in the hallway of the department. A sample of the professional pledge is included in Appendix D.

One aspect of the orientation process, whether it be a prerequisite task independent of a specific course or an assignment in a first-semester introductory course, should be the requirement that new students read the institution's graduate catalog, the program's student handbook, and the applicable profession's code of ethics. Many clinical graduate programs also require that new students submit a signed document verifying that they have received, have read, and agree to abide by the policies of their training program as described in these documents. The signed verification of understanding agreement should be placed in the student's permanent file. This exercise ensures that the student has been informed of the expected standards of conduct and the processes of remediation and gatekeeping. A sample verification of understanding agreement is included in the Appendix E and can be modified according to the program's objectives. This process also validates the informed consent of each student to engage in the program with known conditions of remediation and dismissal.

During the first semester of the program, new students' understanding of program expectations are also reaffirmed by the departmental community. Information about program and professional expectations can be clarified for students through interactions with their faculty advisors, course instructors—especially core faculty members—and assigned peer mentors. When all program-related constituencies are well informed of the professional and personal standards for students defined by both the program and the profession in general, entering students receive a consistent message that is affirmed by all participants in the training process. This includes core program faculty, adjunct faculty, site supervisors, program staff (who have been educated about the program's training standards), current students, and alumni. In effect, the culture of the graduate program in relation to expectations for interpersonal, intrapersonal, and professional behavior is strongly established over time and across the community and is consistently communicated to new students entering the program and the related mental health profession.

Informing Continuing Students

In addition to being good practice, most accrediting entities for training programs within the mental health fields require ongoing systematic assessment of student progress as discussed in detail in Chapter 9. Ensuring that students are familiar ahead of time with evaluation processes, assessment forms, and/or rubrics that will be used allows them to understand what is expected of them and how they will be evaluated. Evaluation procedures present many additional opportunities to remind trainees of standards regarding personal and professional competency. The assessment rubric can be structured so that during a standard evaluation conducted with all student trainees, such as an evaluation of student skill development at the end of a counseling skills course, it lists the specific criteria for personal and professional behavior being measured at that particular point in training. In this way, students not only see where they fall along a continuum of performance but also are reminded of the standards they are expected to achieve. Similarly, when students require constructive feedback on classroom assignments, especially those that involve peer interaction or professional conduct, the instructor can include direct written reference to the associated standards contained within the student handbook. The student is then able to compare to the published standards what he or she has produced or exhibited. Ideally, the instructor's feedback also contains suggestions for continued development in the areas mentioned. If a supervisee's assessment reveals the need for a more formal level of critical feedback or remediation, it is vital that the written documentation again communicates in detail the problematic behaviors and the expected standards for personal and professional conduct as presented in Chapter 8. Throughout the evaluation process, the importance for both faculty and postdegree supervisors of documenting each step in writing cannot be overemphasized (Homrich, 2009).

Standards that are specific to a particular course or expected throughout all courses can be reiterated by means of course syllabi; however, course syllabi should never be the only location for expectations for students' personal and professional conduct. For instance, all course syllabi utilized in a training program may include a section defining the behaviors associated with professionalism in the classroom that will contribute to students' weekly participation points. For example, the syllabi for courses taught in the beginning and middle of the training progression might state the following:

> **Professionalism:** As requirements for this course as part of a professional training program, students are expected to consistently demonstrate professional behavior; this criterion is counted toward your participation grade. This includes but is not limited to the following:
>
> - Being on time to class and with assignments
> - Respectful interactions with students, faculty, and staff
> - Proactive engagement in the learning process and completing assignments
> - Being organized and prepared for the learning experience, especially in class and in work accomplished in student groups
> - Managing paperwork, documentation, and technology effectively
> - Managing personal crises effectively
> - Managing personal information (your own and others') appropriately and respectfully
>
> To receive full credit for participation, you must adhere to the "Professionalism" expectations listed above, participate actively and constructively in class, adhere to professional ethics codes and professional codes of conduct, and in general contribute positively to the class culture.

Practicum and internship course syllabi associated with the final stages of training may address standards more closely aligned with skill development, the maintenance of one's own mental health, anxiety management, and observation of appropriate interpersonal boundaries across settings (Homrich, 2009).

Faculty Supervisor–Supervisee Contract

As students enter their first clinical course, it is recommended that they also sign an additional supervision contract in conjunction with their faculty supervisor that reiterates programmatic and clinical expectations and policies—previously published in the graduate catalog or graduate student handbook—pertaining to student behavior, evaluation, remediation, and discipline. See Notes From the Field 7.1 and Appendix F for sample supervision contracts.

Field Site Supervision Agreement

The same principle of enacting a specific agreement or contract between a faculty supervisor and supervisee applies to implementing a written understanding with the field site agency and field site supervisor. This contract or agreement details what is expected of all parties involved, including the faculty and site supervisors, agency administration, and practicum student. This agreement is another location to reiterate expectations of student supervisees. It also clarifies for the student

Notes From the Field 7.1

At the annual conference of the European Branch of ACA some years back, I found myself talking to a fellow attendee and university faculty member about the importance of supervisory contracts. Until that time, I had considered my practicum or internship syllabus to be the only contractual agreement that was needed between the student and myself. In it, I included important elements such as the standards and expectations of the course and of the student's performance in the course, information about my qualifications and supervisory style, ways to contact me outside of normal business hours, methods of evaluation, and more. I was also aware that the *Best Practices in Clinical Supervision* (Association for Counselor Education and Supervision, 2011) allowed for either a written contract or a syllabus to outline the expectations of a supervisory relationship. The gentleman I was speaking with was at the time a member of the ACA Ethics Revision Task Force, charged with updating the evolving code of ethics for the profession. He had also been involved in a lengthy and highly publicized court case in which a dismissed student had brought legal action against his university. In these two roles, he had learned the importance of having an individually signed contractual agreement with each practicum and internship student he supervised. As a result of that conversation, I realized what good sense having a specific contract for the supervisory relationship made: It provided the opportunity for student supervisees to actively understand and agree to the relationship we were creating while also modeling the experience they should have with future supervisors after graduation. Included in Appendix F is the supervision contract that I currently use with my graduate-level supervisees as well as an example of a contract that is used by a professional supervisor. When creating supervision contracts, it is important to seek legal counsel and consider the requirements of all state and federal laws for the supervisory role, which can vary considerably based on jurisdiction (Wheeler & Bertram, 2015).

as well as the educational and agency institutions the expectations of each participant in the training process (e.g., communication among supervisors across organizations). One program created this informational document after a local clinical agency dismissed a practicum student for unprofessional behavior (intoxication while engaged in practicum activities) without informing the graduate program prior to or after the dismissal (a task that was left to the student intern). In investigating the situation, it was discovered that the site supervisor had the mistaken assumption that there was a commitment to the supervisee to maintain confidentiality, as one would for a client. Of course, the opposite is true: Faculty and site supervisors must communicate openly about supervisee progress and work jointly to support students in remedying behavior prior to or immediately after taking independent action, depending on the severity of the situation and the danger to clients or others. Subsequently, a three-way agreement was constructed for future placement of clinical students that included specific expectations informing each participant in the training effort about the roles and responsibilities of the faculty supervisor and graduate program, the site supervisor and supervising agency, and the student supervisee, including standards of the graduate program for student behavior. All parties are required to sign the document prior to finalizing practicum placement, acknowledging that they have been informed of the standards of practice expected not only of the student but also of everyone involved in the student training and development process.

Information Sources of Standards Expected of Students

As mentioned in the previous section, students acquire information about performance expectations for their academic work, clinical skill demonstration, and professional conduct and dispositions from several sources before and after admission. For most clinical programs, these sources include the graduate catalog, the student handbook, and the ethics code of the profession. Some graduate programs also post expectations on websites and include them in supplemental publications, such as clinical guidebooks, or in syllabi. The recommended best practice standard is that, at a minimum, all evaluative criteria and performance expectations should be detailed in either the institution's graduate catalog or the program's graduate student handbook. In either of these documents, the stipulated ethics codes to which the training program subscribes should be cited and/or included in their entirety as an appendix. Of course, the standards and expectations can and should be reiterated or duplicated in clinical guidebooks, in syllabi, on websites, and in other informal and formal information sources; however, the standards that will be part of any student evaluation process—whether they be for academic performance, clinical skill performance, or professional and personal conduct—should be detailed in one of the these primary program documents. In the event of failed student performance, such as an unsuccessful remediation effort that leads to dismissal, the graduate catalog and graduate student handbook should be cited as the official source of information in legal actions. The previously discussed verification of understanding agreement signed by the student will strengthen the program's position of having appropriately informed the student in the event of a legal proceeding. For these reasons, programs should consider reviewing and updating their primary informational documents on a regular basis. The following content may be considered for inclusion, but these suggestions will vary according to individual institutional administrative policies and are not intended to be all inclusive or exhaustive.

Homrich (2009) suggested that a student handbook or catalog include elements such as the following:

- Clearly articulated standards for graduate student performance, including professional conduct and personal behavior expectations . . .
- Evaluation criteria;
- Procedures for ongoing assessment of student progress in meeting performance standards;
- Methods of providing evaluative feedback to students;
- Gatekeeping procedures;
- Student remediation sequence;
- Possible remediation actions;
- Student dismissal criteria and process;
- Appeals procedures; and
- Endorsement policy describing the department's process of recommending students for employment, licensure, and other credentialing. (p. 10)

Additional policy points to add to this list include the following:

- Limits of confidentiality among and/or between faculty members and supervisors
- Professional practice standards of faculty/supervisors consulting with one another
- Mandated reporting conditions and obligations
- Confidentiality standards for client information, including the Health Insurance Portability and Accountability Act
- Any federal and state-specific legal requirements of prelicensure individuals, including students, engaging in clinical practice within the jurisdiction

An institution's or training program's code of conduct may include guidelines and wording that are identical to the standards derived from professional and institutional guiding principles. As mentioned previously, documents such as the code of conduct are valuable places in which to reiterate details of the department's further expectations for student personal and professional behavior, but all information in program-related documents should be clearly articulated in one of the primary documents: the graduate catalog and/or the graduate student handbook. Barlow and Coleman (2003) suggested the following considerations as standards of professional performance:

> These expectations can include respecting confidentiality of clients; treating fellow students, faculty, client, staff and supervisors with respect; honesty, courtesy, fairness and good faith; upholding the Social Work Code of Ethics; refraining from engaging and condoning criminal activities; refraining from engaging or condoning any form of discrimination; and, giving permission for faculty advisor to discuss his/her progress with other faculty members or field instructors. (p. 153)

Furthermore, the graduate student handbook is a suitable place to address the expected scope of student behavior that will be considered when evaluating personal and professional competence in areas of personal and professional functioning outside of institutional or professional association policies. For example, authors from the field of psychology (S. B. Myers, Endres, Ruddy, & Zelikovsky, 2012; Pham, 2014; Wester, Danforth, & Olle, 2013) have attempted to address the complex issues surrounding the inclusion of information and activity derived from social media in student/supervisee evaluations. For instance, is content only included if the trainee was the one to post the problematic or incriminating information? Or might evidence be considered even if a compromising photo was posted online unbeknownst to the trainee? Brew, Cervantes, and Shepard (2013) found that although more than 50% of the counselor education students they surveyed admitted to posting material that they would not want a client to see, after direct instruction intended to enhance student awareness, the researchers found a significant increase in responsible use of social media privacy settings.

A somewhat related point to consider ahead of time and include in written policy is the manner in which a department or postdegree supervisor will handle reports of concerning extracurricular social behavior that may be incongruent with the interpersonal, intrapersonal, and professional expectations of clinicians. These accounts may come from colleagues in the field, from site supervisors, from supervisees' peers, or directly from the supervisee. Again, it is important to have the related policy in writing and to make it widely available. Ultimately, by signing the informed consent, trainees confirm that they are familiar with the written expectations of the program or arrangement and agree to abide by the policies and procedures set forth, including participation in ongoing self-evaluation. The critical point for program faculty is to publish thoroughly defined and described behavioral expectations prior to encountering such behaviors.

Informing Postgraduate Supervisees of Supervisory Expectations and Professional Standards

Initiating the Supervisory Agreement

Postdegree supervisors must also clearly communicate their standards and remedial policies to potential supervisees as early as possible for adherence to due process, and this process can begin before the supervisor and potential supervisee meet for the first time (see Figure 7.2). Professionals who wish to offer supervision services can incorporate their guidelines and policies into various marketing avenues. For instance, a website can have a page specifically devoted to guidelines for expected interpersonal and intrapersonal professional behaviors of supervisees and the remediation processes that may occur in case of

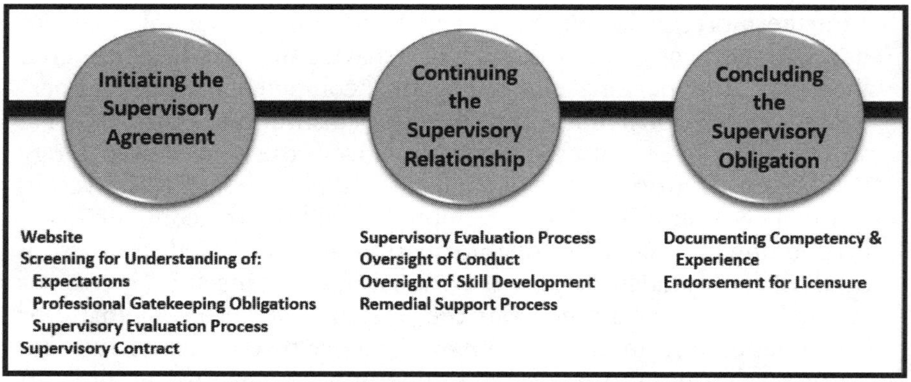

Figure 7.2 • Timeline and Avenues for Informing Postgraduate Supervisees of Supervisory Standards and Policies

deficit. A supervisor may additionally choose to make at least a portion of his or her supervision documents (e.g., supervision contract) publicly available on the website for review.

Prior to engaging in a postgraduate supervisory relationship, supervisors often hold an initial interview with prospective supervisees in order to determine trainer/trainee goodness of fit. It is important for supervisors to screen potential supervisees prior to engagement in order to assess their awareness of and ability to comply with professional standards, whether it be in terms of clinical skill or professional and personal conduct. This is a crucial point in time for supervisors' gatekeeping process because, once locked into a supervisory relationship, supervisors are vicariously and directly liable for the actions of their supervisees.

All policies and standards should be clearly included in the written supervision contract and reviewed prior to beginning the supervisory relationship. The supervision contract acts as the official informed consent between the supervisor and trainee and when comprehensively constructed can help minimize supervisors' risk of liability should a supervisee be accused of malpractice (Wheeler & Bertram, 2015). In fact, written supervision contracts, during both pre- and postdegree supervision, can serve multiple functions, including the following:

1. Clarification of methods, goals, and expectations of supervision
2. Promotion of professional collaboration
3. Reinforcement of ethical principles
4. Documentation of services provided
5. Alignment of supervision with counseling and consultation
6. Establishment of structure and boundaries for trainees
7. Reinforcement of accountability for both supervisee and supervisor (Osborn & Davis, 1996; Osborn, Paez, & Carrabine, 2007; Tanenbaum & Berman, 1990; Welch, 2003)

For postdegree supervisors, the supervision contract serves as the comprehensive location for detailing standards and expectations as well as policies pertaining to evaluation, remediation, and discipline. During the time in which the supervisor is evaluating the trainee as a potential supervisee, the trainee should read through the complete contract and verbalize any clarifications needed in order to make a fully informed decision before entering into the relationship.

Cobia and Boes (2000) suggested including two parts to the supervision contract, one that acts as a professional disclosure statement and another that is individualized to the supervisee. The first portion, developed by the supervisor, includes the "mutual rights and responsibilities of all parties, the parameters of supervision, methods of evaluation, desired outcomes, and potential risks and benefits" (pp. 293–294). The second portion is created collaboratively between the supervisee and supervisor and incorporates learning goals, objectives, strategies, job responsibilities, criteria for evaluation, and other individualized information pertaining to the supervisee (e.g., accommodations requested, feedback preferences, learning style). These may be presented together as one contract or separately as two documents, but each should be signed by both trainee and supervisor after being discussed and agreed on.

Each of the primary professional organizations that dictate the ethical behavior of mental health supervisors (i.e., ACA, American Psychological Association, American Association for Marriage and Family Therapy, Association for Counselor Education and Supervision, Association of State and Provincial Psychology Boards, National Association of Social Workers [NASW], National Board for Certified Counselors) mandate the use of informed consent between supervisors and supervisees. Table 7.1 details particular elements of informed consent that each of these organizations specifically address in their codes of ethics or best practice guidelines for supervision, and these should be taken into consideration when creating the supervision contract.

J. T. Thomas (2007) created "a menu of topics designed to help supervisors identify areas most pertinent to the types of supervision they provide" (p. 226) in an effort to assist with determining the appropriate components of a written supervision contract. These, along with suggestions from other authors (NASW & Association of Social Work Boards, 2013; Wheeler & Bertram, 2015), are included in summarized form in Table 7.2. A supervision contract does not have to include every category from the table; however, the more comprehensive the contract, the better protected the supervisor will be should supervision proceed other than as anticipated. Discussing as many details as possible ahead of time can also help to prevent misunderstandings and conflicts between the supervisor and supervisee (J. T. Thomas, 2007, 2010). Although some categories, such as the supervisor's background and supervisory methods, are somewhat self-explanatory, others de-

Table 7.1 • Supervisory Topics and Standards Addressed in Terms of Informed Consent

Supervisory Standard or Topic	*Source (Code of Ethics or Standard Guidelines)*
Document informed consent	AAMFT (2014), ACA (2014a), ACES (2011), APA (2014), ASPPB (2015), NASW & ASWB (2013), NBCC (2016)
Include specific content for supervision contract	AAMFT (2014), APA (2014), ASPPB (2015), NASW & ASWB (2013)
Communicate elements of supervisor's background	ACES (2011), ASPPB (2015)
Communicate conditions of supervision (e.g., goals, roles)	AAMFT (2014), ACES (2011), APA (2014), ASPPB (2015), NASW & ASWB (2013), NBCC (2016)
Communicate supervisor's responsibilities	AAMFT (2014), ACA (2014a), ACES (2011), APA (2014), ASPPB (2015), NASW & ASWB (2013), NBCC (2016)
Communicate organizational information (e.g., day and time of meeting)	AAMFT (2014), ACA (2014a), ACES (2011), ASPPB (2015)
Use specific supervision methods (e.g., viewing sessions, incorporating self-assessment, live observation)	AAMFT (2014), ACES (2011), APA (2014a), ASPPB (2015)
Communicate fees	AAMFT (2014), ACES (2011), ASPPB (2015)
Communicate documentation of supervision	ACES (2011), APA (2014), ASPPB (2015), NASW & ASWB (2013), NBCC (2016)
Communicate evaluation procedures and/or feedback schedule	AAMFT (2014), ACA (2014a), ACES (2011), APA (2014), ASPPB (2015), NASW & ASWB (2013), NBCC (2016)
Uphold confidentiality of supervisees	AAMFT (2014), ACES (2011), APA (2014), ASPPB (2015), NASW & ASWB (2013), NBCC (2016)
Follow due process and/or complaints	AAMFT (2014), ACA (2014a), ACES (2011), APA (2014), ASPPB (2015)
Address endorsement	AAMFT (2014), ACA (2014a)
Communicate duration and termination of supervision contract	AAMFT (2014), ACA (2014a), APA (2014), ASPPB (2015), NASW & ASWB (2013)

Note. AAMFT = American Association for Marriage and Family Therapy; ACA = American Counseling Association; ACES = Association for Counselor Education and Supervision; APA = American Psychological Association; ASPPB = Association of State and Provincial Psychology Boards; NASW = National Association of Social Workers; ASWB = Asssociation of Social Work Boards; NBCC = National Board for Certified Counselors.

serve additional attention and explanation, specifically standards that define parameters for clinical performance and for interpersonal and intrapersonal behaviors and professional conduct.

The Supervisor's Responsibilities

The supervisor is ultimately responsible for the actions of the supervisee while formally engaged in the supervisory relationship (Wheeler & Bertram, 2015). There are occasions, however, when a supervisor

Table 7.2 • Components of a Supervision Contract

Supervisory Topic	*Component*
Supervisor's background	Academic degrees Certifications Clinical specialties Qualifications for being a supervisor Supervision style Theoretical orientation of psychotherapy and supervision
Supervisory methods	Review audiotapes or videotapes, observe counseling sessions, evaluate clinical records and reports, conduct cotherapy, do site visits, require supervisees to submit an ongoing list of clients
Supervisor's responsibilities and requirements	Legally responsible for supervisee's work Delicate balance of clinical collaborator vs. responsibility as evaluator and gatekeeper If limited, state which services supervisor is overseeing interdisciplinary supervision recommendations Under what circumstances do supervisees seek immediate assistance?
Organizational information	Day, time, and place of weekly supervision Process for rescheduling if needed How to contact supervisor Name and contact information for alternative supervisor if unavailable during emergency Mental health emergency procedures (e.g., client with suicidal/homicidal ideation, suspected abuse)
Supervisee's responsibilities	Meet requirements established by employer/training program, relevant ethics codes, rules and laws, and supervisor May attach or reference job responsibilities Review documents and policies governing trainees (e.g., codes of ethics, organizational policies) Inform supervisor of agreed-upon clinical, personal and/or professional issues in a timely manner
Agency protocols	Any applicable protocols prescribed specifically by the employing agency (e.g., legal or ethical concerns, abuse reporting, threat of harm to self or others, cautionary treatment directives for clients within high risk categories, record keeping)
Potential supplemental requirements	Possible medical or psychological assessments that may be required if deemed necessary
Confidentiality policies	May depend on: State and provincial law; policies of the academic program, training site, or employer; relevant professional ethics codes; specific policies established by the supervisor Circumstances in which the supervisor is obligated to breach confidentiality Who will have access to supervisee's information? Faculty consultation policies (if applicable) Special limitations to privacy (e.g. online supervision)

(Continued)

Table 7.2 • Components of a Supervision Contract *(Continued)*

Supervisory Topic	*Component*
Documentation of supervision	What types of records will be kept regarding supervision? May include: Forms for recording narrative descriptions of supervision meetings, hours logs, meeting dates, evaluation forms, etc. How documentation may be accessed and by whom Length of time documentation will be maintained Methods for securing documentation
Financial policies	Clarify all financial obligations from the beginning (if applicable) Cancellation policy for supervision meetings
Risks and benefits	Examples of potential risks include: emotional discomfort of being scrutinized, disclosures may appear in a performance evaluation or be communicated to program faculty, and may need to report unethical conduct to an outside authority Examples of potential benefits include increase supervisee's understanding of self and enhance clinical effectiveness, and helps to guard against ethical and legal errors
Evaluation	Explain potential evaluation methods (e.g., oral, written form, narrative, self-evaluation) Describe particular skills and responsibilities that will be evaluated Include copies of forms when possible Give a schedule for evaluation and feedback
Complaint procedures and due process	How might the supervisee address dissatisfaction with the supervisor during session? What formal and/or informal avenues will the supervisor provide to assess the supervisee's ongoing satisfaction with supervision services? Who can the supervisee contact if he or she does not feel safe discussing the issues directly with the supervisor? Describe due process procedures (may also reference a student handbook or organization's policy manual)
Professional development goals	Specific learning goals the supervisee may have above and beyond general professional development This may be included in the contract or detailed separately
Endorsement	Verification of hours worked and time spent in supervision Potential methods for expressing concerns about supervisee's ability to competently perform professional functions
Duration and termination of the supervision contract	Define adequate notice of termination by either party Examples of reasons supervision may be prematurely terminated May include a probationary period with the option to extend

Note. Data from National Association of Social Workers & Association of Social Work Boards, 2013; Thomas, 2007; Wheeler & Bertram, 2015.

is only contracted to oversee specific types of services (e.g., play therapy, psychological testing, a specific group of clients seen by the supervisee). J. T. Thomas (2007) recommended that when this is the case, the distinction be clearly stated in the supervision contract in order to clarify liability. The supervisor will also want to explain the balance that will be necessary between being a clinical collaborator in the areas of supervision and serving as evaluator and gatekeeper.

Best Practice Standards in Social Work Supervision (NASW & Association of Social Work Boards, 2013) highlights the possibility of interdisciplinary supervision in which the supervisor identifies with a particular mental health field (e.g., social work) and the supervisee belongs to another area (e.g., clinical mental health counseling). Although most of the time interdisciplinary supervision will address practice issues that are shared among the mental health fields, NASW suggests that supervisors have a responsibility to recognize their limitations and "refer that supervisee to a member of her or his own profession for practice-specific supervision or consultation" (p. 11) when appropriate. When entering into interdisciplinary supervision, addressing this possibility in writing from the beginning can allow the supervisee to identify another professional who can be used as a consultant in advance of the need. This may also prompt a valuable discussion about the particular differences between the two fields.

It is the supervisor's responsibility to communicate how and under what conditions a supervisee is expected to seek immediate assistance or consultation. Although the supervision contract may not contain an exhaustive list, providing broad categories as examples can help a supervisee decide whether it is appropriate to disturb the supervisor outside of normal business hours. J. T. Thomas (2007) offered the following list of possible situations in which a supervisor may wish to be consulted immediately:

- Disputes with clients or impasses in the therapy;
- Allegations of unethical behavior by clients, colleagues, or others (e.g., a client's family members);
- Threats of a complaint or lawsuit;
- Mental health emergencies requiring immediate action;
- High-risk situations; cases in which clients evidence suicidal thoughts, gestures, or attempts or a significant history of attempts; or cases in which clients present with a history of, propensity for, or threats of violence;
- Contemplated departures from standards of practice or exceptions to general rules, standards, policies, or practices;
- Suspected or known clinical or ethical errors and related countertransference;
- Contact with clients outside the context of treatment;
- Legal issues, such as possible reporting obligations related to suspected abuse of a child or vulnerable adult or ethical violations by other professionals. (p. 227)

Furthermore, it is essential that the supervisee be given the contact information for an appropriately trained colleague or two as substitute consultants when the supervisor is not available.

Continuing the Supervisory Relationship

Postdegree supervisors are expected to conduct ongoing evaluation of their trainees and incorporate relevant portions of behavioral expectations into their assessment documentation. J. T. Thomas (2007) highlighted the valuable point that some supervisee problems are rarely evident in the beginning but may develop over the course of supervision despite intentional screening efforts. A supervisee may have difficulty managing stress or may begin to experience symptoms of vicarious trauma as he or she begins to build a larger caseload of clients. Perhaps it comes to the supervisor's attention over the course of time that the supervisee appears to be under the influence of substances while in supervision. In any of these cases, given that the responsible supervisor avoids acting as the supervisee's personal counselor, it may be warranted to refer the supervisee for personal counseling services and/or evaluation. For example, a trainee began demonstrating poor coping skills and mental health issues as she was faced with an unwanted divorce in her personal life. She reported high levels of anxiety and sadness, panic attacks, difficulty sleeping, and an inability to focus on clients during sessions. Although the supervisor initially attempted to focus on coping skills and methods that would help the supervisee center herself prior to and during clinical sessions with clients, it became evident that she needed more intensive personal therapy. The supervisor decided that the supervisee would, among other interventions, be required to attend personal counseling. After consultation with her administrative supervisor at her site of employment, it was also determined to be in the best interest of her clients that the supervisee take a leave of absence while she learned to process and cope with her changing family dynamics. This was of course very impactful for the supervisee in that it also pushed back her date of licensure. When the possibility of referral to a personal counselor or other adjunctive services is made known to supervisees from the very beginning and stated in the supervisory contract, the potential for conflict is reduced (J. T. Thomas, 2007).

Aside from personal issues, the supervisor may find that the supervisee lacks necessary skills or demonstrates shortcomings in ethical judgment and might decide to refer the supervisee for remedial training. This may include a workshop or course in ethics or a conference specifically focused on implementing a particular theoretical orientation with a population of clients, among many other alternatives. Most of the services or evaluations that a supervisor may require are not available free of charge. Consequently, it is recommended that faculty and professional supervisors include the possibility of referral for further training in their supervision contracts and also clarify that any associated financial burden will be the supervisee's responsibility.

Carefully presented, this type of intervention with a postdegree supervisee would receive a successful response; however, the supervisee might simply choose to terminate the supervisory relationship and locate a new supervisor. If this occurs, the supervisor, as a legally identified gatekeeper of the postdegree training process, is challenged to act responsibly. This may include notifying the supervisee in writing of the observed behaviors, standards violations, and concerns about continuing with clinical practice without rectifying the problematic situations; refusing to sign a letter or form of endorsement for licensure for the hours completed by the supervisee while under the supervisor's oversight and informing the supervisee of bases for this decision; notifying the subsequent supervisor of concerns about the supervisee's clinical performance and professional conduct; and/or notifying the state licensure board about the actions of the supervisee and the supervisor's concerns about the supervisee as a future clinician. All of these actions should be documented in writing and include the supervisee in the notification process. Moreover, listing these potential reporting actions in the supervision contract from the beginning enhances the presence of due process.

Confidentiality Policies

Similar to clients, supervisees are entitled to their right to confidentiality with some exceptions (American Association for Marriage and Family Therapy, 2014; American Psychological Association, 2014; Association for Counselor Education and Supervision, 2011; Association of State and Provincial Psychology Boards, 2015; NASW & Association of Social Work Boards, 2013; National Board for Certified Counselors, 2016). The same exceptions that apply to clients also pertain to supervisees (e.g., suspected abuse of a minor or vulnerable adult, suicidal or homicidal intent, court order); however, other potential limitations are specific to the supervisory relationship. These limits to privacy may be "dependent on variables including state or provincial law; policies of the academic program, training site, or employer; relevant professional ethics codes; and the specific policies established by the supervisor" (J. T. Thomas, 2007, p. 227). In the supervision contract, it is critical to include the known limits to confidentiality and any foreseeable ways in which information derived during supervision may be used and/or shared with others. For example, a supervisor may discover the need to report a supervisee's unethical behavior to an outside authority in some extreme cases, as described previously. In addition, when multiple supervisors are involved with a supervisee, coordination of services will likely prove beneficial to the supervisee's development. This is understandably the case in predegree supervision when there is a faculty and a site clinical supervisor; however, this also may apply when supervisees contract for postdegree supervision outside of their organizations of employment. In either of these instances, supervisors are wise to detail the consultation schedule they expect to have with other supervisors and the types of information that may be shared between them. Once agreed on, "disclosures of information beyond those outlined in the initial informed consent require the supervisee's authorization" (p. 228).

Concluding the Supervisory Obligation

All supervisees initially enter into the supervisory relationship with the ultimate expectation that their supervisor will endorse them at the end of the supervision period. After all, this is the reason mental health trainees undergo supervision: to further develop their skills and clinical abilities as they complete another step in training and progress toward greater independence and freedom as a helper. The ultimate goal of years of supervision is to develop a trainee's ability to self-supervise as an autonomous professional. Most of the time, supervisors are able to confidently provide verification of completion of supervisory requirements of the state or jurisdiction governing postgraduate experience and to endorse the supervisee as ready for licensure, certification, or the next step in training. However, despite the supervisor's best efforts to remediate issues, in some instances, the supervisee may not be deemed professionally competent by the end of the requisite supervision period.

> Therefore, supervisors may want to address this possibility in a supervision contract. Stating what they will do if they become concerned about the individual's professional functioning and obtaining the supervisee's agreement to participate in supervision with this understanding will prepare the supervisee and may offer some legal protection for the supervisor should the supervisee later object. Supervisors may indicate, for example, that they will certainly verify that the supervisee participated in the supervision and the hours worked but that if concerns persist, they will also attach a letter describing those concerns. (J. T. Thomas, 2007, p. 229)

The *ACA Code of Ethics* (ACA, 2014a) speaks directly to supervisee endorsement by asserting that "regardless of qualifications, supervisors do not endorse supervisees whom they believe to be impaired in any way that would interfere with the performance of the duties associated with the endorsement" (Standard F.6.d.). Consequently, supervisors should provide in advance examples of situations in which they would refuse to endorse a supervisee. In her study, C. M. Miller (2010) found that more than 28% of the postdegree counseling supervisors she surveyed had refused to endorse at least one supervisee for licensure in the past. The reasons provided for refusal included ethical concerns (e.g., boundary concerns, dishonesty), impairment (e.g., troubling personal characteristics, lack of professionalism), skills deficits, commitment and motivation concerns, and noncompliance with supervisory recommendations. Consistent with due process, the trainee should be well aware of the supervisor's concerns prior to having endorsement withheld. It is important that the supervisee understand and agree from the outset of the supervisory relationship to the potential consequences of impairment or the inability to remediate concerns.

Either party may terminate the supervision contract prematurely and for a variety of reasons. Because there are often consequences to early termination, the *ACA Code of Ethics* (ACA, 2014a) dictates that both supervisees and supervisors provide "adequate notice" (Standard F.4.d.) in advance of ending the supervisory relationship. The *Code* further states that "reasons for considering termination are discussed, and both parties work to resolve differences" (Standard F.4.d.). Supervisees will be unable to provide counseling services to their clients until a new supervisor is secured, so some supervisors attempt to give 2 weeks' notice when possible. Although some causes of early termination may be unpredictable (e.g., serious health complications), in the written contract, the supervisor has an opportunity to outline categories of supervisee behavior that will likely result in early termination. Some examples that could be given include (a) noncompliance with supervisory recommendations, (b) an inability to remediate problematic behaviors within a reasonable period of time, (c) severe skill and conceptualization deficits, and (d) legal or ethics violations.

Conclusion

From the very beginning, each stage of the training process provides a variety of avenues to clearly and repeatedly communicate standards and policies to trainees. Spelling out these requirements and offering periodic reminders supports the trainee's right to make informed decisions and protects the training program or supervisor by ensuring due process. Taking the time to create comprehensive contracts for postgraduate supervision serves to prevent future conflicts between the expectations of the trainee and the supervisor. Although supervisors with well-defined contracts may still, on occasion, encounter trainees who do not perform to predetermined standards, selecting the follow-up course of action is made easier by knowing that potential avenues were clearly stated from the beginning and agreed to by all parties.

Key Points and Best Practices

- The importance of clearly informing students and postgraduate supervisees of the policies and standards that define the expectations for their personal and professional conduct cannot be overemphasized. Furthermore, there are numerous locations in which supervisors can publish these standards and policies in order to make them widely available to potential and current trainees.
- The supervisory contract serves as the comprehensive informed consent document between a postgraduate supervisee and his or her supervisor.

- The primary professional organizations that dictate the ethical behavior of mental health supervisors contribute valuable elements for consideration when creating the supervisory contract.
- Among other tasks, comprehensive supervisory contracts serve to reduce misunderstandings in cases such as the need for significant remediation, ultimate termination of a contract, or refusal to endorse the trainee for licensure.

Chapter 8

Standards for Personal Behavior and Professional Conduct

Kathryn L. Henderson

When initiating a professional relationship with a trainee, a general expectation of clinical educators and supervisors is the trainee's successful completion of training requirements, be it graduation or endorsement for licensure or certification (Bernard & Goodyear, 2014). However, not all trainees progress smoothly through their journey with success; some will experience challenges in demonstrating competence in the behaviors necessary and integral to the role of becoming a clinician. As gatekeepers, faculty and supervisors are responsible for recognizing these behaviors and evaluating all trainees for competency to demonstrate the behaviors necessary to enter the profession.

Although traditional academic achievement and clinical counseling microskills and techniques have been defined to assess student performance (Ivey, Ivey, & Zalaquett, 2014; Young, 2017), defining personal and professional behaviors integral to the role of the clinician is a topic more vast and varied. Although progress is under way within the clinical fields to define the behavioral competencies necessary to be a mental health professional (Duba, Paez, & Kindsvatter, 2010; Henderson & Dufrene, 2013; Homrich, DeLorenzi, Bloom, & Godbee, 2014), a need still exists for empirical research to elucidate and clarify this vital topic.

This chapter focuses on the personal and professional behavioral competencies at the heart of gatekeeping and remediation. Conceptual literature and existing empirical research will be reviewed with accompanying philosophical and ethical considerations to guide practice. Personal and professional behaviors are discussed that scholars have suggested as professional competencies for students to demonstrate. As faculty members and supervisors seek to define their own standards or expectations of students, this chapter may serve as a resource that reviews the breadth of the literature. The chapter also may be helpful when educating other colleagues or shareholders within an agency or a university setting, such as risk management, human resources, or legal affairs, about the behavioral expectations of the clinical mental health field and how they may differ from those of other disciplines.

Literature Across Clinical Professions

When seeking guidance on defining behavioral competencies from official or widely accepted sources, the main resources tapped are professional codes of ethics and accreditation standards. Although these resources address the necessity of evaluating trainees' personal and professional competence, they do not provide definitions or descriptions of what constitutes competence. Instead, these resources broadly address "an individual's overall capability or demonstrated ability to perform as a professional [clinician], whereas competencies refer to components of performance" (Kaslow et al., 2004, p. 708). For example, the Council for Accreditation of Counseling and Related Educational Programs (CACREP; 2015) instructs faculty in its 2016 accreditation standards to establish an assessment process that includes the "identification of key professional dispositions" (p. 18) that will be used to evaluate students. Faculty are then expected to use the data obtained from this assessment process in the remediation and dismissal of students. Part of the challenge in defining these professional dispositions or competencies is the inconsistency inherent in the scenario: Because CACREP leaves defining these competencies to training programs, many different programs have created their own distinctive standards, and hence, a universally accepted set of explicit competencies does not exist (Henderson & Dufrene, 2012; Homrich, 2009; Jacobs et al., 2011; Trimble, Stroebel, Krieg, & Rubenstein, 2012).

The inconsistency inherent in the dialogue on professional dispositions contributes to the challenges faculty and supervisors face when developing gatekeeping policies and behavioral expectations for students. (See What Would You Do? 8.1.) Quite simply, there are many dispositions and behaviors to consider for inclusion as expectations for trainees with very little empirical research. This challenge is unique, given that traditional counseling microskills and techniques (e.g., using open vs. closed questions; reflecting content, feelings, and meaning) have been identified, are widely accepted, are taught in training programs (Ivey et al., 2014; Young, 2017), and are subsequently evaluated to determine minimal mastery (Swank, Lambie, & Witta,

What Would You Do? 8.1

A dilemma of professional conduct related to social media occurred when a student, Aaron, posted on Facebook his recent low grade on an assignment from a certain course. The student complained at length about the grade as unfair and unreasonable, especially because he had made up the volunteer practice client persona he had utilized for the assignment, noting that the professor had not figured out that the client was not real. This student had friended other students from the counseling program, who viewed this post. Several students were upset by both the unprofessional behavior displayed toward a faculty member as well as the apparent academic dishonesty of inventing a client rather than securing an individual volunteer to serve as a practice client per the assignment guidelines. One student who saw the online post decided to report this incident to the faculty member who taught the course. When the concerned student went to print Aaron's post, the post was gone and had been removed. The student proceeded with reporting the incident anyway. After the meeting, the faculty member met with Aaron, who admitted to the wrongdoing and expressed understanding of his actions as a violation of the university's academic honor code. The faculty created a remediation plan focused on behavioral competencies of conflict resolution, ethical decision making, and appropriate communication of emotions. Faculty consulted with their administration regarding the academic dishonesty violation and their concern over pursuing remediation while at the same time filing a formal violation of academic honesty with the Office of Student Affairs.

McAdams et al. (2007) shared the challenges that arose in their experience in this case when simultaneously pursuing both avenues—the Academic Honor Council within the Office of Student Affairs and remediation within the department according to professional standards—involving different policies and campus offices. The Office of Student Affairs agreed to document the academic honesty violation and not pursue its policy in lieu of the remediation plan, with the agreement of all involved parties.

What would you do?

What is your perspective on pursuing both violation of academic honesty through student affairs and formal remediation within the program?

If you needed to find out who to consult with at your institution to determine an answer, do you know which person or office that would be?

Discuss Aaron's use of social media to complain about his experience in a faculty member's course. What specific personal and professional competencies might be tied to his choices?

Consider the same scenario but with a different response from Aaron: What if he denied any wrongdoing?

At this point, it would be his word against the other student's.

What would be your response as the faculty member?

2012). In addition, research on the common factors of counseling that correlate with positive client outcomes has established the efficacy of what are regarded as the *core conditions:* warmth, empathy, and the therapeutic relationship (Lambert & Barley, 2001). The personhood of the therapist is at the foundation of facilitating the core conditions (D. J. Martin, Garske, & Davis, 2000; Procidano, Busch-Rossnagel, Reznikoff, & Geisinger, 1995; Shirk & Karver, 2003), which speaks to the central importance of personal characteristics that are conducive to the therapeutic role. However, defining which personal and professional characteristics are fundamental to the ability to facilitate the core conditions remains unfinished. Concurrently, no cohesive body of empirical research establishes the specific personal and professional qualities a clinician must have to function effectively as a professional. Even ethics codes and professional standards are assumed knowledge, not supported by research.

In general, scholars across the mental health disciplines have primarily considered personal and professional behaviors from the lens of dismissals (Busseri, Tyler, & King, 2005; Fly, van Bark, Weinman, Kitchener, & Lang, 1997; Huprich & Rudd, 2004; Li, Trusty, Lampe, & Lin, 2008; Mearns & Allen, 1991; Olkin & Gaughen, 1991; Rosenberg, Getzelman, Arcinue, & Oren, 2005; Vacha-Haase, Davenport, & Kerewsky, 2004). The lens of dismissals is important because it affects the language used to describe the behaviors: as negative inabilities not demonstrated by trainees or competencies that have not been met, rather than as neutral or positive expectations for trainees to demonstrate. The importance and nuance of language is explored further in this chapter. For a detailed review of behavioral reasons for student dismissals, refer to Chapter 9.

Considerations When Constructing Competencies

As faculty and supervisors develop the behavioral competencies to be expected of their trainees, several factors bear consideration. These competencies will be at the center of the program's gatekeeping policies and procedures; the same competencies stated in program policies should be consistent with the assessment instruments selected for trainee evaluation and be the anticipated focus of remediation plans (Gilfoyle, 2008). The ever-present consideration of due process must also be taken into account, as students need to be aware in advance of the behavioral competencies on which they will be evaluated (McAdams, Foster, & Ward, 2007). Thus, these behaviors will be part of student handbooks, websites, and orientations and referenced in syllabi. Thus, the identification and selection of competencies is a serious endeavor that has far-reaching implications for institutions, programs, agencies, gatekeepers, and the students and supervisees of which these behaviors are expected. (See What Would You Do? 8.2.)

Protecting the best interests of several different constituencies is also a consideration when constructing behavioral competencies. These

What Would You Do? 8.2

The week before graduation, a faculty member received an e-mail from a student in her course that contained a forwarded message. The forwarded message was from a fellow student, Sheila, and was e-mailed to all students in the graduate program. The message contained photos taken by Sheila using her cell phone to record the final exam, which was proctored in a computer lab on campus. In the forwarded message Sheila wrote that this was her parting gift to her fellow students, as she was due to graduate the next week. Faculty members consulted with university stakeholders regarding the scenario and their options. Despite this egregious violation of academic honesty, Sheila had earned strong grades and had no previous incidents of problematic behavior. She was viewed by the faculty as a "great student." The final decision was to allow Sheila to graduate, with the faculty member of the course failing the student for the exam, resulting in an overall grade of C for the course. Faculty members in the program were given the discretion of whether to endorse Sheila for licensure or to provide letters of recommendation.

What would you do?

What is your reaction to the university's decision to allow the student to graduate without remediation?

What might the department/faculty do to prepare proactively for encountering a future incident such as this?

If you were a faculty member at this institution, what would you decide regarding endorsing Sheila for licensure or providing letters of recommendation?

groups can serve as guideposts as faculty reflect on which competencies they consider to be fundamental and necessary for trainees to possess in order to enter the profession. For instance, the following question may guide reflection: Does this behavioral competency protect the best interests of *current and future clients?* This question may be asked with consideration for each of the following constituencies:

- Current and future clients
- The student or supervisee
- Other trainees (i.e., the potential effect on other students)
- The reputation of the profession and professional standards
- Faculty and supervisor decision making (an example of one consideration is whether defining a competency [e.g., receptivity to feedback] will decrease the subjectivity that might otherwise interfere with evaluating trainee competence, as how one evaluator might approach operationalizing that competency could be different from how another evaluator might do so without a concrete and specific definition)
- The reputation of the program for producing competent clinicians

How each affected constituency is impacted by a trainee's behavioral competence rests at the foundation of the behaviors selected for policies. The behavioral competencies included in policies set a standard for which trainees will be held accountable, not only as skilled clinicians but also on personal and professional characteristics inherent to being successful as mental health professionals.

The Mechanics of Language

Constructing and defining standards for the personal and professional behavior of trainees requires reflecting on the mechanics of the language used to describe the behaviors. A key consideration is describing the behaviors as competencies to demonstrate rather than deficiencies to avoid. Competencies are established as characteristics, knowledge and skills, or abilities that trainees are capable of demonstrating (Homrich, 2009; Kaslow, 2004). The competencies should be measurable and observable and described in simple, clear language. A goal is to avoid vagueness, generalizations, and possible subjectivity in interpretation. The aim is for all individuals, when reading the competencies, to arrive at an objective understanding of the expectations associated with that specific behavioral competency. Actual implementation of competencies in the program or agency setting might reveal language used to describe the behavioral competencies that causes confusion, at which point the behavioral competencies should be revised as needed based on applied experience. It is important to note that faculty and supervisors are strongly recommended to obtain the review of their institution's legal, administrative, and/or risk management team prior to implementation. As discussed in Chapter 6, it is key that all stakeholders be in agreement about supporting behavioral standards in advance of launching the standards with trainees.

The flip side of the competency perspective is the perspective to avoid: that of diagnosis. Virtually all supervisors and educators in the mental health professions were initially trained as practitioners. That training and identity is at the core of faculty and supervisors who teach and supervise new professionals. However, the orientation to diagnosis must be set aside when assessing trainees' behaviors in the context of gatekeeping. Scholars caution faculty and supervisors to avoid the pitfalls and dual relationship of diagnosing trainees (Gilfoyle, 2008; Kaslow et al., 2007). Consider this rationale: Diagnosis seeks to understand the impetus for a behavior, to understand the reasons behind an individual's current lived experience and choices. However, in our role as gatekeepers, we are asked not to pinpoint the impetus for a behavior but instead to determine how that behavior is related to the professional competencies expected of all trainees. In essence, we are asked to turn off the skill that for many clinicians becomes ingrained and habitual over time: seeking to understand the basis for behavior. (See What Would You Do? 8.3.)That idea, after

What Would You Do? 8.3

Two master's students e-mailed their professor, who was also their advisor, requesting to meet about concerns related to another student, Heather. When the three met, the two students shared that they were upset with what had happened at a recent social event sponsored by the clinical program's student organization. The professor had not attended this event and asked them to review their concerns. The students shared that Heather, who was enrolled in a practicum with them, had talked at length about several clients by name with students who were in their second semester of the program and hence not enrolled in any clinical classes. Heather had left the social gathering early, and after her departure, the students with whom she had been talking began looking up the clients she had discussed on social media on their cell phones and passing the phones around for others to view the clients' social media pages. Doctoral students had also attended this event and seemed to be aware of what was transpiring. No one had intervened, and the two students expressed concern about the ethical implications of what had happened. The professor shared his concern with them and stated that he would need to consult with other faculty members. The two students asked to remain anonymous and to not have their names revealed. They worried that other students would view them as tattletales.

What would you do?

If you were the professor, how would you respond to the students' request to have their identities remain confidential?

What behaviors do you think need to be addressed with Heather? By whom?

What behaviors should be addressed with the second-year students who looked up the clients on social media?

Would you address the issues of concern with all students or only those involved?

Do you believe the doctoral students had a responsibility to act that was different from that of the master's students?

Who should address the concerns brought forth in this case?

How might identified issues be addressed with Heather, the second-year students, the doctoral students, and/or all students in the clinical training program?

How does the setting in which this incident occurred (an off-site party sponsored by the clinical student organization) impact your choices? Or does it?

all, is at the core of the work we do with clients as mental health professionals. However, supervisors and faculty members are not in the role of personal therapists. Ethically speaking, that role is separate and distinct and one that we are not permitted to adopt with trainees (American Counseling Association [ACA], 2014a). Our focus must remain instead on how trainees' behaviors impact their ability to successfully demonstrate the professional competencies or behaviors that are necessary to enter into the mental health professions.

Personal and Professional Behaviors as Professional Competencies

In addition to the gatekeeping literature, emerging empirical research has examined personal and professional behaviors from the perspective of competencies expected of students and remediation rather than deficiencies associated with dismissals. The results of three studies (Duba et al., 2010; Henderson & Dufrene, 2013; Homrich et al., 2014) are reviewed here for your consideration as helpful resources for developing your own behavioral standards for trainees. As discussed earlier, the evolving dialogue and terminology that are used to discuss this topic are varied; that variety is reflected in these studies and the language used to construct their samples and research questions. For detailed information, please refer to the full studies.

In their study, Duba et al. (2010) examined the "nonacademic" personal characteristics used by faculty members to assess graduate students. Henderson and Dufrene (2013) studied the perceptions of Association for Counselor Education and Supervision members and the behaviors they considered to most often need remediation with master's students. The work of Homrich et al. (2014), which identified and ranked standards of conduct in clinical training programs, is reviewed first as a contributor's perspective shared by one of the coauthors of the seminal research study and a chapter author of this book, Leigh D. DeLorenzi. DeLorenzi also reviews additional research that focuses on competency-based student dismissals in Chapter 9. In addition to the empirical research, the field of psychology has strived to define competencies for personal behavior and professional conduct, which are briefly reviewed here.

• Contributor's Perspective •

Proposed Standards of Conduct in Clinical Training

Leigh D. DeLorenzi

Based on a broad survey of constructs acquired from publications across the helping professions, Homrich et al. (2014) sought profession-wide consensus in determining a list of specific professional, interpersonal, and intrapersonal behaviors in defining the range of acceptable to unacceptable trainee functioning. The study, the only one to solicit input on proposed standards, surveyed 82 counselor educators from CACREP-accredited programs who had also served as supervisors, who rated the importance of behaviors expected of graduate students. Three categories defined in Chapter 2—professional, interpersonal, and intrapersonal behaviors—were arranged by participants in order of perceived significance and are presented here.

Professional Behaviors

The list of professional behaviors in Table 8.1 reflects those most commonly endorsed by counselor educators (Homrich et al., 2014, p. 132) as either important or extremely important (i.e., a mean score falling between 4.5 and 5.29), as Items 1–8 show. Items that fell between neutral and somewhat important for this category (i.e., a mean score falling between 4.0 and 4.49) were Items 9–11. All items were framed positively and prefaced with "Graduate students in counseling are expected to. . . ."

Interpersonal Behaviors

The list of interpersonal behaviors in Table 8.2 reflects those most commonly endorsed by counselor educators (Homrich et al., 2014, p. 133) as either important or extremely important (i.e., a mean score falling between 4.5 and 5.21), displayed as Items 1–6. Items that fell between neutral and somewhat important for this category (i.e., a mean score falling between 4.0 and 4.49) were Items 7–9.

Intrapersonal Behaviors

The list of intrapersonal behaviors in Table 8.3 reflects those most commonly endorsed by counselor educators (Homrich et al., 2014, p. 134) as either important or extremely important (i.e., a mean score falling between 4.5 and 5.22), shown as Items 1–4. Items that fell between neutral and somewhat important for this

Table 8.1 • Professional Behaviors Expected of Graduate Students

Rank and Item	*M*
1. Respect the privacy and confidentiality needs of others.	5.29
2. Understand and maintain the ethical guidelines for counselors as published by the profession.	4.98
3. Engage actively in learning, training, and/or experiential processes and opportunities for personal and professional development.	4.78
4. Prioritize interests of clients over self-interests when providing professional services.	4.76
5. Remain open to ideas, learning, and change.	4.55
6. Fulfill obligations promptly, consistently, reliably, and according to expectations stated by professor or supervisor.	4.55
7. Cooperate with remediation plans and endeavor to adjust or improve behavior.	4.55
8. Engage in productive supervision and consultation with colleagues and peers.	4.52
9. Maintain sensitivity to role differences and power dynamics that may exist in relationships and settings, and manage them appropriately.	4.24
10. Follow the procedures and policies of the graduate program.	4.16
11. Seek professional consultation with regard to recognized personal areas of growth.	4.15

Table 8.2 • Interpersonal Behaviors Expected of Graduate Students

Rank and Item	*M*
1. Respect the autonomy and beliefs of others and refrain from imposing one's personal beliefs on others.	5.21
2. Exhibit sensitivity to the individual and cultural identities of others and display cultural competence by acting respectfully and skillfully in interactions with others.	4.89
3. Communicate with clients and colleagues respectfully and professionally using appropriate verbal and non-verbal language.	4.67
4. Exhibit awareness of and respect for appropriate interpersonal boundaries.	4.62
5. Establish and maintain effective and functional relationships personally, professionally, and therapeutically.	4.58
6. Demonstrate genuineness, empathy, and interest in the welfare of others.	4.53
7. Act with awareness of how personal actions impact others.	4.41
8. Display sensitivity to the feelings, thoughts, and needs of others.	4.32
9. Behave with professionalism appropriate to the situation or setting.	4.02

category (i.e., a mean score falling between 4.0 and 4.49) were Items 5–10.

The purpose of this study was to obtain profession-wide input from faculty and supervisors in the mental health counseling profession about expectations for trainees. The identification and ranking of the standards offers a starting point for programs to formulate their own standards of conduct.

• • •

In related research, Duba et al. (2010) studied the nonacademic criteria used by community counseling programs to assess and retain master's students. The work of Duba and colleagues was conducted before implementation of the 2016 CACREP Standards for counselor education programs, which are reflected in the language of community counseling students. Under the current 2016 CACREP Standards (CACREP, 2015), the community counseling and clinical mental health

Table 8.3 • Intrapersonal Behaviors Expected of Graduate Students

Rank and Item	*M*
1. Exhibit awareness of personal beliefs, values, needs, strengths, and limitations, and understand their potential influence on personal and professional performance.	5.22
2. Accept responsibility for actions and problems.	4.88
3. Manage personal mental health, emotional problems, stress, and/or interpersonal issues effectively.	4.86
4. Demonstrate personal and professional integrity in stated thoughts and actions.	4.52
5. Maintain openness to and respect for differences in ideology.	4.46
6. Communicate information truthfully and accurately.	4.40
7. Participate in self-reflection and self-exploration.	4.36
8. Exhibit maturity and professionalism in reactions and behaviors.	4.32
9. Refrain from allowing use of behavior- or mind-altering substances to impede professional functioning.	4.25
10. Solicit, consider, and respond thoughtfully to constructive feedback from others.	4.07

counseling tracks were combined into one, henceforth called *clinical mental health counseling*. Also, as examined in earlier chapters, the term *nonacademic* has since fallen out of favor because of the inaccurate connotation that these behaviors are not considered expectations necessary to complete degree requirements. Professional conduct and appropriate behavior are components for degree completion and considered part of the academic requirements. In their study, Duba et al. conducted phone interviews with 30 faculty members from CACREP-accredited community counseling programs who were randomly selected from a national sample. Participants were asked to share how their programs evaluated students on five elements of the 2001 CACREP Standards retention policy: (a) individual interpersonal relationships, (b) interpersonal relationships in small groups, (c) openness to self-examination, (d) personal development, and (e) professional development (Duba et al., 2010, p. 156).

Across the five CACREP elements, three themes resulted: "Interpersonal interactions in academic and professional settings; Personality; and Professionalism (behaviors, skills, and knowledge)" (Duba et al., 2010, p. 157). Examples of specific criteria for the first theme of interpersonal interactions for each of the five CACREP elements are summarized in Table 8.4. Table 8.5 summarizes examples for the second

Table 8.4 • Summary of Examples and Results for Theme 1

Example	*Result*
Individual interpersonal relationships	Collaborates Assertive, respectful, and ethical Willing to work with diverse cultures
Interpersonal relationships in small groups	Assertive but cooperative Aware of personal boundaries Accepts and provides respectful feedback Contributes to safe environment Willing to work with diverse cultures
Openness to self-examination	Receptive to feedback Uses feedback Reflects and responds appropriately to material from class Aware of impact on others Demonstrates interpersonal skills
Personal development	Works well with others Nondisruptive and respectful
Professional development	Academic performance in courses, motivation Progresses in therapeutic behavior and conceptualization Follows the *ACA Code of Ethics* Aware of diversity issues Knows theories of change, basic microskills, and treatment planning Demonstrates leadership and professional advocacy

Note. From Duba et al., 2010. Theme 1 = interpersonal interactions in academic and professional settings.

Table 8.5 • Summary of Examples and Results for Theme 2

Example	*Result*
Individual interpersonal relationships	Is flexible, caring, and uncritical Open to new ideas and self-examination Exhibits balance in personal and professional life Aware of personal strengths and weaknesses
Interpersonal relationships in small-groups	Manages conflict Open to feedback Open to personal development Exhibits helpfulness
Openness to self-examination	Able to self-reflect Aware of personal values and issues Not addicted to substances Aware of personal strengths and limitations
Personal development	Aware of unhealthy relationships Takes risks and develops cognitive and social skills Maintains personal and professional balance Aware of personal strengths and weaknesses
Professional development	None

Note. From Duba et al., 2010. Theme 2 = personality.

theme of personality, and Table 8.6 offers examples for the third theme of professionalism.

Note that some behaviors are repeated in each of the three themes. This suggests that the scholars achieved saturation in the data sample as well as suggests the possibility of the universality of that particular behavior.

Table 8.6 • Summary of Examples and Results for Theme 3

Example	*Result*
Individual interpersonal relationships	Follows ethical codes Accepts and receives feedback Identifies personal challenges that affect abilities Establishes rapport with clients
Interpersonal relationships in small-groups	Open and respectful Follows ethical codes Uses feedback and shows improvement in group skills
Openness to self-examination	Accepts realistic expectations of client change Seeks assistance from supervisors Is self-confident in ability Understands role of obstacles in counseling
Personal development	On time and attends all classes Completes assignments on time Is self-assured in skills Is professionally involved Consults with faculty when needed
Professional development	None

Note. From Duba et al., 2010. Theme 3 = professionalism (behaviors, skills, and knowledge).

The final study (Henderson & Dufrene, 2013) was grounded in the perspective of remediation, which can be part of the gatekeeping process. These behaviors regarded as most often needing remediation may be included as competencies prior to the onset of observed problems. Members of the Association for Counselor Education and Supervision, a division of ACA, were surveyed and asked to rank which behaviors out of 34 they found most often in need of remediation with counseling students. The 34 behaviors were compiled following an exhaustive review of the literature on gatekeeping and related topics in the mental health professions. Participants (n = 607) ranked five behaviors as most often needing remediation: receptivity to feedback; basic counseling skills; boundaries with clients, supervisors, and/or colleagues; openness to self-examination; and advanced counseling skills (Henderson & Dufrene, 2013). Participants were also asked to rate the behaviors that they thought could be remediated on a Likert-type scale. A factor analysis conducted on the Likert-type ratings resulted in five distinct factors among the behaviors: Personal Competencies, Professionalism, Personal Challenges, Honesty, and Clinical Competencies (Henderson & Dufrene, 2013). The following list illustrates onto which factor each of the 34 specific behaviors loaded. One behavior, academic performance, did not load onto a factor.

Factor 1: Personal Competencies

- Receptivity to feedback
- Integrating feedback
- Ability to deal with conflict
- Maturity
- Flexibility
- Cooperativeness
- Interpersonal skills
- Ability to express feelings
- Awareness of impact on others
- Acceptance of personal responsibility
- Expression of empathy
- Openness to self-examination
- Capacity to handle stress

Factor 2: Professionalism

- Boundaries with clients, supervisors, and/or colleagues
- Confidentiality
- Representation of credentials
- Professional responsibility
- Procedural compliance
- Consultation with other professionals
- Documentation and paperwork compliance

Factor 3: Personal Challenges

- Substance abuse
- Symptoms of a personality disorder
- Symptoms of anxiety
- Symptoms of depression
- Symptoms of another mental health disorder partner relationship concerns
- Financial concerns
- Physical illness

Factor 4: Honesty

- Academic honesty
- Ethical behavior
- Integrity

Factor 5: Clinical Competencies

- Basic counseling skills
- Advanced counseling skills
- Multicultural competence

The three research studies summarized here offer a broad review of behaviors for faculty and supervisors to consider as standards for trainees. Commonalities clearly exist among the results of the studies and are apparent when the studies are considered together. Future research could compare the existing empirical research, such as through a meta-analysis, to offer a more refined set of behaviors for the field's consideration. These studies are distinct from others in that they focus on positive standards for students to demonstrate or remediate rather than a negative lens of student dismissals. When educators and supervisors are creating standards expected of all trainees in their department or agency, these studies may be helpful in identifying and narrowing down which behaviors are regarded as essential competencies for students or supervisees.

Within the field of psychology, a massive effort was undertaken to determine professional competencies considered foundational and fundamental to the role of psychologists (American Psychological Association [APA], 2006). A task force was established in APA on the assessment of competence in professional psychology. An overview of this undertaking is described in Chapter 1. Three broad domains of competencies emerged from these proceedings, one of which focused on personal behavior and professional conduct (APA, 2006; Fouad et al., 2009). Scholars have developed extensive tools for establishing benchmarks and ways of assessing competence within these domains (www.apa.org/ed/graduate/competency.aspx; APA, 2006; Fouad et al., 2009; Kaslow et al., 2009). A summary is provided here of the competencies that fall within the foundational domain, which comprises personal behavior and professional conduct. For a detailed analysis of the competencies with accompanying behavioral descriptions, please see Fouad et al. (2009).

- Professionalism (integrity/honesty, deportment, accountability, concern for the welfare of others, professional identity)
- Reflective practice/self-assessment/self-care (reflective practice, self-assessment, self-care)
- Relationships (interpersonal relationships, affective skills, expressive skills)
- Individual and cultural diversity (self and other as shaped by individual and cultural diversity, interaction of self and others as shaped by individual and cultural diversity, applications based on individual and cultural context)
- Ethical legal standards and policy (knowledge of ethical and legal standards, awareness and application of ethical decision making, ethical conduct)

Codes of Ethics as Guides for Standards

The research reviewed thus far in this chapter includes many behaviors that are addressed in codes of ethics that are expectations of trainees, such as professional boundaries with clients and confidentiality. Rather than review *in toto* all ethical behaviors, which are examined in detail in books and courses focused on ethical and legal issues, this section focuses on ethical behaviors that have been highlighted as emerging in the field or central to gatekeeping. For example, technology and social media are the focus of a new section in the most recent revision of the *ACA Code of Ethics* (ACA, 2014a). The 2014 *ACA Code of Ethics* also addresses ethical behaviors related to cultural competence, which were at the locus of two lawsuits brought against counselor education faculty. The two lawsuits are reviewed in On the Legal Side 8.1.

Cultural Competence as a Standard

Two court cases involving counselor education programs involved students who were dismissed because of challenges with cultural competence (see On the Legal Side 8.1 for a review of the lawsuits and suggested further reading). The 2005 version of the *ACA Code of Ethics* (ACA, 2005) was central to both lawsuits, as both counselor education programs sued were accredited by CACREP, and hence the programs and all of their students were required to follow the *Code*. The discourse involved in both lawsuits included rhetoric from opposing sides regarding their interpretation of the *Code* and the sections on cultural competence, "do no harm," and personal values, with interpretations of the *Code* as vastly different by the different parties. As a result of apparent gray area in the 2005 *Code* that resulted in multiple and opposing interpretations of the ethical expectations of all counselors, the ACA Ethics Revision Task Force focused on clarifying the language in the 2014 *Code*.

The current *ACA Code of Ethics* (ACA, 2014a) contains specific guidance on the intersection of cultural competence and ethical practice.

On the Legal Side 8.1

Two legal cases were brought against counselor education faculty in approximately the same timeframe in different regions of the United States. Both have been the subject of many scholarly articles and conference presentations. Although the overarching issues of these two court cases are similar—both involving master's students dismissed for lacking cultural competence with lesbian, gay, bisexual, transgender, queer, or questioning clients—the details of each case are quite different. As students of the law are aware, a court case dwells in the details. Thus, please refer to the recommendations for further reading at the end of this section for in-depth analysis and rendering of these complicated lawsuits.

Keeton v. Anderson-Wiley. J. Keeton was a master's student enrolled in the school counseling track at Augusta State University (now Augusta University; *Keeton v. Anderson-Wiley*, 2011). During her first year as a master's student, she expressed her personal beliefs founded in her religious identity regarding same-sex relationships as morally wrong both in the classroom and outside of class with other students and with faculty members. Keeton said that she would tell her future clients/students that same-sex relationships are wrong; help them change their "choice" to engage in same-sex relationships; and, if unsuccessful in changing them, refer them for reparative/conversion therapy to change their sexual orientation. Faculty informed Keeton that to do so would be to impose her personal values on clients, which is unethical according to the *ACA Code of Ethics* (ACA, 2005). Faculty engaged Keeton in a discussion about ethics and the need to leave personal values outside of the clinician's work with clients. Keeton claimed that she was told she would need to change her personal values, a statement that was later not upheld in testimony provided by school officials or in documentation. Keeton was offered the opportunity to complete a remediation plan prior to enrolling in her practicum to remediate her cultural competency with lesbian, gay, bisexual, transgender, queer, or questioning populations, which, if not completed, would have resulted in her dismissal from the program. Claiming that Augusta State University faculty members violated her free speech (including religious freedom), Keeton sued to prevent her dismissal from the program (with a separate preliminary injunction). The preliminary injunction was denied by the district court, the student appealed, and the appeals court upheld the decision of the lower court. Keeton's claims of violation of free speech were dismissed at the district court level in 2012 (Hutchens, Block, & Young, 2013).

Ward v. Wilbanks. At Eastern Michigan University, J. Ward was also a master's student on the school counseling track. In the process of completing her practicum, Ward was assigned a new client who identified as gay. Ward requested that her supervisor refer the client to a different counselor because the client's sexual orientation conflicted with Ward's personal values; if this was not possible, she stated that she would counsel the client on other topics and not on issues related to sexual orientation. Faculty members regarded her request as violating the *ACA Code of Ethics* and initiated their gatekeeping policy (Kaplan, 2014). According to their

(Continued)

On the Legal Side 8.1 *(Continued)*

policy, the student could choose between a remediation plan, voluntary withdrawal from the program, or a formal hearing. Ward chose to pursue a formal hearing with faculty, which examined the concerns brought against Ward and resulted in her dismissal from the program (Hutchens et al., 2013). Ward sued following her dismissal, claiming violation of her First Amendment rights. The district court found in favor of the university (*Ward v. Wilbanks*, 2010), and Ward appealed. The appellate court reversed the lower court's decision, which opened the avenue to continuing to pursue her complaint against Eastern Michigan University (*Ward v. Polite*, 2012). Rather than continue to engage in legal action, the parties settled (Kaplan, 2014).

For further reading, please see the following:

- Appellate court decision in *Keeton v. Anderson-Wiley: Keeton v. Anderson-Wiley* (2011)
- Appellate court decision in *Ward v. Polite: Ward v. Polite* (2012)
- Ethical implications of *Ward v. Wilbanks:* Kaplan (2014)
- Outcome implications from both lawsuits: Hutchens et al. (2013)

Although the necessity to be culturally competent is not new to this *Code* (it was infused throughout the 2005 *Code;* Remley & Herlihy, 2014), the 2014 *Code* expands the discussion of culture and diversity throughout the separate sections and for the first time includes culture in the preamble. The *Code* now defines clearly the values of the counseling profession, including promoting social justice and honoring diversity and multicultural approaches (Kaplan & Martz, 2014). The presence of the profession's values in the preamble is aimed at avoiding misinterpretations of the *Code* that isolate one standard in particular without also considering the full spirit of the *Code* (Kaplan & Martz, 2014). Another key revision centered on personal values. The mandate for counselors to avoid imposing their personal values on clients is not new; however, the 2014 *Code* clarifies that when a counselor encounters a values conflict with a client that centers on cultural issues, it is the counselor's responsibility to seek training to expand his or her cultural competence to avoid discriminatory practice or avoid imposing his or her values on the client (Martz & Kaplan, 2014). Hence, clinicians are required to be culturally competent and to seek "knowledge, personal awareness, sensitivity, dispositions, and skills pertinent to being a culturally competent counselor in working with a diverse client population" (ACA, 2014a, Standard C.2.a.; see also Hermann, Spurgeon, & Watts, 2014). This clarifies that counselors' personal values do not supersede their obligation to be culturally competent and that all counselors must extend the boundaries of their cultural competence when necessary (Hermann et al., 2014). The Ethics Revision Task Force furthermore articulated the role of personal values and referrals, stipulating that ethical referrals are made when the counselor lacks clinical competency rather than when he or she lacks cultural competency (Martz & Kaplan, 2014). The following list summarizes the key standards from the *ACA Code of Ethics* (ACA, 2014a) focused on cultural competence:

- *Preamble, p. 3:* Professional values of the counseling field, including diversity and social justice
- *Standard A.4.b.:* When a values conflict exists, the counselor must seek training on cultural issues
- *Standard B.2.b.:* Referral option included in the 2005 *Code* for end-of-life scenarios removed
- *Standard C.2.a.:* Requirement to be culturally competent
- *Standard C.5.:* Nondiscrimination expanded to include prospective clients
- *Standard C.7.c.:* Clarifies ethical treatment modalities and not using harmful practices, such as conversion/reparative therapy, even when requested
- *Standard E.5.b.:* Consider culture and diversity when conceptualizing and diagnosing clients
- *Standard F.2.b.:* Supervisors address diversity and culture in the supervisory relationship
- *Standard F.11.c.:* Counselor educators infuse culture into students' training

• Contributor's Perspective •

Ethical Use of Social Media as a Standard

Page L. Thanasiu

A thorough examination of the inherent legal and ethical concerns associated with incorporating expected standards for social media behavior is beyond the scope of this chapter; however, it should be addressed from the perspective of due process. If a department or supervisor decides to consider behavior directly or inadvertently discovered through social media or other online social networking sites in the evaluation process, prospective trainees must be clearly informed of this prior to beginning the program or supervisory relationship.

There is a compelling argument to be made that trainees "should understand that posting material online is akin to disclosing it in public" (Wester, Danforth, & Olle, 2013, p. 148) and that, given the ease of access to online information about individuals, the lines separating the personal and professional realms are becoming increasingly blurred. Training programs have encountered dilemmas such as students publicly posting information that (a) implicates them in illegal activities, (b) displays unprofessional behavior, (c) implies very poor coping skills and mental well-being, and (d) violates the confidentiality of a client or peer (Myers, Endres, Ruddy, & Zelikovsky, 2012; Pham, 2014; Wester et al., 2013). There is also the emerging boundary concern about trainees improperly using Internet searches and social media outlets to acquire information about or interact with clients. These concerns are addressed within new standards in the *ACA Code of Ethics* (ACA, 2014a) Section H: Distance Counseling, Technology, and Social Media but may not be included in the ethics codes of all mental health professions. Social media behavior and encounters may lead faculty to recommend creating pragmatic and transparent policies that allow departments and supervisors to take action when such situations arise and identify social media activity as part of the evaluation process for personal and professional conduct. (See On the Legal Side 8.2.)

Wester and colleagues (2013) and Pham (2014) provided valuable elements to consider when crafting standards and expectations for students and supervisees. For example, the emphasis should focus on behaviors that reflect the core competency of professionalism, and in keeping with due process, a trainee must have an opportunity to defend and contextualize any online content that the supervisor/program finds problematic. Wester and colleagues (2013) suggested specific wording for a policy that includes an introduction (which acts as the informed consent portion), an explanation of the reasonable right to privacy, evaluation criteria, and clarification of the evaluation process. Pham described a policy that focuses as well on using online information to evaluate trainees but also emphasizes instructing all trainees

On the Legal Side 8.2

Review the article by McAdams et al. (2007) that recounts the court case brought by a former student against The College of William and Mary for being dismissed from her counseling program. An additional resource is a podcast that can be accessed on CounselorAudioSource of a recorded interview with McAdams discussing the same court case (see www.counseloraudiosource.net/resources/CAS023.mp3).

1. Reflect on the behaviors displayed by the student that led to the faculty's intervention and eventual decision to dismiss.
2. As an exercise, list the behaviors and compare the behaviors to the assessment instrument used by your program or practice.
3. Are all of the behaviors included in your assessment instrument or not?
4. What behaviors do you believe should be identified as standards in a clinical training program?
5. What sources of information will you use to identify the behaviors?

in appropriate use of social media that promotes professionalism as demonstrated by Brew, Cervantes, and Shepard (2013). In addition to the categories outlined by Wester and colleagues (2013), Pham's proposed policy includes (a) appropriate professional online behavior, (b) technological competence and rules for online safety and protection, and (c) tips for responding to social networking requests from clients.

• • •

Conclusion

The subject of the personal behavior and professional conduct necessary for competent clinical practice is currently evolving. This important subject matter has been complicated by the lack of empirical research examining the topic, which is only now beginning to emerge from scholars across the mental health professions. Faculty members and supervisors are encouraged to consider best practice, ethics codes and professional standards, and literature from the joint mental health fields when developing their own standards for professional and personal behavior that will be codified in policies as formal expectations of trainees. Greater specificity and concrete description will aid both trainees in knowing expectations up front as well as faculty and supervisors in consistently assessing for competence in personal behavior and professional conduct.

Key Points and Best Practices

Best Practice Suggestions for Developing Standards

As reviewed here, identifying standards can leave room for subjectivity and individual interpretation, which can become very burdensome during a remediation or gatekeeping process. Trainees need to know specifically what is expected of them and how it will be measured by those assessing them—faculty, supervisors, academic programs, or field sites. Please refer to Chapter 9 for a thorough review of the factors to consider in assessment. In constructing standards for personal behavior and professional conduct, the following suggestions are offered:

- Consider relevant research and literature in the clinical professions, particularly accreditation standards and ethics codes, and be willing to consider the literature of related mental health professions.
- Draw from evidence-based practice wherever possible, realizing that research connecting specific, individual clinician qualities with therapeutic client outcomes is absent.
- Review (state) licensure regulations to identify any professional conduct or behavior expectations that should be reflected in training standards.

- Phrase from the perspective of the trainee ("Students will . . ." or "The supervisee is expected to . . .") versus listing behaviors.
- Describe standards in terms of behavior that is observable and measurable.
- Write behavioral standards in sentence constructions that use positive, active voice (such as "Demonstrate receptivity to feedback") rather than negative or passive voice.
- Link behavioral standards directly to the assessment instruments used to evaluate trainees, and define parameters for acceptable and unacceptable demonstration of each behavior.
- Define each standard with enough specificity to reduce subjectivity or variability in interpretation. For examples, refer to Chapter 9 or the counselor education websites of The College of William and Mary (see the student handbook at http://education.wm.edu/academics/space/cebulletinboard/cehandbook/index.php) and The University of Texas at San Antonio (see fitness to practice at http://education.utsa.edu/counseling/fitness_to_practice/).
- Consult with all relevant stakeholders in your practice or institution (see Chapter 6).
- Widely disseminate drafts of standards for feedback from relevant stakeholders, including trainees, and document efforts and feedback.
- After implementation, revise standards on a regular basis based on practice.
- Include an overarching statement that provides the rationale for standards of conduct (i.e., gatekeeping responsibilities; duty to protect current and future clients; responsibility to protect a functional learning or working environment for others; protecting the reputation of the institution and standards of the profession for training, graduating, and licensing competent clinicians).

Chapter 9

Evaluating Trainee Professional Performance

Leigh D. DeLorenzi

When I was in grade school, it was easy to identify the kids with bad behavior. They were always the loudest, most disruptive, most reactive, and most rule resistant. My teachers worked hard to juggle their multiple roles in the classroom, able to function as both educator and behavior-shaper simultaneously. The inherent hierarchy of power in the room yielded a simple equation: Grownups made the rules, and kids followed the rules or faced the consequences.

By contrast, the identification of and intervention with problematic trainees in mental health preparation programs can be complex, confusing, and at times downright intimidating. Trainees with problems of personal competence (Homrich, 2009) are not always easy to spot, and therefore educators and supervisors cannot rely solely on their intuition. Instead, they must plug in, intimately and intensely, to dozens of trainees at once and preemptively evaluate them, over and over again, using several different measures and while working closely with other evaluators. Without a dynamic system of documented evaluation, there can be no intervention or remediation. Simply put, evaluation is a gatekeeper's roadmap for what comes next.

Introduction to Dynamic Assessment

The measurement and evaluation of personal and professional conduct helps programs monitor student growth, determine training efficacy, advance the profession, and safeguard the public (Kaslow, 2004). One primary goal of measuring and evaluating personal and professional conduct is to ensure that trainees are meeting the minimum criteria for developing the necessary skills, attitudes, values, and behaviors to function effectively as mental health professionals. Another important goal is to inform trainees about their progress, give them constructive structured feedback, and indicate the criteria necessary to meet professional expectations for performance. Although the majority of graduate students meet or exceed the minimum benchmark for dispositional competency, a small percentage of trainees either take longer to meet the competencies, need direct intervention in order to meet exit criteria, or fail to meet these criteria all together (Busseri, Tyler, & King, 2005; Cruise & Swerdlik, 2010). Before remediating problems of professional competency, gatekeepers across the helping professions are mandated by laws, ethics codes, and accreditation standards to base their actions on a variety of formal and informal assessments. This scientist–practitioner model emphasizes the need for empirical support to inform professional decision-making processes (Belar & Perry, 1992; Busseri et al., 2005).

The American Psychological Association (APA) Commission on Accreditation (2015), the *ACA Code of Ethics* (American Counseling Association [ACA], 2014a), and the Council for Accreditation of Counseling and Related Educational Programs (CACREP) standards (CACREP, 2015) all explicitly link evaluation practices as the starting point for all gatekeeping activity. CACREP recently amended its latest iteration of accreditation standards to reinforce dispositional evaluation as a required data-driven decision-making practice. Specifically, the CACREP standards now require accredited programs to (a) identify key professional dispositions, (b) measure student professional dispositions over multiple points in time, and (c) analyze the data regularly. In light of the ever-expanding emphasis on evaluating personal and professional conduct, a well-endorsed, structured, and developmentally progressive assessment plan is necessary. Thus, this chapter seeks to outline a dynamic system of trainee assessment, define the range of acceptable and unacceptable trainee behaviors, and describe the specific benchmarks or gateways for formal and informal trainee evaluation.

The Challenge of Evaluating Behavior

Despite the publication of several gatekeeping and remediation models (Baldo, Softas-Nall, & Shaw, 1997; Bemak, Epp, & Keys, 1999; Homrich, 2009; Kress & Protivnak, 2009; Lumadue & Duffey, 1999; Wester, Christianson, Fouad, & Santiago-Rivera, 2008; Wilkerson, 2006), there are no universally adopted or standardized methods for evaluating dispositions across all training programs. As a profession, clinical training is still in its infancy in terms of developing clearly defined expectations for standards of conduct accompanied by solid gatekeeping assessment tools, which contributes to the challenge. Currently, only a handful of assessment instruments measure and identify specific areas of interpersonal and professional competence. The few notable examples of valid and reliable assessment instruments that do exist (e.g., Hatcher et al., 2013; Swank, Lambie, & Witta, 2012) are still in the early stages of adoption across the helping professions and therefore have yielded only preliminary research findings on strategies, psychometrics, and implications of their use. This ambiguity surrounding the proper way to navigate the complex, confusing, and time-consuming process of gatekeeping, along with the scarce research and few available evaluation measures (W. B. Johnson & Campbell, 2004), leads to increased gateslipping (Gaubatz & Vera, 2002). Thus, researchers across the helping professions agree that mental health training programs need to do a better job of assessing the suitability of trainees for the profession (Belar et al., 2001; Homrich, DeLorenzi, Bloom, & Godbee, 2014; Kaslow, 2004; Kaslow et al., 2006, 2007; Roberts, Borden, Christiansen, & Lopez, 2005).

Given that the first literature on gatekeeping emerged more than 30 years ago, what is taking the clinical professions so long to iron out the kinks of evaluation practices? In a word: terminology. Fluctuating trends and beliefs about the proper ways to define worrisome professional and interpersonal functioning of trainees have led to inconsistencies in structured policies for evaluating personal and professional performance (Hensley, Smith, & Thompson, 2003; Homrich, 2009). The frequent updating of terms accepted across the helping professions to describe qualities that characterize an individual's interpersonal interaction style (e.g., *impairment, psychological fitness, nonacademic functioning, personal and professional competencies, dispositions*) is fueled by the ever-changing literature and the judiciary (Elman & Forrest, 2007; Forrest, Elman, Gizara, & Vacha-Haase, 1999; Homrich, 2009; Kress & Protivnak, 2009; Vacha-Haase, Davenport, & Kerewsky, 2004). Seemingly vague terminology makes the standardization of observable behavior difficult, resulting in inconsistent enforcement of standards (Bhat, 2005; Brear, Dorrian, & Luscri, 2008; Forrest et al., 1999; Homrich, 2009; Kutz, 1986). However, more recent attempts to encourage a profession-wide consensus are beginning to close the gap in widely defined behavioral terms that might be arranged in the form of a scale for testing (Christensen, 2015; Homrich, 2009; Homrich et al., 2014). For example, CACREP (2015), which defines standards for counselor education programs, requires programs to identify and assess students' professional dispositions throughout the graduate program in which they are enrolled. As mentioned in a previous chapter, *professional dispositions* are defined in the glossary accompanying the 2016 CACREP Standards as "the commitments, characteristics, values, beliefs, interpersonal functioning, and behaviors that influence the counselor's professional growth and interactions with clients and colleagues" (CACREP, 2015, p. 5). These broad categories of functioning are undefined and, as stated, not measurable, which thus continues the profession-wide dilemma of defining and evaluating common expectations for trainee conduct.

Determining Checkpoints or Gateways

In order for senior members of the profession to ensure that beginning clinicians are ready to enter the profession, educators and supervisors must engage in repeated formal and informal evaluation of trainees to determine developmental progress and the attainment of minimal acceptable performance standards at the conclusion of training. The evaluation process can begin at or even before admission (Homrich, 2009; J. Miller & Koerin, 2002) and requires attention to all aspects of student performance. This includes measures of personal and professional conduct evaluated at regular intervals across student training (Crawford & Gilroy, 2012; Ziomek-Daigle & Christensen, 2010). An assessment of personal and professional conduct is considered one part of a comprehensive, cumulative evaluation of the trainee and is rarely the sole basis for admission or dismissal.

Formal Versus Informal Evaluations

The assessment of dispositional functioning takes many forms, through both formal instrumentation and information observation. Combining formal and informal evaluation provides a multilayered approach to supporting student learning and development (Homrich, 2009; Kaslow et al., 2007). Opportunities for informal evaluation can emerge in observations of the following:

- The context of every course
- Advising meetings
- E-mail, text, and phone interactions with the trainee
- Activities related to field experiences (e.g., practicum and internship)
- Interpersonal exchanges with faculty, supervisors, peer students, and colleagues
- Interactions in professional settings (e.g., association meetings, conferences, informal program-sponsored gatherings)
- Meetings with trainees when problematic behavior is first noticed to explain expectations and guide students to correct issues prior to remediation

Formal assessments are ones that occur at regular intervals and include structured and/or guided instruments or discussions about a trainee's performance and functioning. Formal evaluations that target personal and professional conduct include but are not limited to the following:

- Annual performance reviews
- 360-degree or multisource assessment
- Competency evaluation rating forms
- Consumer surveys and/or client outcome data
- Site supervisor evaluations
- Self-evaluations in comparison to supervisor evaluations

Specific evaluation information is presented later in the chapter along with guidelines for selection and implementation.

Critical Points in Graduate Training Programs

Although ethics and accreditation bodies mandate regular trainee evaluation and feedback, they fall short of providing guidelines on exactly when these evaluations should occur. For example, Section F.6.a. of the *ACA Code of Ethics* (ACA, 2014a) mandates that "supervisors document and provide supervisees with ongoing feedback regarding their performance and schedule periodic formal evaluative sessions throughout the supervisory relationship." Similarly, CACREP (2015) opts to allow programs to self-determine when these same formative and summative trainee evaluations should occur based on their unique values, training philosophies, program missions, and priorities. A review of the literature reveals several examples of effective checkpoints or gateways within the program timetable. Although a minimum grade point average, fulfillment of comprehensive exams, a successful thesis/dissertation defense, and program candidacy are common examples of gateways reflecting academic functioning, the following checkpoints are presented here as ideal opportunities for measuring personal and professional conduct.

Preadmission

If regular checkpoints are gateways toward professional competence, then the preadmission phase is the first threshold. The recruitment, enrollment, and retention of academically and clinically capable, professional, well-functioning, diverse trainees is an outlined expectation of both ethical and accrediting bodies across the helping fields (ACA, 2014a; CACREP, 2015; Ziomek-Daigle & Christensen, 2010). Because the research shows that some students arrive at a training program with significant personal problems that have the potential to impact their effectiveness as professional helpers (Lafrance, Gray, & Herbert, 2004), programs should attempt to provide advance access to performance expectations—including expectations for professional, interpersonal, and intrapersonal conduct—so that potential applicants can better make conclusions about their personal compatibility with published policies (Gilfoyle, 2008; Homrich, 2009). Explaining the gatekeeping role through graduate catalogs, student handbooks, and/or published codes of conduct (e.g., Homrich et al., 2014) prior to the application process also has the added benefit of reducing liability risks in matters of gatekeeping-related dismissal cases (Gilfoyle, 2008). For example, graduate programs should make clear to prospective applicants which ethics codes they align with as well as expectations for trainee compliance with conduct defined in those ethics codes. Making links to ethics codes readily accessible from the program's website can also encourage applicants to explore whether they are able to meet expectations for respecting client values or cultural factors, for instance. Programs can further fortify the entryway by alerting potential applicants to the values of the program, providing education about how personal issues might impact helping professionals, and encouraging prospective applicants to visit the campus and meet with key faculty prior to submitting their application. Faculty intuition, informal evaluations, and student self-evaluations are the first baby steps on the long road of measuring competencies and conduct.

Admissions

Just as screening is a crucial first step in group therapy preparation, so too are thorough and well-developed admissions screenings of prospective trainees crucial in the helping field. Research demonstrates that in group therapy, the simple act of discussing goals, behavioral expectations, and roles with potential group members allows the group process itself to be more effective (Corey, Corey, Corey, & Callanan, 2015; Yalom & Leszcz, 2005). Looking beyond an individual's potential to perform scholastically, the evaluation method for examining a person's interactional style most commonly occurs during admissions interviews (Swank & Smith-Adcock, 2014) or through structured essays "inquiring about the applicant's interpersonal style, resolution of a difficult situation, response to a values statement central to the program, or attitude toward self-care and wellness" (Homrich, 2009, p. 9). Furthermore, "challenging admissions questions are more likely to reveal intrapersonal and interpersonal concerns, such as boundary confusion, story inconsistencies, attitudes toward individual differences of others, and ability to balance the emotional challenges of the profession" (p. 10). Criteria related to personal and professional competence have historically been attended to least in the admissions process (Lafrance et al., 2004). More recent studies reveal several admissions mechanisms in place to monitor "non-academic characteristics" of applicants related to dispositions (Swank & Smith-Adcock, 2014, p. 48).

In their study on gatekeeping during admissions, Swank and Smith-Adcock (2014) found that faculty-administered assessments of interpersonal skills, writing samples, informal meetings, and group and individual interviews were commonly used evaluation methods for assessing dispositional characteristics of the applicants. Specifically, these methods helped programs evaluate an applicant's:

- Ability to reach consensus when in groups;
- Awareness of his or her coping styles and wellness practices;
- Awareness of personal strengths and weaknesses (self and others' view);
- Ability to receive and incorporate feedback;
- Boundaries, flexibility, and risk taking;
- Personal challenges faced and methods for overcoming them;
- Feelings and experiences related to working with people from diverse backgrounds;
- Problem-solving ability;
- Verbal and nonverbal skills;
- Ethical thinking and behavior; and
- Engagement with others.

After a close examination of each applicant packet, faculty members typically come together to discuss, evaluate, and in some cases score applicants using rating forms (e.g., the Carkhuff Rating Scale; Carkhuff, 1969) against formalized program admission criteria. Other programs have matriculation procedures in place that allow faculty more time with and exposure to applicants who do not meet all admissions requirements. Among the programs sampled by Swank and Smith-Adcock (2014), this probationary period typically ranged from 3 to 20 hours of coursework and involved close monitoring and evaluation of probationary applicants for goodness of fit and performance in the program (i.e., academically, interpersonally, and behaviorally), after which time applicants were either fully admitted, placed on further remediation, or denied admittance. Despite these efforts to reliably assess professional dispositions and screen for psychological issues during admissions, participants in the study reported difficulty implementing adequate screening procedures (e.g., personality assessments) because of legal concerns.

Continuing Students

Once students matriculate, it is critical for programs to institute an ongoing assessment process focusing on the academic, clinical, personal, and professional competence of students. Ideally, this assessment process occurs at regular intervals, involves multiple measures rated by various evaluators, and is transparent to trainees. Hensley et al. (2003, p. 225) found that programs that conducted evaluations of potentially impaired students on an "as-needed basis" had an increased likelihood of failing to identify students until the end of their matriculation in the program (e.g., practicum, internship). Homrich (2009) further emphasized that evaluation procedures must be "consistently applied to all enrollees in order to fulfill the protected right of due process" (p. 11).

Examples of efficient methods for evaluating the personal and professional dispositions of matriculated students include the following:

- An initial progress review at the end of the first semester
- Faculty-rated annual performance reviews
- Faculty-rated program candidacy reviews
- Supervisor-rated performance reviews at midpoints and at the conclusion of fieldwork
- Dispositional assessments within clinical coursework
- Additional meetings initiated after reports of problematic behaviors are observed

Specific assessments within each of these categories are discussed later in the chapter.

Critical Points in Pre- and Postdegree Supervision

Ethics codes related to endorsement mandate that supervisors "not endorse supervisees whom they believe to be impaired in any way" (ACA, 2014a, Standard F.6.d.). Furthermore, certification and licensure boards rely on training programs and supervisors to affirm that students have successfully completed their coursework and clinical hours for graduation, licensure, and certification. This may apply in particular to school counseling students who seek certification versus licensure or supplemental certifications in specialty areas in conjunction with licensure in other professions. These prelicensure checkpoints are designed to prevent trainees who exhibit problematic intrapersonal, interpersonal, or professional behaviors from potentially causing harm to future clients and to prevent gateslipping into a postgraduate or postlicensure clinical position in which their conduct is not monitored as closely. Homrich (2009) recommended that programs and supervisors engage in careful reflection on trainee conduct prior to responding to endorsement requests rather than applying a "one-size-fits-all comprehensive endorsement" for all graduates (p. 14). For postgraduate qualified supervisors, it is also helpful to include a specific clause within the supervisory contract on gatekeeping benchmarks related to personal and professional functioning, expounding on conditions that may prevent a supervisor from continuing to work with trainees.

Hence, several critical points within pre- and postdegree supervision require careful attention to the personal and professional conduct of students and alumni. Across the helping professions, these evaluation checkpoints aid programs and postdegree clinical supervisors in determining readiness for (a) practicum, (b) internship, (c) entry-level practice, and (d) professional licensure and/or certification. Careful documentation of trainee functioning is helpful and can include faculty or supervisor narratives from student-of-concern reports, remediation plans, or evaluation results from a student's permanent file. This prevents crucial information on student functioning from being lost when faculty or supervisors leave an academic institution. Documentation is also required in the event a clinical supervisor decides not to endorse a supervisee for failure to meet the minimum standards of performance as defined by ethics codes and legal statutes. This documentation is typically required as an attachment to the supervisor attestation form for endorsement to the state.

Defining the Range of Trainee Functioning

Ineffective Versus Harmful Behavior

Whereas classroom functioning and the demonstration of clinical skills are easier to define, identify, and measure and can provide sound data for supporting student dismissal, dispositional functioning is more difficult to define, identify, or use as a basis for dismissal. As discussed previously, a lack of universal terms and differing opinions about the extent to which educators and supervisors within the clinical professions should be intervening are partly to blame (J. Miller & Koerin, 2002). Despite the fact that training programs and supervisors rely heavily on intuitive professional judgment when evaluating trainee appropriateness for the field (Bernard & Goodyear, 2014), intuition cannot and should not stand alone. Instead, gatekeepers should evaluate trainee competence on standard criteria established by the profession. In their final report on assessing competencies within professional psychology, Kaslow et al. (2006) asserted that "competencies must be conceptualized as generic and developmental abilities in which knowledge, skills, dispositions, self-perceptions, motives, beliefs/attitudes are considered as dimensions of holistic abilities rather than discrete dimensions of performance" (p. 99).

But how can programs distinguish between unhelpful and harmful personal and professional conduct? Lamb et al. (1987) defined problematic behavior as surfacing in one or more of the following categories:

> (a) An inability and/or unwillingness to acquire and integrate professional standards into one's repertoire of professional behavior, (b) an inability to acquire professional skills in order to reach an acceptable level of competency, and (c) an inability to control personal stress, psychological dysfunction, and/or excessive emotional reactions that interfere with professional functioning. (p. 598)

In addition to examining and evaluating specific behaviors, it is important to assess for certain mediating conditions that elicit more serious remedial action. In an attempt to differentiate problem behaviors from "impairment" along the continuum of trainee competence, Lamb et al. (1987, p. 598) described problem behaviors as those that require remediation but that are not necessarily unexpected or excessive for professionals in training. Conversely, they defined impaired functioning as:

- Lacking trainee acknowledgment, understanding, or corrective action when a problem is identified;
- Not merely reflecting a skill deficit that might be improved with further training;
- Negatively impacting the quality of services delivered by the trainee on a consistent basis;
- Transcending multiple areas of professional functioning;
- placing disproportionate demands on the time and efforts of faculty and/or supervisors; and
- Unresponsive or unchanging despite ongoing feedback, remediation efforts, and/or time.

More recent studies offer more detailed descriptors for behavioral misconduct, including a lack of interpersonal skills, ethics violations, pervasive resistance to corrective feedback, and inappropriate boundaries (Busseri et al., 2005; Henderson & Dufrene, 2012; Russell & Peterson, 2003). Some researchers cite other examples of ineffective dispositional functioning as problems with affect regulation or emotional control, poor awareness of boundaries, substance use, poor personal wellness and stress management, unethical behavior, deficits in cognitive functioning, unmanaged or harmful countertransference, poor clinical decision making, and the misuse of power or respect toward clients (or colleagues) who identify differently than the trainee. Common categories and examples of behavioral misconduct are summarized in the following section (Bemak et al., 1999; Forrest et al., 1999; Haynes, Corey, & Moulton, 2003; Homrich, 2009; Olkin & Gaughen, 1991).

Examples of Behavioral Misconduct

Unethical Behavior

Unethical behavior includes a failure to honor and uphold the ethical guidelines of ACA, APA, the American School Counselor Association, and/or the International Association of Marriage and Family Counselors in either the classroom or practice setting. This includes the following:

- Failure to respect or maintain the confidentiality of peers and/or clients if an assignment, classroom discussions, the course structure (i.e., a group class), specific classroom activities, and/or client sessions explicitly require it
- Failure to uphold confidentiality and/or privacy
- Failure to exhibit cultural competence by respecting individual differences in interactions with others
- Failure to support the individual rights and dignity of others
- Failure to maintain the records and documentation necessary for rendering services

- Failure to respect the autonomy and beliefs of others and/or imposing one's personal beliefs on others
- Failure to maintain professional boundaries with clients
- Failure to use appropriate judgment to respond to situations
- Engaging in inappropriate or harmful transfer or termination with clients
- Engaging in practice outside of one's boundaries of competence
- Engaging in acts of fraud
- Engaging in inappropriate or sexual dual relationships with clients
- Engaging in counseling relationship(s) with friends or family members
- Engaging in discrimination of clients based on race, religion/spirituality, gender, gender identity, sexual orientation, marital/partnership status, language preference, socioeconomic status, immigration status, or any bias proscribed by law

Resistance to Feedback

- Minimally open to or dismissive of feedback
- Minimal to no effort demonstrated toward improving areas flagged as needing improvement

Prioritizing Needs of the Self Over the Client's Needs

- Failure to place the needs of the client over one's own personal needs and interests, for example, in the areas of scheduling, session conduct, treatment planning decisions, availability, and/or responsiveness to the client

Unprofessional Appearance

- Failure to maintain a professional appearance (including hygiene and attire) appropriate for the setting

Ignoring or Disregarding Program Policies

- Failure to follow the procedures and policies of the graduate program
- Failure to engage in productive supervision and consultation with colleagues and/or peers
- Failure to fulfill obligations promptly, consistently, reliably, or according to expectations stated by the professor or supervisor
- Failure to support the learning processes of others, for example, during classes and/or group supervision settings
- Failure to engage actively in learning, training, and/or experiential processes and opportunities for personal and professional development

Inappropriate Use of Technology

- Failure to use technology appropriately and ethically in all situations while respecting others who are present or affected
- Using cell phones, tablets, or laptops in class or in session to engage in activities that fall outside the scope of appropriate use (i.e., texting, social media, pornography)

Inappropriate Interpersonal Boundaries

- Engaging in verbal or physical harassment
- Inappropriate anger outbursts
- Failure to establish and maintain effective and functional relationships with colleagues or clients
- Disregard for the boundaries or needs of another
- Inability to recognize, or refusal to acknowledge, harmful countertransference emerging in client relationships

Emotional Instability

- Failure to express feelings respectfully or professionally, either verbally or in writing
- Failure to respond to personal discomfort with thoughtful consideration for self and others
- Failure to interact with appropriate emotional self-regulation
- Resistance to learning techniques for managing stressful personal issues effectively

Poor Personal Wellness

- Failure to adopt personal wellness practices that allow one to function effectively in his or her role as a student and/or counselor
- Failure to seek, create, or engage in opportunities to appropriately fulfill personal/emotional needs
- Using behavior- or mind-altering substances that impede professional functioning

Capacity for Openness

- Minimally open to or dismissive of feedback
- Failure to maintain openness to and respect for differences in ideology
- Resistance to examining personal reactions
- Failure to demonstrate openness to ideas, learning, and change

Immaturity

- Poor self-awareness or self-control
- Little to no awareness for how one's personal actions affect others
- Failure to take responsibility for behavior

Lack of Integrity

- Acts of dishonesty or disrespect
- Failure to communicate respectfully and professionally by using appropriate verbal and nonverbal language
- Communicating information untruthfully

Inflexibility

- Failure to adapt to the changing needs of the environment

- Resistance to opportunities for self-reflection and self-exploration
- Resistance to examining personal reactions

An Uncooperative Attitude

- Failure to compromise and collaborate effectively with others
- Avoidance of and/or resistance to professional consultation with regard to recognized areas of personal growth
- Failure to resolve interpersonal conflicts with peers/colleagues in a timely, professional manner
- Failure to exhibit professionalism in reactions and behaviors
- Failure to cooperate with a remediation plan

Apathy/Indifference

- Failure to demonstrate genuineness, empathy, and interest in the welfare of others

Insensitivity

- Failure to display sensitivity to the feelings, thoughts, and needs of others
- Failure to provide helpful, nondefensive feedback to others when appropriate

Low Capacity for Self-Examination

- Lack of awareness for how one's personal actions affect others
- Failure to exhibit awareness of personal needs
- Failure to exhibit awareness of one's personal strengths and limitations
- Resistance to opportunities for self-reflection and self-exploration

An Unmanaged Mental Health Diagnosis

Presenting with an unmanaged mental health diagnosis that impedes professional functioning, including but not limited to a diagnosis of any of the following:

- Personality disorders
- Anxiety disorders
- Depressive disorders
- Eating disorders
- Psychotic symptoms

Concerning Partner Relationships

- Engaging in harmful or violent interpersonal relationships that impede one's ability to function effectively as a student and/or counselor

This list is designed to provide concrete examples of potential misconduct and is not intended to be an exhaustive or all-inclusive checklist.

Furthermore, the presence of some of these behaviors may not alone be serious enough to warrant remediation or dismissal. Although more research is needed to help gatekeepers distinguish between behaviors that require immediate intervention and those that might benefit from continued observation, recent research has attempted to clarify some of these distinctions and is discussed in Chapter 8.

Factors Identified as Grounds for Dismissal

Ethical, accreditation, and judicial bodies support differing interpretations of how personal and professional competence are best evaluated in the context of an academic clinical training program, and therefore programs have some leeway in determining how dismissal decisions are made (Busseri et al., 2005; McAdams, Foster, & Ward, 2007). Beyond issues of poor academic performance and deficient clinical skills, issues related to unethical behavior or insufficient interpersonal abilities are common reasons for dismissal (Forrest et al., 1999). However, because dismissal proceedings can be stressful and confusing for faculty and students, they can also be the most avoided gatekeeping intervention (Gaubatz & Vera, 2006; Homrich, 2009; McAdams et al., 2007). A variety of factors are linked to these concerns, including (a) emotional stress, (b) difficulty reaching consensus among faculty or supervisors, (c) lack of access to sufficient objective data, (d) the time and effort required for documenting, (e) reluctance to document problems or initiate dismissal, and (f) anxiety about lawsuits (Busseri et al., 2005). Faculty and supervisor hesitancy to engage in a thoughtful, structured protocol for remediation can also stem from fears of overreacting or hopes that problems will resolve on their own with time (McAdams et al., 2007), thus avoiding the need to confront the problematic behavior.

Fears of legal reprisal for dismissal are frequently cited in the literature as a rationale for avoiding gatekeeping action. Specifically, training programs worry that trainee conduct-related dismissal may be overly subjective, impulsive, retaliatory, disparate to academic performance, and/or prejudicial toward the student (Lamb et al., 1987). McAdams et al. (2007, p. 213) described the "dismissal decision dilemma," stating that programs often choose to retain an unfit student to absolve the program of litigation risk while violating their ethical responsibility to protect the public, or they terminate the unfit student and place the well-being of their program at risk. In a discussion of their court case, McAdams et al. (2007) emphasized the link between their structured professional performance evaluation protocol and the successful litigation outcome for their program, stating that the evaluation "provided a grounded framework for decision-making in situations when faculty objectivity might easily have been impaired by intense emotion" (p. 220). Thus, in situations in which programs fail to uphold ongoing evaluation and feedback as part of their due process requirements in dismissal decisions (see Chapter 3), litigation fears may be warranted.

To reduce legal risks associated with dismissal, policies linked to personal and professional conduct should be developed in collaboration with other faculty and administrators and subsequently made available to all trainees via program handbooks. Included in these policies should be structured evaluation systems that directly tie inappropriate and/or unprofessional conduct to ensuing disciplinary actions (Kaslow et al., 2006; McAdams et al., 2007; Papadakis, Hodgson, Teherani, & Kohatsu, 2004). Regularly administered dispositional and competency-focused evaluations ensure that programs assess, document, and intervene with students in a fair and equitable fashion. Furthermore, in matters of dismissal, all faculty should be involved in the evaluation and decision-making process so that trainees understand that remediation and dismissal decisions are based on recommendations of the entire faculty and do not result from a relational conflict with a single professor (Gilfoyle, 2008; Homrich, 2009). Greater attention needs to be paid to the gatekeeping function when students are assessed as having competence problems that cannot be effectively remediated (Kaslow et al., 2006; Vacha-Haase et al., 2004).

Measuring and Evaluating Conduct

The following sections provide guidelines for selecting and administering a variety of specific evaluation methods for assessing personal and professional conduct.

Selecting Assessments

A structured, well-organized, and consistent system of ongoing evaluation is fundamental in determining whether a counselor-in-training is equipped to continue on the journey toward independent practice (Homrich, 2009). The literature across the helping professions outlines important principles for the selection and utilization of evaluation methods. In the field of professional psychology, conferences and task forces dedicated to assessing the competency of clinicians-in-training (e.g., Kaslow et al., 2007) concluded that assessments should be multitrait, multimethod, and multi-informant and should measure individual differences in competence in a variety of domains, considering behavioral domains independently of academic domains (Busseri et al., 2005). Programs have adopted a variety of evaluation methods for determining clinical suitability, including faculty and/or supervisor performance evaluations, treatment outcome assessments, peer reviews, and valid/reliable assessments for evaluating competencies. The following principles of assessment lay the groundwork for selecting proper measures.

A Climate of Transparency

Prior to implementing an assessment protocol for your organization, it is helpful to establish a climate of transparency. The ideal program climate is one that fosters trust, understanding, and clarity (V. A. Foster & McAdams, 2009; Kaslow et al., 2007). In their article on transparency and performance assessments, V. A. Foster and McAdams (2009) stated that faculty hesitancy to discuss or enact professional performance assessment policies can lead to a negative, critical, pejorative climate rather than a climate in which students perceive competency assessment as a helpful and necessary component of training for a career in helping. Furthermore, they stated, "A relationship seemingly exists between the level of faculty members' willingness and ability to execute their professional performance assessment mandate and the positions that students will ultimately assume regarding their personal responsibility for gatekeeping within the counseling profession" (p. 275). Therefore, a culture of transparency is best created through the thoughtful establishment of fair and accessible expectations and procedures and consistent, uncensored dialogue between faculty evaluators and students. Professional performance standards and expectations should be available to students through multiple venues, including new student orientations, annual student meetings, advisor meetings, program websites, student handbooks, course syllabi, and electronic course sites like Blackboard (V. A. Foster & McAdams, 2009).

Developmentally Informed Assessment

Faculty members and supervisors must be able to differentiate between a student who is capable of meeting the minimum training requirements and a student who is not. However, given the rigorous, triggering, and emotionally intense nature of mental health training programs, some academic, emotional, and behavioral difficulties are to be expected. Just as supervision and education are not one-size-fits-all approaches, neither is the assessment process. Not only do trainees in the helping fields enter training programs and the accompanying fieldwork experiences with varying capacities for learning new information and demonstrating proficiency with clinical skills, a diverse student body will display a wide variety of personal, interpersonal, and intrapersonal functioning. Dispositional assessments therefore should be developmentally sensitive and used along the continuum of counselor development throughout the span of a career, as counselors are ideally expected to improve and become more skillful with time and experience. Because students gain competence at different rates, developmentally informed assessments should take the form of continuously changing individual competence profiles reflecting both the strengths and weaknesses of each student (Hatcher et al., 2013). Furthermore, because assessment should adjust to the developmental level and stage of learning of the trainee, a competency assessment used at the beginning of a program may not be appropriate for assessing competence at the end of that program (Homrich, 2009; Kaslow et al., 2007). Homrich (2009) stated,

> Faculty and supervisors should recognize that interpersonal and professional competence is neither a dichotomous nor a static construct, that the developmental processes of students should be recognized and respected, and that conclusions about the potential for growth that are based on trainees' status or previous experiences should be avoided. (p. 15)

After all, the purpose of a training program is to support clinical learning, skill building, and professional development. Only after clinical educators and supervisors carefully and sensitively assess a trainee's dispositions can they provide ongoing guidance as trainees attempt to model dispositions that are appropriate to the field of mental health.

Multi-Informant Assessments

Faculty in training programs are uniquely qualified as gatekeepers in that their ability to evaluate trainees is enhanced by frequent access over time to the trainees in a variety of professional settings (e.g., in the classroom, at the clinical site, and during supervisory sessions). Yet dispositional evaluation must go beyond classroom observations. Although much can be observed about trainee dispositions within the classroom, trainees with problematic conduct have the capacity to make excellent grades (Bernard & Goodyear, 2014). Therefore, a strong working alliance between faculty members and clinical supervisors is needed to gather meaningful data about a person's competence from multiple sources, perspectives, and environments (Kaslow et al., 2007; Turnbull, Gray, & MacFadyen, 1998). Interrater reliability can be difficult to achieve when multiple people are evaluating a single subject without formal instruction beforehand. This is true for both valid/reliable evaluation instruments and open-ended, case-based oral examinations or vignettes. Therefore, steps should be taken to orient and provide training to all core faculty, adjunct faculty, and site supervisors using a multi-informant evaluation in order to minimize threats to reliability.

Competency-Based Evaluation

Gatekeeping difficulties emerge when programs fail to enact written policies and procedures related to evaluation or when faculty struggle to achieve consensus on how student competencies should be measured and/or applied when making dismissal decisions (Forrest et al., 1999). Thus, researchers across the helping professions have emphasized the need for competency-based evaluation of trainees. Similar to academic and skill-based evaluations, personal and professional conduct should be conceptualized as competency-based student learning outcomes. This approach allows gatekeepers to define and evaluate behaviors from a prevention-focused and positive viewpoint—not just through the lens of deficit remediation (Henderson & Dufrene, 2012). Furthermore, competency-based education allows programs to document students' achievement of competence over time, providing earlier and more effective remediation when performance falls below expectations. Once competencies are identified by programs, they stand (or falter) based on the strength of assessments being used. Specifically, stated Hatcher et al. (2013), the success of competency-based education is contingent on the degree to which the program is set up to assess specific, developmentally based competencies that guide student learning and track student progress and the degree to which the program uses assessment results to improve its approach to developing students' capacity to successfully attain identified competencies.

Important Diversity Considerations

Trainee competency assessments, like all other assessment measures, should be sensitive to individual and cultural differences, such as those listed in the ACA and APA codes of ethics (i.e., differences in age, gender, gender identity, race, ethnicity, culture, national heritage, religion, sexual orientation, disability, marital/partnership status, language preference, immigration status, and socioeconomic status). Just as with clients, trainee behavior may be an extension of the individual student's cultural experiences, gender socialization, religious training and beliefs, and other life experiences (Bemak et al., 1999; Homrich, 2009). Furthermore, trainees are more likely to acknowledge their limitations and areas for improvement if cultural contexts and socialization experiences are considered with assessment results (Forrest et al., 1999). As V. A. Foster and McAdams (2009) pointed out:

> Students who are members of underrepresented groups (e.g., people of color; students for whom English is a second language; gay, lesbian, and transgendered persons; those with disabilities) may feel vulnerable to unfamiliar policies that are perceived to reflect dominant culture constructions of professional performance and competence. (p. 273)

Therefore, when reviewing evaluation or assessment results of students whose cultural identity or socialization experience conflicts with program conduct or behavior standards, programs might consider enacting the following procedures. First, faculty and supervisors should meet regularly to discuss the program's philosophy regarding these types of conflicts before, during, and after they arise. Gaining consensus on protocols for addressing conflicts will enhance trainer cohesion so that conflicts are responded to in a consistent manner. Second, although programs should intervene in a timely manner, they must also take their time to carefully and thoroughly evaluate the circumstances. It is important for gatekeepers to listen to student feedback regarding dispositional evaluations that they deem unfairly biased toward the dominant culture. Faculty and supervisors should carefully note such feedback and discuss whether evaluations or assessments are a good fit for every student. This might mean that a program's battery of dispositional assessments is constantly being evaluated and periodically replaced with assessments more sensitive to various cultural identities and socialization experiences.

In addition, the student's advisor, supervisor, program chair, or professor or the entire faculty might invite the student for a meeting with the sole purpose of gathering accurate information regarding such conflicts. Rather than an opportunity to jump into disciplinary or remedial action, this meeting should instead be seen as an opportunity to hear the student's point of view and/or clarify any misunderstandings. It also serves as an excellent springboard for future interventions, communications, assessment revisions, or remediation plans involving the student, if necessary. Last, as with all remedial scenarios in gatekeeping, students must be given the opportunity to learn about why, for example, a particular conflict is potentially problematic for mental health professionals working with clients. If students are willing and able to learn about the ethical standards related to behavioral benchmarks, they must be given the chance to integrate what they have learned. This can take time, and therefore faculty should be willing to extend certain timetable expectations in these scenarios. It might take a full year or 2 years to document improvement in these areas for certain students, whereas other students without these cultural or socialization backgrounds might integrate new behaviors within a semester. However, if a student is resistant to feedback or explicitly states that he or she refuses to learn other ways of behaving in line with ethical behavioral standards, faculty should document the student's decision and move forward with the next phase of remediation.

Formative and Summative Assessment Feedback

In a series of publications outlining principles, recommendations, and toolkits for assessing trainee competencies (Kaslow et al., 2006, 2007, 2009), scholars agree that assessments should be mutually informative and composed of both formative and summative evaluation. Although formative and summative assessments are separate measures, they can and should interact with and inform each other. For example, results from one summative assessment might provide information for self-improvements in a future formative assessment during the next stage of the training process (Donaldson, 2003; Kaslow et al., 2007). Furthermore, formative and summative assessments are not merely tools to be kept in confidential folders, locked away in the filing cabinets of program trainers. These assessments are equally, if not more so, designed to benefit the trainee.

Formative assessments provide ongoing, developmentally informed, and thoughtful feedback to the trainee in order to deepen learning and foster directions or goals for growth. Examples of formative assessments might be case presentations, skills evaluations such as live/recorded performance ratings, and/or feedback on dispositional functioning, to name a few. Summative evaluations, by comparison, are outcome measures depicting some endpoint of learning and may take the form of annual reviews, end-of-semester site supervisor evaluations, a degree conferral, completion of an internship, endorsement for licensure, or receipt of a board certification.

Both types of assessments should highlight areas of strengths, weaknesses, and/or deficits falling below the minimum threshold for a particular stage or state of performance in a given domain (Kaslow et al., 2006). Moreover, results of both formative and summative assessments should directly inform training plans and remediation efforts for each individual student. Programs should also refrain from using formative assessments as summative assessments. This requires programs to utilize a variety of targeted measures instead of the same broad measures over and over again and ensures that multiple professionals provide independent, thoughtful, accurate, and routine evaluations of all trainees (Homrich, 2009).

Specific Types of Assessments

Four common categories of competency assessment for trainees entering the helping professions were presented by Kaslow et al. (2006): (a) measures of knowledge, (b) measures of decision making, (c) measures of performance and professional attributes, and (d) integrated assessments of practice-based skills and tasks. The first two categories, measures of knowledge and measures of decision making, usually take the form of either multiple-choice, short-answer, essay, or standardized tests or oral/written/videotaped vignettes for which a trainee has to explain decisions based on a particular case presentation. These measures are effective for evaluating academic functioning and are familiar to professors evaluating student learning within content areas. Personal and professional conduct are more effectively assessed using the last two categories of assessment listed above using annual reviews, faculty or supervisor evaluations, portfolios, 360-degree evaluations, and/or structured assessment instruments to evaluate dispositions. These assessments allow multiple raters to evaluate functional performance, such as the trainee's level of professionalism, interpersonal communication skills and implementation, ability to work with others, self-awareness, emotional intelligence, and ethical decision making, among other personal and professional qualities. Many instruments measuring these domains are scored on a Likert-type scale indicating whether the target (or expected) skill, behavior, or disposition is deficient, developing, or present based on the developmental level of the student and program expectations (Homrich, 2009). Table 9.1 outlines a variety of specific assessment instruments used to assess the dispositional characteristics of trainees.

Table 9.1 • Assessment Tools Used to Measure Dispositions

Tool and Dispositional Items/Constructs	*Type*
360-Degree Evaluation (Lockyer, 2003) Questionnaire-based assessment method in which trainees are evaluated by peers, clients, and coworkers on key performance behaviors, including the following: • Personal and professional awareness • Recognizes personal limitations • Seeks supervision when needed • Insight about personal issues that affect treatment • Respectful interactions with staff • Timeliness, organization, and preparation • Managing personal crises effectively • Follows stated rules/regulations • Ethical behavior • Demonstrates multicultural competence	B
Annual Performance Reviews Annual qualitative faculty and supervisor evaluations assessing: • Professional behaviors (i.e., attire, timeliness) • Openness to feedback • Multicultural competence • Interpersonal functioning • Emotional stability • Self-care • Ethical behavior	S
Basic Skills Evaluation Device (BSED: Nelson & Johnson, 1999) This instrument has a section on "professional conduct," defined as: • Initiating and maintaining appropriate contact with other professionals. • Maintaining a personal professional image. Avoiding publicly denigrating or criticizing colleagues. • Consulting with professionals and others involved with cases appropriately, with appropriate signed releases, and in a professional manner, always keeping the client's welfare foremost. • Handling unexpected and crisis situations with poise and skill, using consultation when appropriate. • Punctuality with therapy sessions and other professional meetings. • Following clinic policies in setting and collecting fees	F
Client Outcome Data • Surveys or qualitative client feedback on dimensions of counselor professionalism.	F
Competency Benchmarks in Professional Psychology (APA, 2012) • Professionalism –Integrity –Deportment –Accountability –Concern for the welfare of others –Emerging professional identity –Multicultural competence –Ethical, legal, and professional conduct –Reflective practice/self-assessment –Self-care –Interpersonal skills –Affective skills –Expressive skills	B

(Continued)

Table 9.1 • Assessment Tools Used to Measure Dispositions *(Continued)*

Tool and Dispositional Items/Constructs	*Type*
Counseling Competencies Scale–Revised (CCS-R; Swank, Lambie, & Witta, 2012)	B
Counseling dispositions and behaviors:	
• Professional ethics	
• Professional behavior	
• Professional & personal boundaries	
• Knowledge & adherence to site policies	
• Record keeping & task completion	
• Multicultural competence	
• Emotional stability & self-control	
• Motivation to learn and grow/initiative	
• Openness to feedback	
• Flexibility & adaptability	
• Congruence & genuineness	
Counseling Self-Estimate Inventory (COSE; Larson et al., 1992)	F
• Multicultural competence	
–Working effectively with clients different from trainee	
–Maintaining nonjudgmental stance with clients	
–Avoiding imposing values on clients	
–Ability to bridge cultural differences	
• Awareness of values	
–Reflecting on personal attitudes and values that may impact counseling relationship	
Counselor Skills Personal Development Rating Form (CSPD-RF; Torres-Rivera, Wilbur, Maddux, & Smaby, 2002)	F
• Emotional sensitivity (empathy)	
• Multicultural competence	
• Awareness of personal biases	
Criteria of Nonacademic Characteristics (Duba, Paez, & Kindsvatter, 2010)	B
This instrument evaluates the following constructs within (a) individual contexts, and (b) small group contexts:	
• Interpersonal interactions in academic and professional settings	
• Personality	
• Professionalism (behaviors, skill, and knowledge)	
• Student openness and self-evaluation	
Demonstrated Multicultural Counseling Competence (DMCCC) Measure (Sehgal et al., 2011)	F
• Multicultural competency (knowledge and practice)	
Family Therapy Skills Checklist (FTSC; Briggs, Fournier, & Hendrix, 1999)	F
• Preparedness for supervision	
• Incorporating supervisory feedback	
• Ethical behavior	
FIASCO Rubric (Christensen, 2016)	B
• Flexibility	
• Integrity	
• Awareness	
• Stability	
• Compassion	
• Openness	
Interpersonal Professional Relationships Competency Rating Form (APA, 2012)	B
• Empathy, compassion, & desire to be helpful	
• Experience and use of affect	
–Emotional self-awareness	
–Emotional maturity	

(Continued)

Table 9.1 • Assessment Tools Used to Measure Dispositions *(Continued)*

Tool and Dispositional Items/Constructs	*Type*
Interpersonal Professional Relationships Competency Rating Form *(Continued)*	
• Affect tolerance	
–Effectively managing emotions	
–Tolerates ambiguity	
• Effective boundary management	
• Recognized effects on self and others	
• Respectful interactions with others across cultural differences	
• Effective interpersonal skills in challenging situations	
• Open to feedback	
• Cooperation and collaboration	
• Expressive skills	
• Awareness of and commitment to interpersonal competence	
Personal Characteristics Evaluation Form (Frame & Stevens-Smith, 1995)	F
• Flexibility	
• Positivity	
• Cooperativeness	
• Willingness to accept/incorporate feedback	
• Ability to deal with personal conflict	
• Accepting personal responsibility	
• Appropriate emotional expression	
• Awareness of impact on others	
Professional Counseling Performance Evaluation (PCPE; Kerl et al., 2002)	B
• Professional responsibility	
• Competence	
• Maturity	
• Integrity	
Professional Performance Review Policy Standards (McAdams et al., 2007)	F
• Openness to new ideas	
• Cooperativeness with others	
• Ability to deal with conflict	
• Initiative and motivation	
Professional Qualities Evaluation (Lewis and Clark Psychology Department, 2016)	B
• Professional responsibility	
–Ethical/legal behavior	
–Appropriate interpersonal interactions	
–Openness to other viewpoints	
• Competence	
–Awareness of limitations	
–Takes responsibility for deficiencies	
–Basic cognitive, affective, sensory, and motor capacities to respond professionally to peers, professors, and clients	
• Maturity and attitude	
–Demonstrates appropriate self-control	
–Behaves honestly, fairly, and respectfully	
–Demonstrates awareness of personal beliefs and the effect of these on work	
–Ability to receive and incorporate feedback	
–Appropriate levels of self-efficacy	
–Engages in effective conflict resolution when conflicts arise	
–Positive, flexible, solution-oriented attitude	

(Continued)

Table 9.1 • Assessment Tools Used to Measure Dispositions *(Continued)*

Tool and Dispositional Items/Constructs	*Type*
Professional Qualities Evaluation *(Continued)*	
• Integrity	
–Refrains from making false, misleading, deceptive statements	
–Avoids potentially harmful dual relationships	
–Respects rights, dignity, and worth of all people	
–Demonstrates multicultural competence	
–Considers impact of actions on well-being of others	
• Social and self-awareness	
–Knowledge of own intersecting identities, and how these may affect the counseling relationship	
–Awareness of worldview, and how this informs definitions of normality-abnormality	
–Demonstrates ability to monitor personal well-being, attitudes, or problems and to accept mentoring, supervision, and remediation when they interfere with program standards.	
–Maintains humility and uses privilege to promote social equity	
Self-assessments/reflections	F
• Qualitative self-assessments on dimensions of professional, interpersonal, and intrapersonal behavior.	

Note. B = both formative and summative; S = summative; F = formative.

Conclusion

As an industry, the mental health professions are still in the early stages of developing, researching, and implementing valid and reliable gatekeeping assessment instruments. Currently, only a handful of valid and reliable assessment instruments exist that measure and identify specific areas of interpersonal and professional competence. More time, testing, and development are needed to ascertain the effectiveness of assessment tools as they are adopted across the helping professions. Accrediting bodies and ethics codes for the clinical professions explicitly link to evaluation practices as the starting point for all gatekeeping activity. Solid assessment practices help programs to monitor student growth, determine training efficacy, advance the clinical professions, and safeguard the public. (See What Would You Do? 9.1.)

Key Points and Best Practices

- There are several critical checkpoints at which programs and postdegree supervisors should evaluate trainee personal and professional conduct. Through marketing and advertising, programs should seek to make their mission and program standards clear from the preadmission stage. Once admissions are under way, faculty gatekeepers should assess personal and professional conduct through interviews, writing prompts, and experiential activities, scoring structured dispositional evaluations of each applicant. Faculty gatekeepers should formally and informally assess

What Would You Do? 9.1

Caroline was a 27-year-old Cuban American female who was admitted to a graduate program in clinical mental health counseling. She recently transferred into the program from another university because her husband wanted to move closer to his ailing mother. In her first semester, she scheduled several meetings with her advisor to discuss concerns she was having with professors and peers in the program. During those meetings, she told her advisor that she perceived her professors as "mean and unqualified" and noted that at least two of her classmates "should never have been accepted into the program because they are really stupid." The advisor attempted to get more details from Caroline on her experiences with peers and professors in the program, but the student was unable to give many concrete examples and spoke only in disparaging generalities, unable to consider positive qualities. The advisor periodically checked in with Caroline's professors to assess how she was doing, and they all raved that she was one of the top performers in the class.

Toward the end of the first semester, Caroline frequently showed up unannounced to her advisor's office and asked to talk about her personal issues related to hating her mother-in-law and the challenges she was facing conceiving her first child. After suspecting that Caroline had misaligned the advisor as her personal therapist, the advisor suggested that she consider seeking personal counseling to help her deal with some of these hardships. The student voiced resistance to seeking counseling because she was "afraid the counselor will make her look at painful memories from her past." She then disclosed a long history of severe abuse and trauma, including psychologically abusive parents, several rapes in high school and college, and three or four suicide attempts since the 12th grade.

During the week of her final exams, Caroline called her advisor late in the evening almost every night, presenting with suicidal ideation and panic attacks related to the content of some of her course readings and exams. "I can't read this stuff! It's really upsetting for me, and I get so distraught that I think about dying if I have to read another sentence or get up in front of my class and do my final presentation on these topics." She further stated, "You're the only person I trust and the only person I want to talk to. If I didn't have you to call, I don't know how I would survive."

What would you do in this situation?

What specific problematic dispositions are present with this student?

What methods of assessment might be helpful in defining and tracking her problematic dispositions?

What next steps should you take as her advisor?

the dispositions of students who matriculate at regular intervals, including after their first semester, during annual reviews, during candidacy reviews, through 360-degree evaluations, and through structured dispositional instruments. Structured gatekeeping efforts and evaluations should not cease after graduation but should continue during postdegree supervision that commences with clearly written expectations in the supervisory contract and designated assessment points over the course of the supervisory relationship through to endorsement and licensure. (See Notes From the Field 9.1.)

- Faculty and supervisor gatekeepers should use formal and informal assessments to evaluate and track key professional, interpersonal, and intrapersonal behaviors. Because dismissal can be challenging when students are performing well scholastically but struggling with personal and professional conduct, documenting and providing regular feedback to trainees is crucial. The same holds true for the endorsement of supervisees to continue training and/or attain licensure.
- A climate of transparency is helpful because faculty and supervisor hesitancy to discuss or enact professional performance assessment policies can lead to a negative, critical, pejorative climate rather than a climate in which students and supervisees perceive competency assessment as a helpful and necessary component of training for a career in helping.
- When selecting a suite of evaluation instruments that align with specific program goals and professional standards, gatekeepers should ensure that formative and summative measures are developmentally informed, multi-informant, competency based, and considerate of the developmental level and cultural diversity of trainees.

Notes From the Field 9.1

During application reviews for prospective students in a graduate program for marriage, couples, and family counseling, an application was flagged for further discussion by program faculty. The published standards and mission of the program strongly emphasized social justice advocacy and multicultural competence as a key factor of the program's identity. The applicant was a 46-year-old African American woman with a high grade point average, strong scores in standardized testing, excellent letters of recommendation, and impeccable writing skills. Yet two faculty members noted concerns after reading her essay and experiencing her during the interview. Her resume reflected 15 years of volunteer experience related to her role as a pastor's wife. She mentioned several times in her essay that her reason for wanting to pursue a graduate degree in mental health was to "enhance my ability to bring hearts and minds to Jesus Christ."

During the interview, all applicants were asked one question related to counseling people of different religious backgrounds and/or value systems. She answered, "The Bible tells us what the truth is, and I would try to help my clients see that truth if the opportunity presented itself in session." Using the program's constructed Personal Qualities Evaluation Checklist as the dispositional evaluation at admissions, faculty rated the applicant as deficient on the item "The student respects and values cultural, individual, and role differences, including those due to age, gender, race, ethnicity, national origin, religion, sexual orientation, disability, language, and socioeconomic status." The program chair noted, "The applicant demonstrated less sensitivity and open-mindedness to persons from other cultures and expressed a desire to change others based on her personal values," and recommended that she only be admitted on the condition that she was able to demonstrate an ability to value various perspectives.

The faculty decided that they needed to better assess the applicant's willingness to learn about and practice multicultural competence as defined by various program standards, laws, ethics, and accrediting bodies across the helping professions. Thus, the faculty required the applicant to respond to the following writing prompt:

> The mission of our graduate program is to prepare counseling students to be the best counselors they can be. Our program is unique in that it encourages learning about and participating in social justice advocacy for marginalized individuals and groups of people who do not share equal power in society because of their immigration status, race, ethnicity, age, socioeconomic status, religious heritage, physical ability, gender identity, or sexual orientation. The curriculum of each and every class is built around a central tenet of social justice advocacy and multicultural competence. This "infusion" means that in each class students are building their personal awareness, knowledge, and skills to help prepare them for effectively working with clients across the spectrum of every race, ethnicity, spiritual identity, class, gender identity, and sexual orientation.
>
> Students are expected to identify and become aware of their own personal beliefs and life experiences and then learn to separate those beliefs

(Continued)

Notes From the Field 9.1 *(Continued)*

and experiences from the work they do with clients. Trainees must be able to affirm their clients' views, especially when the client has a different set of behaviors and beliefs from the counselor. In addition, in several classes, students make presentations on ways to advocate for different marginalized groups. For example, they don't just educate their peers on issues relevant to counseling lesbian, gay, bisexual, transgender, and queer clients (e.g., a presentation on the ethical issues associated with certain religious reparative therapies), they call lawmakers and attempt to shape policy through legislative advocacy. Faculty and supervisors in the helping professions are legally and ethically mandated to only endorse students who are willing and able to demonstrate multicultural competence.

There are a multitude of ways each student fulfills this requirement that is individualized and monitored by faculty in great detail. For more information on the expectations and process, please review the attached student handbook, which outlines the definitions and expectations associated with becoming a multiculturally competent future practitioner in our program. Please also review the attached dispositional assessment that students must pass in order to progress in the program. Pay special attention to the "social and self-awareness" section of this assessment for details on how multiculturally competent dispositions are evaluated.

The faculty would very much like to learn more about your opinions, views, interests, or experiences regarding social justice advocacy within counselor education. Specifically, please write an explanation (a couple of paragraphs) of how you plan to support and affirm clients from all social identities and cultural contexts, especially those clients with religious or spiritual traditions, sexual orientations, or gender identities different from your own. We routinely invite prospective applicants interested in master's degrees in marriage, couple, and family counseling to evaluate whether our program's commitment to multicultural and social justice principles and practices is a good fit for them as well.

After receiving the prompt, the candidate thanked the faculty for the information and opportunity to learn more about the program mission, standards, and evaluation practices. She also chose to remove herself from consideration and instead opted to enroll in a nearby graduate program for Christian pastoral counseling.

Chapter 10

Designing Remediation Plans and Interventions

Kathryn L. Henderson

This chapter contains an in-depth review of the purpose of remediation with key issues to consider throughout the remediation process. Methods for approaching remediation with students are reviewed along with the role of remediation plans in the gatekeeping process. Remedial interventions used in plans are discussed with considerations for recommended practice. Implications for policies and procedures are examined, and a sample set of policies is provided. Best practice suggestions for creating remediation plans are reviewed.

Remediation Defined (or What's It All About?)

Remediation represents a direct and active effort by faculty and supervisors to provide a trainee with an opportunity to achieve success on a competence the trainee has either (a) yet to master at a basic level though provided with opportunities to do so (i.e., through traditional classroom strategies or informal comment) or (b) demonstrated challenges maintaining mastery at a basic level. Remediation typically occurs as a part of the gatekeeping process (Frame & Stevens-Smith, 1995; Kerl, Garcia, McCullough, & Maxwell, 2002; Lumadue & Duffey, 1999; McAdams, Foster, & Ward, 2007; Ziomek-Daigle & Christensen, 2010) with the accompanying goal of only endorsing supervisees or graduating students who have demonstrated clinical competence and do not pose a risk to client welfare (American Counseling Association [ACA], 2014a; Council for Accreditation of Counseling and Related

Educational Programs, 2015). The decision to begin a remedial intervention typically follows a series of proactive steps. These include widely circulating a set of behavioral and conduct competencies trainees are expected to fulfill, communicating a published gatekeeping policy to students that includes procedures for assessing students' personal and professional competencies, and faculty or supervisors providing informal feedback to a student struggling with one or more competencies over time and/or across settings. A lack of change in student behavior after these preventive actions typically leads to consultation among colleagues about ongoing concerns and whether to initiate the program or agency's formal remediation procedures. The specifics about how this process unfolds are very individualized and vary from case to case; however, the primary goal is to establish the foundation for a formal and structured intervention when informal attempts at correcting a trainee's behavior fail and when concerns about conduct become serious enough to raise the question of whether the individual is capable of working with clients safely and effectively.

An important big picture aspect of remediation is the basic intention for it to be a constructive experience that provides an opportunity for the trainee to learn or grow successfully in specifically defined ways. Key issues that were addressed earlier in this book must be considered throughout the remediation process. One key factor is related to due process: Remediation must not be punishment, nor should it be arbitrary or capricious in nature (Gilfoyle, 2008; McAdams & Foster, 2007). Punishment is connected with disciplinary consequences typically associated with academic dishonesty and honor code violations. Thus, the intent to punish is considered separate and distinct from remediation (McAdams & Foster, 2007). Given the specter of punishment, the process of remediation can often be intimidating or frightening for students and supervisees, sometimes resulting in defensiveness instead of being received as helpful. After all, the definition of *remediation* is an action intended to remedy a problem situation. Emphasizing the purpose of remediation as an opportunity for success can assist with establishing the expectation of a constructive experience while also empathizing with students' scenario and struggles.

Another key issue throughout the remediation process is striving to clearly define behavioral expectations for students to achieve in a measurable manner. Clarity regarding the behavioral expectations that faculty and supervisors need to see demonstrated can ease trainees' fears and concerns about the process. Keep in mind that emerging research has indicated that the majority of students are uninformed about the gatekeeping policy of their programs (J. M. Foster, Leppma, & Hutchinson, 2014; V. A. Foster & McAdams, 2009; Parker et al., 2014). For this reason, remediation procedures, both informal and formal, should begin with a review of the expectations for trainees; the remediation policy and procedures, including details of what will happen in what timeframe; and each participant's role and responsibilities in the process. The idea of being transparent from the beginning is key to creating a constructive experience with a hopeful outcome (V. A. Foster & McAdams, 2009).

Providing frequent and clearly stated feedback to trainees is a fundamental element of remediation. A supervisor or faculty member's evaluative role is central to the remediation process. Evaluating and informing trainees about their progress or lack of advancement toward remedial goals as circumstances unfold supports the formative feedback process of providing students with the opportunity to address any concerns as they arise. For student supervisees who are completing a practicum or internship while engaged in a remediation process, frequent communication between the site supervisor and assigned faculty members is imperative and should be documented and shared with the trainee.

A final key aspect of remediation to consider encompasses the limits of remediation—essentially, what remediation it is *not*. Not all remediation plans will end with success. Recognizing the boundaries of the roles of faculty members and supervisors is vital to recognizing the limits of remedial intervention. Although faculty members or supervisors can provide an opportunity for a student or supervisee to be successful through remediation, the decision of what to do with that opportunity rests exclusively with the trainee. Many faculty and supervisors also wear the hat of well-trained mental health clinicians and might have clinical impressions about what is impacting a trainee's performance. However, it is important to remember that in the gatekeeping relationship the role of educator and supervisor does not also include therapist; ethically speaking, clinical educators and supervisors cannot also serve as trainees' personal therapists (ACA, 2014a). The role of personal therapy in the remediation process is examined at length in this chapter, but note that faculty and supervisors who provide therapy or any type of mental health evaluation to trainees are engaging in inappropriate dual relationships. Rather than focus on potential mental health diagnoses and symptoms, Gilfoyle (2008) recommended focusing on trainees' observed behaviors instead of interpreting or analyzing those behaviors.

Macrolevel (Big Picture) Guidelines for Remediation

Empirical research on gatekeeping and remediation is slowly emerging; however, there is a general paucity of clear instructions or professional standards for approaching remediation with students (Rust, Raskin, & Hill, 2013). Although some ethics codes, accreditation standards, and licensure laws require that faculty and supervisors evaluate trainees, very few describe a remediation process for problematic behavior. Only the counseling profession specifies in its accreditation standards and ethics code expectations that remediation will occur in gatekeeping (ACA, 2014a; Council for Accreditation of Counseling and Related Educational Programs, 2015). Yet even these sources do not explicate what is entailed in the remediation process. An examination of the conceptual literature reveals scholars who have offered recommendations and guidelines for how to remediate students (see Dufrene & Henderson, 2009; Gilfoyle, 2008; Kaslow et al., 2007; Kress & Protivnak, 2009; McAdams & Foster, 2007; Rust et al., 2013). Several of these authors were informed by experience with ethical and legal cases, such as McAdams et al. (2007) at The College of William and Mary, who wrote about lessons learned from a court case that resulted from dismissing a student, and Gilfoyle (2008), the general counsel for the American Psychological Association, who described potential legal issues arising from clinical training cases. The common thread that unites many of the guidelines is the principle of due process. Due process, a legal consideration that is necessarily infused throughout gatekeeping practices and procedures, is examined in detail in Chapters 2 and 3. The implications of due process specific to remediation procedures are reviewed here.

Summary of Due Process Considerations for Remediation

- McAdams and Foster (2007) emphasized establishing routine student evaluations on the personal and professional criteria included in a program or agency's gatekeeping policy and informing trainees in advance about evaluation procedures. This mirrors the proposals from Kaslow et al. (2007) that remediation be adopted with a spirit of full disclosure and that all students be informed of routine evaluations and potential outcomes of the evaluations, such as remediation or dismissal.
- The perspective conveyed throughout remediation should be positive, with interventions that are intended to be corrective, not punitive (Kaslow et al., 2007; McAdams & Foster, 2007).
- Consider the standard of substantive due process by selecting remedial interventions that address a compelling interest or obligation, such as protecting client welfare. Avoid remedial endeavors that could be considered arbitrary or capricious in nature (Gilfoyle, 2008; McAdams & Foster, 2007), which is the primary argument for a legal challenge.
- Create remediation plans that equal or match the severity of the trainee's observed challenges in performance (McAdams & Foster, 2007). If the plan seems too severe to address the targeted deficiency, the plan could be considered punitive and, hence, not remedial in nature.
- McAdams and Foster (2007) stressed the importance of documentation during the remediation process. In the eyes of the

law, if it's not documented, it didn't happen. Written notes summarizing the content of student meetings is an example of documentation; e-mail is also a form of documentation. After a student meeting, e-mailing all parties who attended with a follow-up acknowledgment of the meeting that includes a brief summary of the discussion or decisions made can create official documentation. Another option is to audio-record student meetings when possible and with the consent of meeting attendees and the guidance of the organization's legal counsel.

Please see Appendix G for sample documentation.

Suggested Approaches to Writing Remediation Plans

After faculty or supervisors have recognized a trainee's continued challenge achieving a competency problem despite receiving informal feedback and consulted with others in the training milieu, the next step typically involves meeting with the trainee and initiating a period of formal remediation. Central to the remediation process are remediation plans. Reflective of due process considerations, plans are drafted by faculty or supervisors and discussed with trainees, which provides an opportunity for trainee input or collaboration before implementation (Gilfoyle, 2008; McAdams & Foster, 2007). Guidance from scholars provides a set of suggested approaches for constructing remediation plans (Dufrene & Henderson, 2009; Gilfoyle, 2008; Kaslow et al., 2007; Kress & Protivnak, 2009; McAdams & Foster, 2007):

- Devise written remediation plans that follow a structure.
- Outline the observed, objective facts of the student's scenario that demonstrate competency problems or behavioral deficiencies.
- Demonstrate how those competency problems are not aligned with established standards for student personal and professional behavior according to the evaluative criteria in the gatekeeping policy.
- Identify remedial goals. Write the goals in the positive voice as an expected competency to be gained rather than a behavior to stop, similar to the approach for creating behavior management plans. In other words, describe in behavioral and observable terms what the trainee will do rather than what he or she will not do.
- Specify the methods prescribed for the trainee to achieve the goals. Remedial interventions ideally should be measurable and concrete tasks that can be documented (e.g., receiving a certificate from attending a workshop, achieving an observable increase in implementing feedback received from a supervisor). See the discussion on interventions in this chapter for details.
- Include the timeframe for the duration of the plan, with dates for progress reports and/or a scheduled follow-up evaluation(s)

of the student's progress in achieving the remedial goals. If deadlines are necessary, they should be clearly stated along with expected outcomes at each point.

- Have all individuals present at the remediation meeting sign the remediation document, then distribute the finalized document to all attendees and place it in the student's file.

Please refer to Appendix C for sample remediation plans provided as example correspondence following up on a remediation meeting.

Remedial Interventions

Although recommendations for remediation plans have contributed to defining the remediation process, identifying and evaluating remedial interventions to include in plans from an empirical stance remain relatively unexplored (Forrest, Elman, Gizara, & Vacha-Haase, 1999). See Notes From the Field 10.1. Table 10.1 summarizes the scant research on the use of remedial interventions. A small pool of remedial interventions used in graduate programs and supervision has been theorized by scholars, including the following: (a) personal counseling, (b) increased (more frequent) supervision, (c) repetition of academic courses, (d) repetition of practicum or internship, and (e) dismissals from graduate programs (Bradey & Post, 1991; Brown, 2013; Elman & Forrest, 2004; Kaslow et al., 2007; Lamb et al., 1987; Olkin & Gaughen, 1991; Procidano, Busch-Rossnagel, Reznikoff, & Geisinger, 1995; Russell & Peterson, 2003; Vasquez, 1999). Of these interventions, the use of personal counseling as a remedial intervention has received the most scrutiny.

Personal Therapy

The use of personal therapy as a remedial intervention is a natural consideration given our role as trained mental health professionals. Of

Notes From the Field 10.1

For examples of remediation plan templates, consider referring to the following resources:

- The American Psychological Association Competency Initiatives in Professional Psychology website (American Psychological Association, 2017b) contains a remediation plan template under the heading "Resources Related to Students With Competence Problems."
- In their article "Professional Development Plans to Remedy Problematic Counseling Student Behaviors," Kress and Protivnak (2009) include a sample remediation plan in Appendix C.
- The suggested elements of a remediation plan are reviewed in the article "A Framework for Remediation Plans for Counseling Trainees" by Dufrene and Henderson (2009).

Table 10.1 • Programs Surveyed Using Intervention in the Remediation Process

Research Study	*PT*	*IS*	*RPI*	*RDC*	*TU*	*WEAC*	*AW*	*LA*	*FD*	*AOP*
Bradey & Post (1991)[a]	.23	.43[e]								
Brown (2013)[a]	Yes	Yes	Reduced				Yes	Yes	Yes	
Fly, van Bark, Weinman, Kitchener, & Lang (1997)[b]		.05[f]					.03		.22	
Olkin & Gaughen (1991)[c]	.77	.40	.64	.70	.32	.38		.62		
Procidano et al. (1995)[b]	.28	.12					.18	.11	.39	.23
Russell & Peterson (2003)[d]	≥.50	≥.50		≥.50	≥.50	≥.50		≥.50		

Note. Values are percentages unless otherwise indicated. Reduced indicates reduced practicum and internship. Yes indicates this intervention was reported in the study. PT = personal therapy; IS = increased supervision; RPI = repeating practicum or internship; RDC = repeating didactic cources; TU = tutoring; WEAC = workshops or extra assignments or coursework; AW = advising to withdraw; LA = leave of absence; FD = forced dismissal; AOP = advising to other programs.

[a]Counselor education programs. [b]Psychology programs. [c]Master's degree programs (including psychology, counselor education, and marriage and family). [d]COAMFTE = Commission on Accreditation for Marriage and Family Therapy Education programs. [e]Faculty review. [f]Additional review.

the four clinical professions, only ACA (2014a) addresses the role of personal therapy during remediation. The *ACA Code of Ethics* directs counselor educators to assist students in locating a personal therapist "if counseling services are suggested as part of a remediation process" (Standard F.9.c.). A key word in this quote is *suggested*, which is reflective of what Elman and Forrest (2004) labeled a *hands-off* approach to using personal therapy as an intervention. A hands-on approach to remediation would entail *requiring* personal therapy rather than suggesting it. The lens of the hands-on versus hands-off approach presents a continuum of how to approach designing remedial interventions in general, from prescribed and structured to more flexible and unstructured. Supervisory theory and style will likely play a large role in determining a professional's place on the continuum, along with the trainee's context and any preferences established by supervisor's employers, largely through published procedural standards at the institutional level as well as legal counsel.

Key considerations will impact how personal therapy is used as a remedial intervention:

- How will the counselor be selected who provides therapy to the trainee? By faculty or supervisors? Or by the trainee? Will a list of recommended therapists be provided to the student, or will the student be sent to a public or online list of local providers? How will the cost of therapeutic services be considered if there is no free counseling services available to trainees, as the expense may be prohibitive?
- How much communication will transpire between the faculty or supervisors and the treating therapist? How will the therapist know why the client-trainee is coming to counseling or the extent of the problematic behavior if it is conveyed only through trainee self-report? This question reflects the dilemma of upholding the trainee's expectation of confidentiality of individual counseling sessions while holding the trainee accountable for making measurable progress on behavior changes specified in the remediation plan.
- Will the trainee be required to provide documentation of attendance at therapy? Will the documentation address topic(s) discussed? Will the treating therapist be expected to make a general evaluative statement at the conclusion of therapy regarding the trainee-client's progress in a specified area of concern?
- What happens if the trainee fulfills the requirement to attend the prescribed therapy session but there is no change in problematic behavior?

The complexities inherent in the use of personal therapy in remediation are reflected in scholars' criticism. Kaslow et al. (2007) pointed out the lack of guidelines from an official body regarding how to use therapy in remediation, along with the lack of research regarding its effectiveness as a remedial tool. The issue of confidentiality begets questions about the supervisor's role (or lack of one) in the trainee's therapy sessions, especially regarding goal setting for the sessions, which theoretical approach or interventions might be best to address the student's challenges, and how much programs might be involved in determining whether the trainee has successfully remediated after participation in personal therapy (Olkin & Gaughen, 1991; Schoener, 1999; Vasquez, 1999).

In a qualitative research study, Elman and Forrest (2004) sought to discover how training directors of counseling psychology programs were handling these issues surrounding the role of personal therapy in remediation. They found that the majority of participants were using what the researchers considered a hands-off approach: suggesting or recommending therapy, not communicating with the treating therapist, and not requiring documentation of completed therapy sessions. This approach favors the student's confidentiality as a client. Elman and Forrest (2004) suggested a more hands-on approach to using personal therapy in remediation, which would favor accountability to the program. Recommendations included (a) developing detailed policies for how personal therapy may be used in remediation and communicating those policies to all trainees in advance (Elman & Forrest, 2004; Gilfoyle, 2008; Kaslow et al., 2007); (b) reviewing ethical considerations with the trainee and the treating therapist regarding confidentiality and the limitations or exceptions required by the program for informational purposes in terms of remediation decisions (Gilfoyle, 2008); and (c) determining how the trainee's progress, or lack thereof, during therapy will be communicated to the program to inform the concerns at the center of remediation, along with any required outcomes for trainees to achieve toward meeting remedial goals (Elman & Forrest, 2004; Kaslow et al., 2007).

Other Remedial Interventions

Outside of personal counseling, remedial interventions have primarily focused on more frequent contact with trainees and repeating courses. Please see Table 10.1 for a summary of empirical research on remedial interventions.

Increased Advisory or Supervisory Contact

Requiring more frequent contact with the trainee usually involves increased supervision or periodic meetings with one or more faculty members to track progress (Brown, 2013; Kress & Protivnak, 2009; McAdams & Foster, 2007; Olkin & Gaughen, 1991; Procidano et al., 1995; Russell & Peterson, 2003). For example, if a trainee is completing a clinical practicum or internship within a graduate program, or is engaged in a postdegree supervisory period, more frequent contact could be accomplished by requiring an increase in the number of weekly supervision meetings. A related consideration is designating who is providing the increased supervision, which might include a site supervisor, an academic advisor, a course instructor, a doctoral student supervisor, participation in group supervision, or some combination. In some cases, cross-supervision may be indicated with the addition of a new supervisor to the team to provide a fresh perspective on the individual's clinical functioning. Another consideration is to define what *increased* means (e.g., how often or how many hours per week). For students not yet in their fieldwork, increased remedial contact could mean regular meetings with a faculty advisor (Russell & Peterson, 2003) or with an assigned faculty member not currently teaching the student who provides oversight regarding behavioral concerns. The specifics of the regular meetings should be defined to help with transparency, addressing details such as how often the parties will meet, how long the meetings with last (e.g., 30 minutes), the location of the meetings, the topics to be discussed during the meetings, and expectations of the trainee (such as engagement in the discussion process, production of written lists or reports, or provision of evidence of task completion). Specificity not only makes expectations clear to the trainee, it provides an indicator by which to measure fulfillment of the remedial intervention.

Repetition of Coursework

As a remedial intervention, repeating courses can be divided into two types of courses: (a) clinical courses to develop skills and (b) traditional didactic content courses to increase knowledge and subsequent application to clinical work. As an intervention, the repetition of courses could affect the trainee's final goal (such as graduation) or intended specialization (such as working with a specific clientele; McAdams & Foster, 2007). How often a course is offered by a program is also a consideration: If a course is not offered frequently, perhaps once per year, would the ensuing delay be regarded by the trainee as punishment? Although simply requiring a student to repeat a practicum or an internship is one approach (Olkin & Gaughen, 1991), other approaches entail restricting the trainee's access to these courses until successful remediation has been demonstrated (Biaggio, Gasparikova-Krasnec, & Bauer, 1983) or removing the trainee from clinical courses if concerns arise during his or her time at a site (McAdams & Foster, 2007). Similarly, trainees can be required to repeat academic coursework that has already been completed (Kress & Protivnak, 2009; McAdams & Foster, 2007; Olkin & Gaughen, 1991; Russell & Peterson, 2003), and faculty will have to determine whether this must occur through enrollment in the current program, so core faculty can oversee progress, or whether enrolling in the course at an outside institution is permitted. A related remedial intervention could be to attend tutoring to address specific knowledge areas or skills (Olkin & Gaughen, 1991).

Identification of Desired Changes or Outcomes

Regardless of the structure of an intervention intended to increase knowledge, skill, and/or personal or professional behavior, it is important that supervisors and/or faculty members clearly establish the expected outcome of the remedial intervention at the outset. What specifically is the anticipated result of the experience? Will a specific experience be enough support for the trainee to yield the hoped-for outcome? What will happen if the student or intern completes the assigned intervention (a course, personal therapy, a workshop) but the behavior of concern does not change? It is important for both parties—the student/supervisee and the faculty/supervisors—to have a clear understanding of the outcome expected in terms of behavioral change before a remedial intervention is assigned. It is important to include these expectations in written form within the remediation plan so that all involved in the remediation process understand the desired outcome(s) and the consequences should the remediation plan not be fulfilled.

The anticipated consequence of the plan may include a reflective process by the student as part of the intervention. For example, Kress and Protivnak (2009) suggested as remedial interventions requiring students to complete a reflective journal assignment or research paper focused on their challenges or requiring them to attend a professional development workshop that addresses specific areas of deficit, such as empathy development. Some programs require that a presentation be made to the faculty or supervisory team about what the trainee learned about himself or herself while engaging in the remedial assignments. In some situations, the trainee might be asked to prepare and read a statement addressed to faculty or supervisors acknowledging their initial concerns about the problematic behavior and directly addressing the discoveries and changes the individual made to remedy the conduct.

Student Restrictions

During the process of remediation, a related consideration is restricting student standing or presence in the program. (See Notes From the Field 10.2.) An official leave of absence from the program might be appropriate depending on the situation and its timing within the student's program of study (Biaggio et al., 1983; Brown, 2013; Olkin & Gaughen, 1991; Procidano et al., 1995; Russell & Peterson, 2003). A leave of absence can be beneficial when the student's scenario includes personal life challenges that need to be addressed, such as substance abuse or physical health concerns. Depending on the student's interpersonal dynamics and/or abilities, part of the dialogue might include counseling the student out of the clinical profession and, hence, to withdraw from the program (Biaggio et al., 1983; Brown, 2013; Fly, van Bark, Weinman, Kitchener, & Lang, 1997; Procidano et al., 1995). In the broader context of gatekeeping, a final result could be a forced dismissal from a program if a trainee does not show the improvement

Notes From the Field 10.2

A graduate student was observed engaging in immature interactions and unprofessional conduct with peers in several classroom settings. The behavior was reflective of high school-level conduct: giggling at inappropriate times, distracting others, not engaging in topical discussion in class, and cracking jokes during small-group work that derailed the focus of the conversations. The lack of professional conduct was discussed with the student, and she became more disengaged as her distracting and interrupting behaviors continued. Her faculty advisor expressed concern to the student about her professional maturity level during the practicum placement process, explaining the expectations for professional conduct in a clinical setting. The student reported that she understood the concern and was ready to focus on appropriate conduct in the clinical situation.

Early in the practicum, the field site supervisor concluded that the student was lacking in engagement, clinical curiosity, initiative and focus, and professionalism and suggested to the faculty supervisor that dismissal of the student from the site was the appropriate action. This then occurred. Faculty met with the student to address the seriousness of the dismissal, suspended the student from the practicum until changes in her professional behavior occurred, and reiterated the previously stated concerns about the student's conduct and professionalism by reviewing expectations for professional conduct and observing and defining the behaviors that demonstrated that the student was performing below the standards expected. After a meeting with the faculty, the student was asked to summarize her understanding of the faculty and site supervisors' concerns in a detailed letter to the faculty accompanied by her proposed solutions to the problem areas. The student did so, listing professional conduct, professional identity, conscientiousness about clinical work, defensiveness, and lack of openness to feedback, among others. This indicated that she fully heard the faculty's feedback. The student went on to propose her own remediation plan for correcting these professional deficiencies, which was an impressive demonstration of maturity. She asked for feedback on the plan and assistance in further understanding and implementing changes. This meeting and the student's request for feedback was followed by a letter from the faculty clarifying a common understanding and appreciating her demonstration of maturity by accepting feedback and proposing remedies. The faculty also offered additional strategies supplementing her "treatment plan" (as the student termed it) with a few more directives and suggestions.

Four months later, prior to the upcoming practicum placement period and after one or two interim meetings with her advisor to report on her progress, the student met with the faculty. In a prepared statement, the student described the actions she had taken to address faculty concerns and change her behavior and outlook on professional functioning. She reflected on her increased self-awareness, acknowledging the validity of the faculty's concerns and the discoveries she had made about herself and her behavior. She thanked the faculty for intervening with care and respect, especially her advisor, who had been clear and consistent while also en-

(Continued)

Notes From the Field 10.2 *(Continued)*

couraging her self-exploration and development. At the conclusion of the statement, she reported her realization that her behavior had in part reflected her ambivalence about pursuing the profession of counseling. This student realized that she would be a much better fit for a different career (an allied health profession that included technical vs. clinical skill) and announced her decision to withdraw from the program. The student noted that she was pleased to have made this breakthrough and thanked the faculty for their direction. She withdrew from the program and returned the following semester to attend the graduation ceremony of her previous peer group.

The student in this example was encouraged to receive and consider feedback received by the faculty and formulate her own plan for a series of interventions that addressed the concerns and the changes in behavior that needed to occur to meet the graduate program's standards for professional conduct. Faculty support of this developmental process led to an unexpected, but likely appropriate, discovery and outcome. It is always essential to convey to a student clear and detailed expectations about interpersonal, intrapersonal, and professional behavior followed by specific examples of problematic conduct defined in precise behavioral terms during the feedback process. Depending on the concerns and the student's interpersonal style, it might also be strategic to ask the student what he or she believes needs to occur for the problem to change and to request that the response include descriptions of specific strategies. This allows for trainee collaboration in the change process and buy-in as well. Faculty or supervisors can still supplement a given plan, but suggested interventions for remediation do not have to be top-down proposals, especially for adult learners.

required by the remediation plan. This possibility should be discussed with all trainees at the beginning of the remediation process and the conversation documented in order to fulfill the due process requirements of informing students in advance about potential consequences. The possibility of delay in the program of study and/or dismissal should also be included in all remediation plans. Ideally, a statement of potential restrictions that could occur when students or trainees are unable or unwilling to change problematic professional behaviors will have been published in the graduate catalog, student handbook, supervisory contract, and/or agency handbook for student review prior to program enrollment.

Outcomes of the Remediation Process

In general, the outcome sought from the remediation process is a positive one that entails the trainee successfully completing the remedial requirements and meeting all identified goals. A positive result is the student continuing with coursework or clinical experiences toward graduation or a postgraduate supervisee's endorsement for full licensure or certification. Although these are the desired results, several other potential outcomes might transpire. At times trainees will experience challenges during the remediation process that could pose barriers to the successful or timely completion of the plan. In these cases, the trainee's particular outcome will require a gatekeeper decision. Trainee outcomes and gatekeeper responses are reviewed in Table 10.2.

Challenges and Considerations in Remediation

The lived experience of facilitating remediation can vary greatly and depends in large part on the trainee's response to remediation and the ensuing outcome. (See What Would You Do? 10.1 and 10.2.) Faculty and supervisors need to be mindful of the impact of remediation on the trainee and on the relationships between the trainee, faculty, supervisors, and the program or agency. A trainee's response to remediation may be intense, with strong negative emotions, such as hostility and anger. Recalling the boundaries of the supervisory role and the professional mandate of supervisors and faculty as gatekeepers can be useful in facilitating an empathic and sensitive response while at the same time not agreeing with the trainee's choices that have led to remediation and still holding the supervisee accountable (Henderson & Dufrene, 2015). For example, clinical supervisors and educators can empathize with the struggles a student is experiencing but should not accept these struggles as a rationale for failing to submit tapes or assignments on time or not completing the required hours for practicum. These experiences are often time consuming and psychologically demanding

What Would You Do? 10.1

As a tenure-track faculty member, you are assigned to teach the second semester of Internship. In the third week of the semester, you are notified by one of the master's interns that she has been dismissed from her internship site. Immediately concerned, you request to meet with the student and reach out to the site supervisor. The site supervisor discusses concerns about the intern's basic counseling skills and ethical issues in terms of lacking cultural competence and professional boundaries with clients. You are alarmed and inquire when these concerns began to surface. The site supervisor details extensive discussion with the student's previous instructor for the first semester of Internship. Checking the student's folder, you find no documentation of these concerns; moreover, the student's grade for the prior internship semester is recorded as a high passing grade. When you meet with the student, she acknowledges having been aware of the site supervisor's concerns.

What would you do?

Depending on the potential trainee outcomes in Table 10.2, how would you proceed differently?

Table 10.2 • Trainee Outcomes and Gatekeeper Responses

Trainee Outcome of Remediation	*Gatekeeper Response*
1. Successful cooperation and change: The trainee: a. is motivated to participate in the remediation plan, b. takes initiative to complete all required plan objectives, and c. is assessed as demonstrating the necessary professional competencies identified as goals in the plan.	1. Continuing the trainee in training process: The remediation plan is evaluated at the end of the time period and determined to be successfully completed. The remediation plan is closed, and the trainee moves forward in their training. The outcome is documented and placed in the trainee's file.
2. Cooperation but unsuccessful change: The trainee engages in items: a) and b) (above row); however, she or he is unable to achieve item c) and is not able to demonstrate a basic level of competence on the remediation goals.	2. Stopping the trainee until successful change is demonstrated: This gatekeeper response could involve two different options: a) the timeframe for the remediation plan is extended beyond the original remediation period, or b) a leave of absence for the student is considered. The trainee's cooperation, potential to achieve the goals as demonstrated during the original remediation timeline, and personal life circumstance will impact which option is optimal for each trainee.
3. Lack of cooperation or willingness to participate in remediation: This outcome might present in a variety of ways. The trainee might attend meetings to discuss remediation and agree to the remediation plan; however, the trainee does not initiate the steps required to complete the goals in the plan. Alternatively, the trainee might refuse to participate in meetings or disagree with the need for remediation and refuse to engage in interventions to demonstrate change.	3. Dismissing trainee when remediation goals not achieved: The gatekeeper response to dismiss a trainee is often a difficult one for all involved. Trainee outcome 2 or 3 could result in dismissal.
4. Decision to leave training program or change professional path: At any stage of the remediation process, the trainee might gain insight or attain new self-awareness. Insight can include a lack of fit for a clinical profession, and new self-awareness can include a view of self, interests, and skills previously not realized that leads to pursuit of a different professional path.	

What Would You Do? 10.2

You are a doctoral student who completed a supervision theories course the previous semester. You are looking forward to working with your first supervisee. You are assigned a master's-level practicum student, Kristen, and begin meeting for supervision weekly. Kristen struggles to complete the weekly assignments on time and for two consecutive deadlines does not produce the required recording. She discusses her personal life extensively in supervision and is frequently upset and emotional. You informally address these concerns with Kristen and consult with your faculty supervisor (of supervision). As the next few weeks unfold, Kristen begins missing time at her clinical site and her scheduled supervision meetings.

What would you do?

Depending on the potential trainee outcomes in Table 10.2, how would you proceed differently?

What would you do if Kristen's behavior continued and your supervisor (of supervision) downplayed or dismissed your concerns and discouraged action on your part outside of the supervisory relationship with Kristen?

for all involved, trainees, faculty, and supervisors alike. Faculty and supervisors balance many roles and tasks while also carrying out their gatekeeping responsibilities. Consulting with colleagues fulfills best practice standards and can also lend support and professional connection during a typically stressful experience. Engaging in self-care to strive toward balance and maintaining perspective are ongoing goals of many professionals and are essential during remediation.

Case Study

Using a single case, I consider four potential outcomes based on details of the circumstances. This exercise illustrates possible responses gatekeepers may consider. (See On the Legal Side 10.1.)

Simple Feedback Resulting in Successful Behavioral Change

Warren, a Caucasian male in his late 40s, is a master's student enrolled in a counseling techniques course. In this course, students learn basic and advanced counseling skills and techniques and practice using the skills on one another in role plays during class. The class instructor, Dr. Wellful, an African American female in her late 20s, has observed Warren playing the role of the counselor three times over 4 weeks. Although students typically experience some challenges at the beginning of the semester, after Week 4 most students are demonstrating growth in their skills and applying feedback. Warren has not demonstrated a similar developmental pattern of growth or the ability to apply feedback and becomes visibly emotional and frustrated during

On the Legal Side10.1

Reference the article by Hermann and Herlihy (2006) on the *Bruff v. North Mississippi Health Services, Inc.* (2001) court case. In summary, the *Bruff* case involved a practicing counselor who was employed by an employee assistance program. After Bruff had been working with a client for a while, the client disclosed that she was a lesbian. Bruff informed the client that she could not work with her because her sexual orientation conflicted with Bruff's personal values. Reflect on Bruff's position in the context of the code of ethics for your profession (psychology, counseling, social work, or marriage and family therapy) and/or the legal mandates of your particular state's licensure laws regarding discrimination or imposition of personal values in the context of providing clinical services.

Imagine that you are Bruff's clinical supervisor. What would you do when initially informed about Bruff's scenario and message to the client? How would you approach discussing remediation?

his Week 4 demonstration. At this point, the instructor e-mails Warren to request a meeting to discuss his experience in class.

Warren attends the meeting with Dr. Wellful, who initiates the dialogue by asking Warren how his experience has been so far in the course. Warren apologizes for letting down her down and states that he is aware of feeling paralyzing anxiety during the role plays. He admits that all of the skills he has been practicing during the week fly out of his head. He then becomes so upset in class that he cannot focus when receiving feedback from his peers or the instructor. Warren remembers feeling a similar type of anxiety years ago when he worked in a marketing job that required him to make cold calls to potential customers; he ended up taking medication and quitting the job because of the anxiety. Now he is feeling lost and as if he might not be cut out for a career in counseling.

Dr. Wellful reflects Warren's current concerns and the depth of his emotion. She validates his ability to reflect on his emotions and how his past experience is impacting his current performance in class and validates his willingness to share this experience with her. She shares that everyone has strengths and areas of growth that they bring to the role of counselor and that she has worked with students in the past who have faced similar challenges as Warren. One avenue for self-care and wellness, regardless of one's life experience, is seeking personal counseling. Dr. Wellful discloses the value she found in personally seeking counseling for herself and how positively impactful counseling has been for her. Warren is open to seeking personal counseling, which is available at the student counseling clinic on campus free of charge. He states that he will go straight there after the meeting.

The following week before class, Warren asks to speak with Dr. Wellful in private. He expresses gratitude for her feedback and suggestion of seeking personal counseling. He is now committed to attending counseling regularly and has once again started taking the medication that he took in the past. He was hoping not to need to take the medication ever again, and he realizes that this was negatively impacting his performance in class and the program. He wants to genuinely try to grow in the class and pursue this career. Although he does not want to take the medication long term, he is committed to learning other ways to manage his anxiety. Dr. Wellful encourages Warren's new path and the courage it takes. Warren's anxious behavior in class is noticeably reduced, as demonstrated by his ability to hear and incorporate feedback. This results in improved performance in class during clinical skill role plays and an increase in Warren's confidence in pursuing a counseling career path. Warren successfully passes the class.

Remediation Process Resulting in Successful Behavioral Change

This scenario picks up after Warren meets with his instructor and seeks personal counseling; however, he still does not demonstrate growth in his basic clinical skills in class role plays, despite feedback from both peer students and the faculty member. Dr. Wellful asks to meet with Warren a second time and requests that an additional faculty member attend in accordance with the program's gatekeeping policy. During the meeting, Warren expresses his frustration with his lack of progress in class, which has resulted in the increase in his anxiety. He verifies that he is following through with attending counseling and taking medication. Dr. Wellful approaches the meeting as a brainstorming session to create a remediation plan that will provide Warren with remedial interventions geared toward creating the opportunity for success. She reviews the program's policy and explains how remediation works, along with the possible outcomes of delaying the program of study by repeating courses and of student dismissal, though that option is not expected or currently being considered. Warren expresses his understanding and agreement to participate in a remediation plan.

Warren and the faculty members brainstorm remedial goals and interventions tailored to his challenges. Remedial interventions agreed on include formal assignments to address the development of counseling skills, a wellness plan created by the student, and a required weekly practice schedule of clinical skills to be documented and submitted to Dr. Wellful. In the wellness plan, Warren pledges to attend personal counseling weekly and incorporate anxiety reduction techniques such as mindfulness-based stress reduction practices into his daily schedule. Warren commits to the remediation plan and requests to ask assistance from peers in the program to practice his skills. He also requests access to the program's media library to view therapy sessions by a range of practitioners intended for educational use. Warren follows the remediation plan and begins to demonstrate growth in his counseling skills. Because of his struggle with anxiety and demonstration of clinical skills in the class, Warren asks to retake or audit the course again prior to starting his practicum, which is added to his remediation plan. Warren successfully completes the remediation plan and proceeds in the program to graduation.

Increased Trainee Self-Awareness Resulting in Self-Selecting Out of the Profession

This scenario begins after the remediation plan is created and in effect. Warren commits to the remediation plan, follows through on each remedial intervention, and begins to demonstrate slow growth in his skills. Warren asks to meet with Dr. Wellful and her faculty colleague close to the end of the semester. In this meeting, he reflects on his experience and notes that he is appreciative of having been given the opportunity to find success through remediation. He has not experienced this level of support in his past and feels gratitude for the faculty members' commitment to him as a student. Through personal counseling, though, Warren has reflected on his level of anxiety and the effect it has had on his engaging in the counseling process. He also has examined his career choice and now believes that the responsibilities and dynamics of the counseling role do not fit his interpersonal style. He feels secure in this decision and feels that his other strengths would lend themselves to a more appropriate career match without inciting his anxiety. Dr. Wellful recommends that he seek the services of the on-campus career center. He agrees, decides to end his role as a student in the clinical program, and withdraws from the program.

Forced Dismissal

This scenario also begins after the remediation plan is created and in effect; however, Warren's experience following through on the plan is different. Rather than committing to the plan, Warren begins to stop regularly attending class with Dr. Wellful, avoids engaging in or responding to communication with her, is late in submitting assignments, and receives a few low grades; this pattern emerges in his other courses too. Warren does not initiate communication with his instructors about these occurrences; he also does not take the initiative to complete the remedial interventions.

Two students enrolled in the course ask to speak with Dr. Wellful about concerns they have about Warren. The students report that Warren has discussed using illegal drugs, which he finds more beneficial than the anxiety medicine, and has admitted that he has attended some classes under the influence. He has offered to share the drugs with his peers as his recommended method of managing performance fears. Dr.

Wellful and her colleague consult with all program faculty members about Warren's scenario and request to meet with Warren again.

Warren e-mails a response that contains several complaints about Dr. Wellful, criticizes her personality and teaching ability, and states his disagreement with the remediation plan. He says that he will meet but only with his attorney present, as he thinks he is being discriminated against. Dr. Wellful communicates the university's policy that the university attorney must also be present if a student brings an attorney and that faculty are not permitted to meet with an attorney otherwise. Warren finds this to be further evidence of being discriminated against. He shows up in the program's office suite unscheduled with his attorney present; there are no faculty members on the premises at that time, and Warren becomes anxious and verbally aggressive toward the office assistant as he demands to meet with someone. The office assistant calls the dean's office, who sends a representative over to attempt to address the situation. Warren continues to act in an emotionally agitated manner and threatens that everyone will be very sorry they treated him poorly by "making up" requirements other students do not have. He leaves the building with his attorney. The dean's office contacts the counseling program's faculty members about the incident and says that a campus police report will be filed regarding the verbal threat. Given the escalation of the circumstances, and following the program's gatekeeping policy, faculty members vote on a forced dismissal of Warren from the program. The decision is sent by certified mail and e-mailed to the student, who never responds. (See On the Legal Side 10.2.)

Conclusion

Remediation is a formal and documented process designed to address a trainee's observed performance competency concerns with the goal

On the Legal Side 10.2

McAdams et al. (2007) shared their experiences of being sued by a student who was forcibly dismissed. In their case, similar to the case of Warren, fellow students came forward and spoke with faculty about concerns they had regarding the student at the focus of remediation, expecting that the discussions would be considered confidential. McAdams and colleagues shared about learning the hard way that confidentiality between students and faculty is not guaranteed when a lawsuit has been filed. Students may be required to testify during the deposition process of a court case. It is recommended that faculty and supervisors not promise or guarantee confidentiality to reporting peers. It may be helpful to acknowledge the challenges of this role while educating students about the professional standards for their part in protecting clients and the profession from problematic practitioners, a position they may likely encounter with future colleagues.

of providing the trainee with the opportunity for successful change congruent with the expectations of the clinical profession, program, or agency. Due process considerations provide guidelines to structure the remediation process so that it is conducted in a deliberate and fair manner. Remediation plans represent official documentation of requirements trainees are expected to meet in order to be evaluated as successfully completing remediation and ready to continue with the clinical training process. Remedial interventions are included in plans as measurable and concrete steps a student or supervisee must complete to meet remedial goals. Outcomes of student remediation can range from successful remediation and continuation to graduation or endorsement to forced dismissal from a training program or supervisory contract. Overall, the role of faculty and supervisors as gatekeepers is to provide transparent guidance and feedback to trainees as they endeavor to provide for the best interest of the trainee and the profession.

Key Points and Best Practices

- Approach remediation as a constructive experience to provide a trainee with the opportunity for success. Remember that once you provide that opportunity, it is up to the trainee to decide what to do with it.
- Construct remediation expectations according to due process guidelines, such as by avoiding punitive remedial interventions.
- Write remediation plans that follow a clear structure and incorporate best practices from the field:

  –Summarize a factual scenario that describes the student's competency concerns.
  –Link observed competency concerns to established evaluative criteria.
  –Create remedial goals that are positive expectations for students to accomplish with specific remedial interventions to achieve those goals.
  –Detail the timeframe for the plan with follow-up reports or evaluations.
  –Include a template statement regarding possible consequences of failing to demonstrate competency as required by the plan, such as dismissal.
  –Distribute the finalized plan to all required individuals and obtain signatures.

- When selecting remedial interventions, reflect on the desired outcome and how to tailor the interventions to the student's unique scenario and needs.

Chapter 11

Documentation in Gatekeeping

Theresa A. Coogan

The realm of gatekeeping in clinical training is a function of supervision and includes skill development, content knowledge, and professional identity development. Supervisory oversight encompasses the gatekeeping role in the education and preparation of clinicians. One related task of gatekeeping is documenting the oversight process. The literature in the clinical field is abundant with best practices and models of supervision for clinical trainees (Bernard & Goodyear, 2014; Falender, Ellis, & Burnes, 2013; Stoltenberg & McNeill, 2010). A growing body of literature explores the larger responsibility of gatekeeping in the mental health professions (Behnke, 2005; Bemak, Epp, & Keys, 1999; V. A. Foster & McAdams, 2009; Gaubatz & Vera, 2002; Lumadue & Duffey, 1999; Swank & Smith-Adcock, 2014; Ziomek-Daigle & Christensen, 2010). However, detailed practices for documentation during the gatekeeping process, although repeatedly identified as critical in the literature, have yet to be fully articulated or defined. The aim of this chapter is to offer suggested practices for documentation procedures in gatekeeping situations from the perspective of preventing further complications or ethics violations.

Every agency or organization develops various documentation procedures and protocols to meet its unique record-keeping needs. The data recorded in forms, reports, and correspondence, as well as the policies and/or procedures for handling these documents, are often developed in reaction to precarious situations that have occurred at the agency or organizational level. Often, institutions discover a gap in their procedures when evidence of some action is not recorded. For example, an unexpected legal or administrative challenge arises that reveals a lack of recorded justification for the actions taken by faculty regarding a problematic student. Just as best practices for supervisory procedures have been generalized and shared to inform effective strategies at the larger systems level, documentation models can also be applied to effectively record behaviors, reactions, proceedings, and decisions occurring in gatekeeping processes by the supervisors and faculty involved. This information is relevant for all levels of a clinical training program within higher education and at affiliated training sites.

Clinical supervisors and educators are often wary of the process of documentation, challenged by balancing not enough and too much in the recording of events as well as the time it takes to thoughtfully describe events in written form. In jurisdictions known as *public record states*, this reticence may be increased by available access to records. In the mental health professions, documentation is used for many adaptive reasons to support the ongoing process of tracking clinical work. This same logic and procedures apply to the practices of clinical training and supervision efforts, regardless of institution or jurisdiction-specific policies. Recording the progress of supervisees and students and their interpersonal and intrapersonal behavior and professional conduct in the context of clinical training is especially critical when problematic behavior emerges.

Documenting the details of a trainee's behavior that may compromise client welfare is an essential component of gatekeeping. Documentation expectations of the clinical professions are further explained in the *ACA Code of Ethics* (American Counseling Association [ACA], 2014a) Standards A.1.b., A.6.c., and B.6.; the *Ethical Principles of Psychologists and Code of Conduct* (American Psychological Association, 2017c) Sections 3 and 6; the *NASW Code of Ethics* (National Association of Social Workers, 2017) Section 3.04; and the American Association for Marriage and Family Therapy (2015) *Code of Ethics* Sections 3.5 and 6.4. Supplementing these professions' ethical standards are the documentation and record-keeping requirements established by the licensure and practice laws of regulatory boards in state jurisdictions. Although these standards address documentation requirements affecting client care, the intent and content can be extended to record keeping for tracking the progress of clinical trainees. In addition, various agencies and educational institutions typically have documentation guidelines that can substantiate the acts of informing, remediating, and dismissing students or supervisees.

Understanding recommended procedures for evaluating and recording supervisee or student conduct is a necessary process that enables supervisors, educators, and clinical trainers to fulfill their ethical and legal obligation as professional gatekeepers (Guest, Jackson, & Dooley, 1999). Intentional documentation as gatekeepers also models professional behavior and competence for students and supervisees as they enter the field as practitioners (Gaubatz & Vera, 2006). Having defined practices and procedures to document all efforts taken to assist a student trainee in changing problematic behavior will also aid others, during and after the progression of a gatekeeping case, to understand the details and process of a situation if an administrative or legal review becomes necessary. This is most likely to occur when the program, agency, or educational institution becomes involved in charges of violating agency or institutional policy or when legal challenges are initiated.

Documentation is defined as a record of information about what occurred in a given situation; it is a tangible overview of events and includes evidence such as correspondence, progress evaluations, records of conversations, samples of student work, syllabi, calendars, written observations of behavior, minutes of meetings, policy handbooks, and/or recordings of clinical skill demonstration. Inadequate or nonexistent documentation could result in gateslipping and may undermine the protection of the well-being of future clients as well as the training program itself, especially if the program is accredited. In addition, the respondeat superiors (faculty and/or supervisors) involved in a poorly documented case may be defenseless in responding to an accusation of violation of due process.

Documentation includes all electronic or paper items that authenticate an action or event. The more detailed the documentation, the more useful it is if and when it is needed to establish the history and sequence of a chain of events. For example, during a clinical training program, when indicators of problematic behavior are either overlooked or not documented, the rationale for instituting future remediation efforts to address an accumulation of concerning performance incidents may be undermined or immobilized.

Why Document?

Documentation is a key step in substantiating gatekeeping procedures. It can assist faculty and supervisors in ensuring consistent interventions and remediation practices across trainee situations as well as provide a clear history of the needs and practices of the program, agency, or institution. Gatekeepers are charged with upholding professional standards and appropriately remediating or screening out students and supervisees ill suited for clinical work. However, providing evidence of failure to uphold professional standards is only possible with supporting documentation that clearly demonstrates a pattern of concerning behavior and the attempts to assist the individual in demonstrating acceptable professional conduct.

Documentation is also critical for reporting purposes at the departmental or institutional level. Graduate training programs are typically responsible for reporting program enrollment, retention, and completion information to outside groups such as accreditation bodies, state departments, or licensure boards. Recording necessary details, such as aggregate data on student progression as well as the functioning of individual students, is important to fulfilling the requirements of statistical reporting.

Furthermore, documentation provides not only a track record for a single case but also evidence of practices and results across multiple situations over time. This information can provide institutions and agencies with the opportunity to identify general themes or patterns that might be useful in designing prevention policies. For example, if it appears that the agency repeatedly seems to be hiring graduates seeking supervision for licensure who disregard or are ill informed about ethical practices, supervisors might consult about the root causes of this problem as a risk management strategy as well as for quality control of services provided. The agency may choose to conduct more thorough screening of applicants prior to engaging in supervisory relationships, it might consider the educational institutions from which supervisees have graduated as a determinant of employment, or it could design an ethics training workshop to be required of every new employee to inform supervisees about expectations and standards of practice. Without awareness of themes that emerge from multiple documentation points across time and situations, such proactive interventions would not be possible.

Providing a Timeline

Thorough documentation can be utilized to support developmental plans for trainee growth and change. Written records of progress are helpful tools for gauging whether trainees are advancing as expected in comparison to the program or agency's standards. Reflecting on the historical information accumulated in a student's record can assist the supervisor and supervisee in evaluating progress and identifying goals for necessary areas of growth, a future deadline, or the coming academic year. Even if a student is in good academic standing, clinical educators are aware that training is not centered solely on academics and documentation of progress, and goal attainment is essential for both the development and demonstration of clinical skills and professional conduct.

The recommended practice for training programs is to have a written policy for documenting behaviors or conduct of concern as well as ongoing scheduled evaluation data. Documentation practices and expectations of faculty and supervisors should be proceduralized and all responsible parties informed of the process. This includes adjunct faculty, clinical faculty, site supervisors, and secondary supervisors. Documenting trainee performance and progress, especially when red flags are observed, allows all involved and responsible parties access to a collection of informational data that can reveal patterns, timelines, cycles of progress or lack of progress, administrative or intervention actions attempted, trainee responses, and other details critical to substantiating the initiation of the gatekeeping process.

Promoting Objectivity

Many students and supervisees have learning curves or developmental challenges that can lead to problematic situations. The goal of educators is to support students striving for successful growth in their learning process and advancement as professionals. If behaviors of concern continue to occur without change, documentation will show that pattern objectively, rather than relying on the memories of involved faculty or clinical colleagues. Maintaining records with as much objectivity as possible will assist all involved in the remediation process, which can often occur over an extended period of time. Documentation across relevant interactions and events can also diffuse the influence of one individual's subjective perspective or goals for change—whether that be the student/supervisee or the faculty/supervisor.

Ensuring Consistency

Documenting expectations and progress also assists faculty and supervisors in consistently applying achievement standards across advisees, students, and supervisees, ensuring fairness and, if challenged, proving uniformity of responses across situations. Documentation includes published expectations or program standards documented in a program handbook as a measure for all students; an institution or agency's criteria for policies and procedures found in a graduate catalog or employee handbook or manual; and other published sources of information describing expected behavior, conduct, and performance. Referring to these institutional publications when documenting interventions, such as remediation procedures, supports the evidence that gatekeeping practices are grounded in policy and not opinion based—a critical standard in adjudicating gatekeeping cases in court related to charges of arbitrary and capricious injustices. Documentation also substantiates that the program or agency's policies are informing the gatekeeping process.

When to Document

It is important to understand not only the importance of documentation but also when to initiate documentation. Recording student progression throughout a graduate program is important because it provides a recorded timeline of fulfilled requirements, observed events, and/or concerns raised. (See On the Legal Side 11.1.) Documented behaviors can be preventive and should not be initiated only after a problem is identified; rather, best practice recommendations support

On the Legal Side 11.1

A student dismissed from a graduate training program filed a lawsuit against the university. The attorney representing the student was attempting to establish a basis for arbitrary and capricious action toward the dismissed student and implied age and gender discrimination on the part of the faculty. During a deposition with the faculty member who had served as department chair at the time, the attorney asked details about past students who had participated in remediation processes or who had been dismissed. He asked questions about gender, age, and the standard violations of each student involved. The department chair was not able to recount all of the information in the moment and asked whether she could return the following day with the information after referencing her records. Because of the documentation practices of her program, the information was chronicled, and she was able to construct a chart detailing previous students involved in remediation and dismissal proceedings from the past 10 years, excluding identifying information. Despite intensive questioning, the plaintiff's attorney was unable to establish a pattern of age or gender discrimination given the information documented in the department's records. The lawsuit was amended accordingly.

consistent documentation practices across multiple points in time that can establish patterns of progress or demonstrations of acute or chronic behavior. Throughout a graduate program, most students will encounter universal or routine benchmark points that are worthy of documentation. Examples of routine documentation points include the following:

- The student's application to the graduate program
- Evidence of entering student agreement to abide by program policies and the ethical guidelines of the profession, such as the verification of understanding in Appendix E
- Performance reviews conducted at the conclusion of the first semester, every semester, and/or annually
- Successful completion of a critical course, sequence of courses, or given semester with a minimum specified grade
- Demonstration of a predetermined level of clinical ability during a preliminary skills course or a prepracticum experience
- Demonstration of appropriate interpersonal behavior or professional conduct as evaluated at the conclusion of each year of enrollment in the graduate program

As students or supervisees advance in a clinical training program, documented points of achievement accrue and reveal a pattern of student development. Thus, it is important that the assessment processes and timing of evaluation points be standardized for all trainees throughout the graduate program or field experience. Each program has its own timeline of expected achievements; thus, documentation points should be adapted accordingly.

Maintaining documentation while and after an individual is enrolled in a graduate program is especially helpful when one is subsequently endorsing trainees for graduation, certification, or licensure, especially because not all licenses or certifications in the mental health professions have the same requirements across jurisdictions. When one is endorsing graduates, records maintained over the progression of training, especially in clinical practice settings, provide information needed to determine whether program requirements (e.g., course content) or completed field experiences (e.g., number of clinical contact hours completed) fulfill the requirements for licensure as defined by a given state's regulatory body, not just the regulatory body of the home state where the degree was obtained.

Best practice recommendations for documentation in a training program include having a clear and transparent protocol for recording trainee progress, accessing records, preserving records, determining a length of time to maintain records, and destroying timed-out records. Information describing the program's practices and procedures for documenting may be stored in multiple locations and various means (hard copy and electronic). Many programs will choose to publish procedures in a program or faculty handbook, supporting easy access to this information by core faculty, new faculty, faculty with multiple departmental appointments, and adjunct faculty as well as students. Evaluation processes are commonly discussed with students as part of a mandatory new student orientation to the clinical program and also are published in a student handbook and/or graduate catalog that is typically posted online.

Faculty practices and timelines regarding maintaining documentation should be discussed in the same detail and with regularity among all faculty responsible for preserving the process. New faculty, whether adjunct or core, should be alerted to and educated about procedures for documenting student progress to prevent gaps in data collection. The same holds true for field site placement directors and supervisors. These partners in the clinical training process should be informed about the critical importance of communicating and documenting observations of trainee progress or behaviors of concern at the earliest moment the behavior occurs. Agency field site partners should also be educated about the standardized evaluation instruments and processes they will be expected to utilize at scheduled points in the practicum or internship period. Thus, graduate training programs should have written policies of what, when, where, and how to document, followed by how to maintain those records for easy access by all individuals responsible for teaching, supervising, and evaluating trainees. (See What Would You Do? 11.1.)

The timing of documentation can also be critical in defending program faculty or field site supervisory practices if challenges to policies

What Would You Do? 11.1

Procedures in your program require that all faculty, core and adjunct, contribute information about their observations or evidence of each student's progress, especially issues of concern, in advance of the annual evaluation meeting. The purpose of this procedure is to gain a comprehensive understanding of each student from the professionals with whom the student has interacted. The annual evaluation process includes identifying any actions that need to be taken to inform the student of the faculty's concerns, reviewing program expectations, and establishing a plan for action or further development with the student to change the behaviors of concern. This is typically assigned to the student's advisor to handle as an informal feedback meeting.

One of your advisees was identified as a student of concern during the annual evaluation period at the conclusion of his first year in the program because of some general disruptive behaviors in class that appeared occasionally. Your advisee is now in his second year of the graduate program. This week you learned that he engaged combatively with a faculty member in class and lost his temper with a peer colleague in a class discussion. In this instance, he was unable to manage his emotional reactions and was reported to have verbally attacked other students in class with whom he disagreed. Several students who were negatively affected by this student's behavior approached the department chair to complain about the lack of safety in their classroom due to his intimidating behavior and recounted multiple incidents that led to their fear of speaking up in class.

The faculty met to review and discuss these most recent concerns and to consider how to intervene with the student and address his problematic behavior while also creating a plan to protect the learning environment for other students. Part of the deliberation was whether this was a one-time incident or an indication of a developing problem. A faculty member casually mentioned in the meeting that this same student had "gone off" on him and others during classroom discussions once this semester and again in previous classes he had taught. Neither of these incidents had been addressed by the faculty member, reported, or documented. This information significantly raised the level of concern about this student; however, the multiple missed opportunities to initiate gatekeeping procedures may have reinforced the student's behavior as acceptable. The faculty are now very concerned about your student's inability to control his behavior (intrapersonal problem), interact effectively with peers and resolve conflict (interpersonal problem), and behave in a manner that is expected of a marriage and family therapist (professional conduct).

What would you do?

What would you say to the faculty member who chose to avoid confronting or reporting the student's behavior?

How do you approach your advisee about his pattern of highly problematic behaviors, especially after his pattern of emotional reactivity over time has been overlooked?

What are the due process challenges if the faculty decides that it is necessary to immediately suspend the student from continuing in the program to ensure the safety of others and the integrity of the learning environment?

(Continued)

What Would You Do? 11.1 *(Continued)*

Once this incident is dealt with, what measures are needed within your department and among the faculty to prevent a similar situation from occurring in the future?

or litigation arise. Being able to substantiate that students or supervisees knew of policies in advance and agreed to comply with those policies is very helpful when problems occur. It is important to have a procedure for collecting, dating or time stamping, and maintaining relevant documentation as an aspect of gatekeeping.

What to Document

Progression benchmarks and evaluation points are often determined by the structure of the training program (e.g., cohort vs. rolling enrollment model, a lock-step program of study vs. an unstructured sequence of course enrollment). For all benchmarks, there are important components of documentation, whether housed within the official academic student record maintained by the institution on all matriculated students or informally recorded as working documents within the department during the period when a student is enrolled. One variation in this practice may be for nondegree/nonmatriculated students who are permitted to take courses, although even they should be familiar with relevant program policies in advance of registration, even when there is no reason to conduct ongoing evaluations of them beyond the course. Documentation should be initiated whenever contact occurs regarding concerns about student or supervisee functioning. Appendix G provides multiple samples of documentation of student behavior and faculty action.

All recorded information should include, although not necessarily be limited to, the following:

- The *date*, *time*, and *location* where the interaction or event occurred.
- The names of all *individuals in attendance* at each contact and their role in the interaction. It is important to note that there is a fine line between documenting names and using initials to protect identities. This is a gray area when a possible concern is first noted. It is recommended that gatekeepers use initials until such a time when full names are required for formal remediation and official record keeping.
- A brief *description of the purpose* or rationale for the event or action being documented (e.g., follow-up to a midpoint evaluation by the practicum site supervisor; a meeting to address the interpersonal functioning of a student; an annual advising

appointment to check in on the student's progress academically, clinically, personally, and professionally).

- An update or *review of prior contacts* related to the current action or event, including descriptions and the status of previously identified plans, goals, or outcomes, if relevant. Records should also include a detailed description of the *content discussed* during the contact—what was stated and who stated it—as it is relevant to the purpose of the meeting or issue at hand.
- A description of the *processes that occurred* during the contact—functionally and interactionally. Depending on the interaction, this description might include the trainee's conduct and reactions, such as specific nonverbal observations that occurred, or the tenor of the meeting.
- The basis or *rationale for identifying concerns* (e.g., ethics codes, program standards, the university handbook, university catalog, agency procedures book, state licensing boards).
- The *action or remediation plan* created during the documented contact, if applicable, specifically stating the full names of who will perform what action by what date based on the concern addressed in the meeting discussion. Action plans are usually constructed at the end of a meeting to consolidate the discussion and decisions that occurred and to create a consensus among all in attendance. Creating an action or remediation plan may take multiple meetings, perhaps in different formats (by phone, in person, etc.). It is recommend that gatekeepers use one document for the action plan rather than having one version for the student(s) and one for the faculty/supervisor(s).
- *Distribution of the meeting summary* and/or action plan (if such an outcome occurred). Once finalized, this document should be sent to all involved. Depending on the type of meeting (formal or informal), an e-mail recounting the meeting and/or decision may suffice. For situations that require official notification, a standard letter printed on official letterhead sent via certified mail to the student's home address may be appropriate. An additional formal e-mail may also be sent if the university or agency has adopted e-mail as the official form of institutional communication.
- The *trainee's recourse*, such as an appeals process, in challenging a program procedure or decision. It might be appropriate to include this information when a change in student status is part of a formal outcome notification.
- *Signatures or other written acknowledgment* validating participation in a meeting, receipt of follow-up correspondence, or review by appropriate members in the institutional chain of command. In other words, records should include documentation to prove that the individuals who need to see the information have been provided with access to it.

Similar to clinical case records, documentation practices illustrate for the student or supervisee the appropriate process for addressing concerns as outlined by ethics codes and due process laws. ACA provides the most detailed guidance on gatekeeping practices of the four allied mental health professions. Standard F.6.b. of the *ACA Code of Ethics* (ACA, 2014a) states that supervisors "seek consultation and document their decisions to dismiss or refer supervisees for assistance. They ensure that supervisees are aware of options available to them to address such decisions." This same statement is reiterated in Standard F.9.b.1. as it applies to educators working with students. The only way to verify that these ethical practices occurred is through documentation. Samples of documentation in line with these suggestions are available in Appendix G.

Documenting Trainees' Understanding

Another best practice to ensure that students have received and understand policies and procedures expected of all trainees is to include a verification of understanding procedure as part of the orientation process and at each new stage of the graduate program. Examples of occasions when a written agreement informing trainees of expectations during a forthcoming phase of training is appropriate include entry into the training program, commencement of clinical work, or commencement of a contracted supervisory relationship. Some programs may have other points during the course of training when a new set of expectations for student behavior are initiated. Attaining each trainee's acknowledgment of receiving, reading, and agreeing to the procedures, policies, and expectations published in critical documents emphasizes the importance of the information. The critical documents listed in a verification of understanding or informed consent document may include the graduate program or agency's handbook or catalog, ethics of the profession represented, human resources policy, academic honor policy, or other documents that contain required policies and procedures that participants need to read and for which they will be held accountable. The sample verification of understanding form provided in Appendix E was designed to be issued to entering students at the new student orientation. Asking trainees to read this important information and affirm fulfillment of this responsibility via their signature serves as documented informed consent for enrolling and engaging in the training program or supervisory relationship. The signed verification form should be returned by a designated date to an assigned representative (faculty member, agency supervisor, postdegree supervisor) prior to or at the beginning of enrolling in a training program or starting as a supervisee at a clinical agency field site. Acknowledging receipt of, understanding of, and agreement with information about topics such as student assessment criteria, ethical guidelines, requirements for professional conduct and personal behavior, remediation, retention, and gatekeeping processes as published in training documents informs students and alerts them to the seriousness of program and professional standards.

A similar procedure can be followed at the commencement of fieldwork experiences. It is prudent for training programs to document that students or supervisees have acknowledged receipt of key documents. This verifies that they understand the information and agree to abide by the policies and expectations of the profession and the program in advance of their enrollment or soon after they begin the graduate program.

Agency field sites and site supervisors should similarly document a supervisee's understanding of their organizational policies, expectations, and procedures during the supervisee orientation process. Following initial notification of program/agency requirements, it is recommended practice for training programs at either academic or field sites to document ongoing informational or evaluation processes and outcomes, noting any observations of concern about a student or trainee's behavior when they are first noticed and recording all efforts taken to inform the student of the concerns.

Documentation and Student Privacy

The Family Educational Rights and Privacy Act (FERPA) regulates disclosure of student records and grades. This act includes some categories of documentation within educational institutions and in conjunction with outside partners involved in the training process. Sometimes trainees have the idea that supervisors and faculty members are bound by the same confidentiality mandates provided to a client. It is important to inform students that confidentiality of documentation, discussions, and other disclosures in a training setting cannot be assured because consultation among respondeat superiors, a best practice standard in gatekeeping, may be necessary to monitor student progress. This is best conveyed by a statement in the program's student handbook or policy manual. Despite their need for consultation, it is important for faculty and supervisors to be mindful of federal or institutional rules regarding the confidentiality of records of a trainee or supervisee's performance, both positive and problematic.

Educators and supervisors should consider the general principle of need to know as a guide in protecting the privacy of students to the best extent possible. The sharing of information and documents with colleagues such as site supervisors, adjunct faculty, administrators, and others not directly involved in the student oversight process should only occur when it is necessary to support the educational needs of the student and as it contributes to providing support and/or remedial correction aimed at student success. Others working with the student or supervisee may need to be informed of documented concerns in order to assess student progress, maintain oversight of client care, or support student development. Individuals on the receiving end of information about a trainee should be instructed to maintain student privacy as appropriate.

The line between gossiping about a student and discussing plans for addressing concerns can be very thin, and clinical educators and supervisors are encouraged to model professional behavior in following the need-to-know principle as a guide for their behaviors. When information about a trainee is shared with other members of a training team for purposes of consultation or protection, it is prudent to document who was included in the discussion, what information was shared, and why it was shared. This is the best strategy for maintaining accurate professional records illustrating all efforts taken to support a student. Recording these actions also protects clients, involved faculty member(s), and/or supervisor(s), should their actions be questioned at a future time.

When it comes to engaging in a gatekeeping process or procedure, although it may be tempting to have all individuals initially involved in a situation participate in sharing information, program faculty must identify the primary stakeholders who truly need to be a part of evaluating and addressing the trainee's concerns. A good question to ask is this: Who are the (least number of) individuals who need to be involved in the details of a remedial intervention at this point?

Consider the case of an adjunct faculty member who observes problematic behavior and notifies the core faculty of a student exhibiting interpersonal problems via an e-mail.

- Should the adjunct faculty member be involved in the initial meeting discussing the problems with the student?
- Is it appropriate for the adjunct to be involved in the discussion and decisions about remedial strategies?
- Should core faculty keep the adjunct informed of the student's progress in relation to the remediation plan?
- Is the adjunct faculty member's presence or involvement critical to determining the student's status pending the outcome of the remediation plan?

Often, the only parties who need to sign a remediation action plan are the trainee, the immediate supervisor(s) or faculty member(s) who is (are) directly supervising the remediation process, and any faculty members or supervisors who are assigned to consult on the situation. The individual who reports the initial concern may not need to be a participant in the process of investigating the situation further, developing action or remediation plans, or making decisions about student progression from point to point. At some stage in a disciplinary process, the participation of the department chair or the administrative supervisor/director of the involved organization(s) should be considered on a case-by-case basis while ensuring as much respect and privacy for the trainee as possible. Ultimately, individuals involved should have a clear purpose in supporting the developmental growth and adaptive changes desired from the student/trainee.

When a situation with a student or supervisee begins to become more involved (i.e., moving from informal feedback to the initiation of remediation activities), best practice recommendations are that more than one faculty member or supervisor be present in feedback discussions (McAdams, Foster, & Ward, 2007). Additional faculty member(s) or supervisor(s) can assist in observing and confirming trainee responses, moderate the opinions of others, serve as process observers who notice countertransference or attempts at splitting, or document meeting content from more than one perspective; however, too many participants can result in a range of different opinions that can subvert the development of a consensus for action and confuse the process. Avoiding confusion and lack of consensus may be especially important in the case of future challenges to the outcome of the remediation process.

How to Document

The content of documentation regarding students and trainees should be detailed enough so that someone who did not attend the meeting would understand the purpose of the meeting and the events that occurred. Decisions made at meetings should be clearly articulated in writing. Exchanges that occurred relating to concerning behavior should be described as close to verbatim as is possible. Any observable actions or reactions of significance that are relevant to the presenting issue should be detailed in behavioral terms. It is recommended that faculty members and supervisors always document exchanges with students or supervisees with the assumption that the record may become a piece of legal evidence, just as with client records. Appendix G contains several samples of documentation of student behavior and faculty action.

In objective documentation practices, two primary assumptions inform the goals of the documentation record itself. First, the wording used in the record should concisely and specifically describe the observed behavior, especially as it reflects the concern related to the clinical training program's standards: expectations of trainees, ethics, licensing requirements, safety of clients or others, and so on. The same wording that is used in the record can also be used to follow up with the trainee in a postmeeting letter. Second, the documentation must be thought of as an official or legal document that contains information known to all involved, including the trainee. This is important in fulfilling due process standards (refer to Chapters 2 and 3 for more information on critical terminology).

When meetings are arranged to address a specific concern, it can be helpful to construct an agenda for the meeting that can also serve as an outline for the written record of the meeting. Having an agenda is a particularly smart way to organize content and assign the involvement of all participants to provide for efficiency in task orientation.

Written documentation should be completed during or immediately following an exchange, conversation, or meeting. Once the person assigned to writing the record of a meeting has completed the task, the recorded notes should be sent to those in attendance to correct any misinformation or inaccurately portrayed events before the documentation is finalized. When meeting with a student or supervisee, whether it be for a formal or informal discussion, the gatekeeper should produce a written summary of the critical points of the meeting. In the case of a remediation proceeding, the formal detailed documentation should be sent via e-mail and/or certified mail to the trainee as soon as possible. If documentation is sent via e-mail, it is appropriate to ask all recipients to acknowledge receipt of the message. It is helpful when documentation can be completed and e-mailed to all parties involved within 48 hours. This will allow the content of the meeting to remain fresh in participants' memories so that if any adjustments to language, procedures, reported outcomes, and so on, need to be made, they can be identified quickly. A swift turnaround also allows the student or supervisee the opportunity to clarify information, make an expedient response, or contest the content of the documentation.

Processing of the documentation should be guided by program policies. For example, determining where the information is stored, by whom, and in what format is worthy of consideration. If only one person maintains the documentation on his or her computer, what is the backup system in the event of a technical issue or the absence of that individual? Should data be stored on a secure share drive or Internet cloud system? Who should receive e-mail copies of documentation? When should paper copies of documentation be utilized? These important questions should be considered with an awareness of long-term needs. Developing and implementing policies helps to ensure consistent practices.

Ultimately, documentation is for the benefit of both the clinical training program and the trainee. It is in the best interest of the training program to provide a transparent and consistent process to equitably support students and to manage problematic situations by documenting a timeline of actions and compliance with published policies and procedures and by creating a paper trail in the event of needed follow-up, intervention, or remediation. In addition, it is in the best interest of the student or supervisee to receive concrete evidence of his or her accomplishments in the program and benchmark assessment points (e.g., capstone experiences) and to receive a clear record for planning future goals for optimal student development. Documentation is also important for worst-case scenarios, such as the filing of complaints, appeals, or legal action. When they have proactive documentation, gatekeepers go through these emotionally challenging and time-consuming processes much more easily and with greater confidence.

It is always important to remember the two adages of documentation:

- If it's not written down (documented), it didn't happen!
- Write for the record as if the trainee were reading over one shoulder and an attorney were reading over the other.

Practical Examples for Clinical Educators and Supervisors

Bringing together the when, what, how, and why of documentation is a critical requirement for best practices in the gatekeeping process. The following are universal examples that can be relevant to any clinical specialty area. Faculty and supervisors are encouraged to consider these examples as they apply the components of documentation from a gatekeeping perspective and to consider how these examples may be helpful to the institutions and agencies where they contribute to clinical training efforts.

Each graduate training program has its own style or approach to program management and student development. It is important to remember that the best practice suggestions and benchmarks presented in this chapter and book are meant to be broad enough to assist you in adapting them to best suit your program needs. Regardless of variations in program approaches, documentation points should be consistently followed according to the stated procedures and policies of the department, program, or agency.

The first recommended benchmark for documentation is the application file and the admissions committee's decision, including any reservations that arise about a prospective student. The end of the first semester is the next point in documenting student adjustment, although a formal evaluation of student progress may be deferred to the end of the first year in some programs. The annual evaluation of students should include documentation of the progress of each student academically, clinically, professionally, and personally as related to qualities necessary to function as a clinician. The documentation should include a quantitative rating, qualitative comments about the ratings or emerging concerns, and planned action to support or provide feedback to the student about his or her performance. Documenting evaluation data in a spreadsheet or chart that can be viewed by all in a meeting simultaneously is a helpful strategy. A key to the meaning of quantitative ratings that describe qualitative attributes or criteria should be available to all who are using the rating system. See Appendix H for a sample student progress evaluation rating form and accompanying rubric used for an annual evaluation process completed by faculty for all students enrolled in a clinical program.

A system for documenting student achievement relative to the published standards or expectations of the program must be constructed to prove a systematic pattern of evaluation of and feedback to students. Scheduled evaluation points are required by some program accreditation standards, such as those of the Council for Accreditation of Counseling and Related Educational Programs (2015). The student evaluation process should also include an opportunity for students to self-reflect and report on their perceived development as clinicians-in-training. A self-assessment report could include a standardized evaluation instrument as well as the opportunity to provide a qualitative narrative reflecting the student's efforts in the program. Some additional questions to consider in documenting student progress include the following:

- What skills or strengths does the student use or exhibit?
- How is he or she engaging in the self-reflection process?
- What supports might the student benefit from to optimize his or her successful continuation in the program?
- What areas of continued development does the student need to focus on and further develop (e.g., interpersonal communication skills, critical thinking, analytical skills, self-confidence, helping skills).

A quantitative system for an evaluation process may include a standardized instrument with a rating system or Likert-type scale responses. Scale descriptors such as "working toward," "making progress," "actively working on," or "regularly demonstrated" might be helpful. Chapter 9 discusses methods of evaluating students and supervisees. Both faculty or supervisors and trainees can complete the same evaluation method or form to provide multiple perspectives and comparison points on a supervisee or student's progress.

Once student evaluations are completed, the faculty advisor or supervisor can meet with the student/supervisee to discuss the evaluation, offer feedback, and identify strategies that support areas of needed development and future success. The important points of the conversation should be documented, shared as a follow-up summary for the student in written form, and placed in the student's record. The same procedures can be followed for documenting similar aspects of training events or assessment points.

Ethical Implications for Documentation

Encountering ethical or legal dilemmas is a challenge that reinforces the need to establish preventive and intentional protocols and practices for documentation. Implementing consistent record-keeping procedures assists supervisors, educators, and training programs in clearly and efficiently identifying patterns of behavior, whether those patterns are problematic or adaptive (Jasonson et al., 2008). Documentation also provides evidence of the feedback process, which assists the supervisor or faculty member in supporting trainees who are able and willing to improve by establishing how they were previously successful. This information, when reinforced as constructive feedback based on a documented pattern, can contribute to a trainee's self-efficacy, self-concept, and self-esteem as a future clinician. Alternatively, documentation may provide evidence that reveals that a trainee or supervisee is incapable of or unwilling to change despite feedback and/or attempted remedial interventions. A pattern or timeline of events revealed in a student record can be as important as the content and can also support decisions regarding student or supervisee continuation in a program. Determining a trainee's track record is important in initiating gatekeeping processes based on ethical principles and mandates.

A common reason why many educators and supervisors avoid documenting when they should stems from anxiety that whatever is written may be used against them at some point in the future. It is true that creating a record concretizes an individual's observations, concerns, and decisions; however, faculty and supervisors are encouraged to remember their ethical obligations to evaluate and act on student progress, intervening when necessary. Maintaining records that are objective recordings of observable behavior, and that are affirmed through consultation with and the input of others involved, can help minimize these concerns. Professionalism is an expectation inherent in the ethics codes and standards of the clinical professions (reference Chapter 2 for more information). The components of professional conduct are important for educators and supervisors working to protect and train future practitioners and acting in the best interest of current and future clients (Bernard & Goodyear, 2014).

Ethical decision making is often emotionally charged. One practice for ensuring the accuracy and objectivity of documentation is to have other supervisors or faculty members review the draft copy of a report, meeting description, or proposed correspondence. These consultants may suggest wording to minimize the appearance of emotional reactivity, bias, or judgmental commentary that may emerge on the part of the writer or may clarify important descriptions on which the remedial action is based. Documenting behavior and reactions impartially chronicles valuable information about an individual's pattern of behavior. Collegial review is also a helpful practice in coconstructing records of events from multiple perspectives. Few situations escalate to legal matters; however, assuming the possibility of litigious action encourages a faculty member or clinical supervisor to make intentional efforts to be conscientious in record-keeping efforts routinely.

Another suggested strategy is to incorporate information about the importance of documentation practices into the curriculum, particularly at the doctoral level, when engaging in discussions about gatekeeping and ethical decision-making processes in attending to problematic students. This approach provides the opportunity for future supervisors and faculty members to learn about adaptive and objective documentation practices. Documentation can also be infused into an ethics course, which is typically a standard requirement across all clinical specialty areas. This assists trainees who will become future educators and supervisors in learning about and adopting helpful documentation skills, understanding the importance of establishing clear record-keeping systems, and demystifying the benefits of documentation beyond its application to client records.

Best practices for clinical training are grounded in the frameworks of ethics codes of the profession (e.g., the *ACA Code of Ethics* [ACA, 2014a], *Ethical Principles of Psychologists and Code of Conduct* [American Psychological Association, 2017c]) as well as other professional specialties. For programs that also hold discipline-specific professional accreditations, program standards require documentation to ensure equitable and consistent practices as well as evidence that those practices are being implemented. The Council for Accreditation of Counseling and Related Educational Programs (2015), American Psychological Association Commission on Accreditation (2015), Council on Social Work Education Commission on Accreditation (2015), and Commission on Accreditation for Marriage and Family Therapy Education (2017) are highly regarded resources among training programs because they reflect the desired standards of clinical preparation within the given profession. In these manuals and the respective associations' ethics codes, supervisors and educators can find additional requirements that can be considered best practice standards as they inform the establishment of procedures for data collection, evaluation of the data collected, and documentation of these processes.

Documentation and Due Process

As discussed in Chapters 2 and 3, due process is detailed in the Fourteenth Amendment to the U.S. Constitution and also addressed in state laws. Chronicling events in written form as they occur is especially critical when an outcome results in the dismissal of a trainee from a training program and/or a delay in graduation (e.g., being held back for a semester or a year for additional remediation or additional supervised training) incites litigation. Programs should note that in due process cases, the burden of proof resides with the plaintiff; however, in order to defend the fact that due process was followed, the program or agency must rely on unambiguous documentation to prove that it provided the trainee with ample opportunity to meet the standards of the program or training site (Gilfoyle, 2008; Olkin & Gaughen, 1991) and did not act in an arbitrary or capricious manner. Proving this calls for documentation that substantiates that the trainee was advised of the evaluation process and outcome, was explicitly informed of potential outcomes if the action plan or if remediation criteria were not satisfied, and was given appropriate support and occasion to demonstrate change. Corroborating details must be recorded in writing, not just offered verbally in discussion. Proper documentation efforts also include providing the trainee with a copy or summary of all information gathered, providing evidence that the situation and alternatives were explained, and providing evidence that the timeline of events was consistent with due process procedures.

Conclusion

Clear and transparent documentation procedures throughout the entire training experience—beginning with the admissions process and concluding with graduation or licensure—are important not only to affirm progress or readiness to continue through checkpoints or gates within the training sequence but also to establish a record of problematic situations and the attempted remedies. Best practices in gatekeeping include documenting that evaluation processes were implemented thoroughly and consistently for each student and supervisee across the course of his or her training while also documenting the outcomes of any actions taken to support student development. Having all documentation procedures vetted, institutionalized, and disseminated to all affected participants in advance of implementation contributes to effective and efficient best practices in chronicling student progress. It also models professional behavior that students-in-training can incorporate into their future practices as clinicians, educators, and supervisors.

It is crucial that clinical educators and supervisors who maintain records do so with as much objectivity as possible to assist in fair and just application of the remediation process. The fairness of a remediation or dismissal proceeding might be tested administratively or legally, and timely documentation may be the only source confirming how past events led to the processes or conclusions in question. Maintaining consistent formats for constructing documentation also ensures that practices and policies are grounded in standards or policy, not opinion. Should a situation escalate to the legal realm, having evidence of objective and professionally supported efforts that are fairly and consistently applied to all trainees would be useful in disproving charges of arbitrary or capricious treatment.

Clinical educators and supervisors are reminded that the goal of gatekeeping is not to punish or limit students who experience problematic challenges during their training sequence; rather, the goal is to support students and supervisees in affirming and facilitating their successful professional growth and development to the extent possible. Ultimately, documentation substantiates the processes that occurred over the course of trainees' educational and training experience to support them in their academic, clinical, and professional development and establishes the goodness of fit of trainees for the clinical profession they seek to enter.

Key Points and Best Practices

- Intentional documentation supports best practices for all parties involved—educators, supervisors, and trainees.
- Best practice recommendations for documentation in clinical training programs include having a clear and transparent protocol for recording trainee progress, accessing records, preserving records, determining a length of time to maintain records, and destroying timed-out records.
- Documentation procedures in an agency or institution should be vetted, institutionalized, and disseminated to all affected participants in advance of their implementation.
- Documentation policies should be consistently followed according to the stated procedures of the department, program, or agency.
- Consistent documentation practices across multiple points in time can establish patterns of trainee progress or problematic behavior.
- Including a verification of understanding procedure as part of the new trainee orientation process and again at each stage of advancement into a new level of training (such as proceeding to clinical work) is recommended. This document serves as validation that critical policy information was provided to the trainee in advance and also verifies that the trainee was informed of and consented to fulfill the expectations and requirements of the training program.
- Trainees should be informed in advance that confidentiality of documentation, discussions, and other disclosures in a training setting cannot be assured because consultation among respondeat superiors is a critical aspect of the gatekeeping process.
- When gatekeeping situations with a student or supervisee become more involved (i.e., moving from informal feedback to the initiation of remediation activities), best practice recommendations are that more than one faculty member or supervisor be present during all interactions and meetings with the trainee, especially when gender differences are involved.
- Documentation should be initiated whenever contact occurs regarding concerns about student or supervisee functioning.
- Documentation can be a preventive process that both informs and establishes transparent and equitable practices and policies.
- It is important to remember the two adages of documentation: (a) If it's not written down (documented), it didn't happen! and (b) Write for the record as if the trainee were reading over one shoulder and an attorney were reading over the other.

Chapter 12

Preventing Problematic Behavior in Trainees

Theresa A. Coogan and Alicia M. Homrich

The vast majority of students and supervisees aspire to meet the expectations of their training program, graduate, and achieve licensure and professional employment. Most trainees are capable of achieving this goal and are willing to make the necessary effort and corrections to do so. At times, some students or supervisees struggle more than others. Whether the struggle is small or large, it is the appropriate occasion for experienced members of the profession involved in the training milieu to step in and proactively support trainees' development and achievement potential.

The clinical professions suffer whenever an inappropriate candidate is graduated or licensed. There is the potential for harm to not only clients but also the public's opinion of the helping professions, which can further stigmatize the value of mental health practice. Faculty and supervisors have a vested interest in assisting students and supervisees in performing well. Institutions that graduate or launch effective mental health clinicians enhance their status and potential success for recruiting future trainees who are drawn to programs with high standards. This reputation is affected not only by respectable graduation rates and training outcomes but also by the quality of the graduates or trainees as they integrate into the profession.

Educational programs, faculty, training sites, and supervisors should commit to supporting trainees in becoming effective practitioners who have the skills and professional qualities needed to best serve their clients. Proactively preparing trainees to adopt strategies that promote personal wellness and long-term healthy functioning can help prevent problematic behavior in both the training setting and future professional practice.

Modeling Appropriate Behavior

Students and supervisees observe their faculty and supervisors' interactions and, according to Bandura's (1986) social cognitive theory, imitate the behavior of respected role models. Imitation is based on the trainees' observational perceptions and the interrelated processes of attention, retention, production, and motivation, which lead to integration and enactment of the observed behavior. "According to Bandura's social learning theory, trainees learn essential professional competencies by observing a role model—defined in the medical literature as a person considered to demonstrate a standard of excellence to be imitated" (Jochemsen-van der Leeuw, van Dijk, van Etten-Jamaludin, & Wieringa-de Waard, 2013, p. 26). Elements of client care, including effective communication skills and professional conduct, are examples of modeled behavior that influence a student's development as a clinician. Role models are people who have specific qualities that students and supervisees would like to have or individuals who hold positions that trainees aspire to attain, such as licensed clinician, future faculty member, or supervisor. Role models are considered examples to be emulated based on their professional manner, qualities, and effectiveness as clinical practitioners. Desirable characteristics include responsibility, enthusiasm, compassion, openness, integrity, and positive interpersonal relationships in the professional setting (Paice, Heard, & Moss, 2002). Role models help teach learners the values and behaviors essential to being professional practitioners. They foster the learning process and play a major contributing role in influencing the character, behavior, and professional values of future mental health practitioners.

Faculty members and clinical supervisors are not only experts in content and skills of the profession but also role models for the trainees whose development they oversee. Therefore, professionalism and appropriate behaviors modeled by trainers are critical and must be considered in proactively supporting the development of supervisees and students. This may seem to be a commonsense statement; however, most clinical educators and supervisors can share many stories about colleagues in the field who engage in unprofessional and/or unethical behaviors. In a comprehensive review of the literature across clinical professions, Jochemsen-van der Leeuw et al. (2013) found three categories of attributes of positive role models: patient (client) care qualities, teaching qualities, and personal qualities. Current knowledge of the field, a commitment to excellence and growth, therapeutic skills, and clinical reasoning that reflected a solid basis of knowledge were considered to be the most important qualities of clinical practitioners as role models in the findings of these researchers. In addition,

> a positive role model is compassionate, caring, engaging, and empathic to patients, and is able to build a personal connection with them. He or she is dedicated to the quality of patient care, and centers the care he or she provides on the patient rather than the illness. (p. 28)

Althouse, Stritter, and Steiner (1999) similarly observed that "role models clearly exhibited personal traits which can be described as genuinely nice, caring, warm, and committed to helping others—both their patients and their students.. . . generally aware that students were depending on them for guidance" (p. 118). These quotes highlight the importance of professional conduct and interpersonal qualities in working with clients as role modeling for trainees.

Jochemsen-van der Leeuw et al. (2013) also discovered that clinical educators were positive role models when they used a humanistic style of teaching, created a safe environment for learning, made the effort to establish interpersonal rapport with learners, and adopted a positive attitude toward trainees in general. Supervisors and educators who exhibited enthusiasm for their work and for teaching made themselves available to trainees to support and clarify their learning, encourage critical thinking, make learning exciting, and inspire achievement (Althouse et al., 1999; Jochemsen-van der Leeuw et al., 2013). Clinical educators and supervisors who actively model positive engagement and professional conduct, and who also acknowledge the importance of these qualities as role models, inspire their students and supervisees to integrate these behaviors into their own professional identities. Further specific personal characteristics of positive role models in clinical training settings include patience, self-confidence, healthy self-esteem, honesty, integrity, cooperation, humility, humanism, and leadership ability (Jochemsen-van der Leeuw et al., 2013).

Given that these interpersonal and intrapersonal qualities align with expectations and standards discussed previously in this book, the influence of training professionals as role models is critical. The training environment allows students and supervisees to practice and adopt these professional qualities in a supportive setting as they learn about who they are as clinical practitioners. Educators and supervisors are invited to reflect on their own practice by asking themselves the following question: In what ways am I modeling appropriate professional behavior to my students/supervisees? Although trainees relate to their faculty and supervisors in various ways, modeling is a powerful way to transfer professional and interpersonal values, attitudes, and patterns of thoughts and behavior to students and supervisees (Bandura, 1986). If educators view themselves as role models in the education process, they intentionally develop a learning climate that encourages continuous striving for competence, even when in the not-knowing stages of encountering a new situation. Trainers acting as role models emphasize the development of clinical competence in their trainees in terms of both acquiring knowledge and applying it to the care of clients (Althouse et al., 1999).

The research affirms the ethics codes and accreditation standards of the allied mental health professions, such as the *ACA Code of Ethics* (American Counseling Association, 2014a) and the Council for Accreditation of Counseling and Related Educational Programs (2015) standards, which stipulate that educators and supervisors have a responsibility to provide academic training that includes understanding the professional conduct expected of those practicing within the clinical field. As has been discussed in previous chapters, ethics codes describe professional behavior expected of clinical trainees. In written form, these concepts may seem abstract; however, when they are modeled by seasoned professionals, the reality of professionalism comes alive in the observed operationalization of these important attributes. Supporting positive trainee professionalism from the beginning of training, starting with the influence and instruction of faculty and concluding with the role modeling of clinical supervisors, could help minimize the development of problematic behavior.

Developing Encouraging Working Relationships With Trainees

Effectively and intentionally modeling professional conduct includes demonstrating healthy interpersonal connections, caring, and warmth and offering guidance (Althouse et al., 1999; Jochemsen-van der Leeuw et al., 2013). Trainees are drawn to clinical trainers who demonstrate these qualities and communicate effectively with students. Such trainers actively engage in two-way personal–professional relationships that support the student or supervisee's development as a clinician, often moving into the role of mentor (Paice et al., 2002). According to W. B. Johnson (2002),

> Mentoring is a personal relationship in which a more experienced (usually older) faculty member or professional acts as a guide, role model, teacher, and sponsor of a less experienced (usually younger) graduate student or junior professional. A mentor provides the protégé with knowledge, advice, challenge, counsel, and support in the protégé's pursuit of becoming a full member of a particular profession. (p. 88)

Although not all professional relationships between trainers and trainees will encompass the qualities of mentoring, both role models and mentors can create a learning environment that fosters the prosocial and professional development of students and supervisees. This experience can lead to increased career satisfaction, enhanced development of professional skills and competencies, and future achievement for clinicians-in-training (Bigelow & Johnson, 2001; W. B. Johnson, 2002). When students or supervisees respect their superiors, they are more likely to carefully observe and emulate them. They are also more receptive to advice and feedback (Bigelow & Johnson, 2001), which could potentially result in a reduced incidence of problematic behavior due to lack of guidance or example.

Establishing a positive professional relationship that is intentionally encouraging also allows supervisors and educators to more effectively approach supervisees and students with difficult feedback when their behavior is not up to standards. Trainees are more likely to be receptive to feedback about sensitive topics, such as emotional regulation, when they know the faculty member or supervisor genuinely cares about their success. In these situations, the trainee is more likely to value and respond positively to corrective information. Not all trainees enter graduate programs knowing how to act professionally; thus, supportive and encouraging relationships with caring faculty and supervisors can support changes in behavior and hopefully prevent the need to remediate problematic behavior in trainees.

Positive working relationships within departmental or agency settings that support the efforts of trainees can also reduce the need to engage in gatekeeping processes. Students and supervisees who are encouraged to perform their best work—academically, clinically, and professionally—by faculty and supervisors whom they respect and trust are more likely to respond by doing so. Any training setting that creates a culture of proactive support for excellence "can have positive and sustained impacts on . . . individual practices" (Mintrom, 2014, p. 2). Mintrom (2014) identified the following teaching strategies that promote excellence:

- Guiding work habits that embody transferable skills
- Promoting deliberate practice of learning
- Giving effective feedback
- Creating transparency by clarifying and demystifying expected performance standards
- Scaffolding teamwork among students and/or trainees as they work with their peers toward the goal of excellence

Regardless of learning style and work habits, people are more successful when they are grounded in a positive and nonthreatening environment that prioritizes their success.

Polychronis and Brown (2016) acknowledged that faculty and supervisors must understand that relationships with students and supervisees are ultimately hierarchical because of the evaluative obligations inherent in the role of respondeat superior. This includes the responsibility of gatekeeping. Regardless of the personal–professional working relationships that form through mentoring, teaching, or supervising, supervisors and professors are called on to evaluate trainees and take action if performance is substandard. Engaging intentionally in creating appropriate, meaningful, and supportive relationships with students and supervisees can expedite successful gatekeeping processes when trainees believe that their faculty or supervisors are acting in their best interests when providing critical feedback or implementing necessary remediation activities. Respondeat superiors can utilize their relational skills to create interactions that reflect caring and supportive interpersonal connections. Genuine positive regard for the individual can allow the student involved in remediation to be more receptive to the process rather than defensive, resistant, or noncompliant. When necessary, faculty and supervisors can use their skills as clinicians to work through conflict and model appropriate communication and professionalism, contributing to a supportive environment for change or acceptance of undesirable outcomes. Compassionate personal–professional relationships that support student development while also prioritizing clearly defined gatekeeping obligations contribute to transparency. Notes From the Field 12.1 provides an example of the various roles faculty or supervisors can model during a remediation process.

Fostering Professional Development to Prevent Problems

An aspect of a comprehensive training program is attention to the individual's overall personal development as a professional. Effective clinical education programs encourage trainees to engage in self-reflection to increase self-awareness, participate in self-care, and adopt professional behaviors. These components combined with substantial education about ethics and professional standards can serve as protective factors that prevent the emergence of problematic behavior in trainees as they strengthen their identity and self-efficacy as effective professionals. Although there are different theoretical frameworks in the field of mental health training, a universal perspective across most professions is the value of clinicians knowing and understanding themselves at a deeper level if they are to be effective helpers with their future clients. Supporting the practices of self-awareness, wellness, and the ability to self-monitor is important as trainees engage in their individual professional identity development processes.

Self-Awareness

When practicing clinical and self-reflective skills, students are learning about themselves, how they understand others, their view of the world, and how their cognitive and affective processes may intersect with potential successes and challenges in a therapeutic relationship.

Notes From the Field 12.1

Modeling professional behavior is important even during difficult events when trainees are likely to be extremely anxious or defensive. It is also very important that all faculty and/or supervisors participating in a gatekeeping intervention are in synch about the importance and the goals of the effort. The conflictual nature of gatekeeping actions is often stressful for faculty and supervisors (although not as much as for trainees), yet maintaining a caring and professional demeanor is important not only for the process but also for the opportunity to model how to deal with conflict and other difficult encounters.

It is recommended that faculty or supervisor participants plan for formal remediation meetings in advance. Most important is to identify the purpose of the gathering, the agenda or order of items to be addressed in the meeting, and the expected or potential outcomes. It is also suggested that participants come to an agreement about assuming various roles for the purpose of supporting the student, fulfilling the goals of the meeting, and maintaining the integrity of the gatekeeping process.

In one graduate training program, faculty decide in advance who will take on which functions while allowing themselves the flexibility to shift roles if necessary as the meeting unfolds. Faculty also determine in advance who will introduce a given topic. Possible roles, depending on the situation, include the following:

- *Advocate or ally:* offering support for the student's positions. This might include reflecting the student's perspective, acknowledging the emotional difficulty of the moment, offering encouragement for the student's strengths or successful past efforts to address the problem, and so on. This role is usually assumed by the faculty member who has the most positive working relationship with the student. It does not include siding with the student or supervisee; rather, it is about being an ally in the meeting so that the individual does not feel overwhelmed by the power differential inherent in the gatekeeping experience.
- *Historian:* recounting the events that brought the student to this point in the gatekeeping process.
- *Reviewer of expectations:* reminding meeting participants of ethics codes, program standards, institutional or department policies, and the purpose of gatekeeping.
- *Process observer:* noting the interactional dynamics occurring in the meeting that are going well or resulting in an impasse, such as reactions that either affirm or contradict the problematic functioning of the student. The process observer can serve as timekeeper, noting the points in the meeting when it is appropriate to move on to the next agenda item, such as toward a conclusion.
- *Mediator:* observing points of conflict or dilemmas and proposing possible solutions in relation to those points of divergence.

(Continued)

Notes From the Field 12.1 *(Continued)*

- *Enforcer:* implementing the functional details of the program's gatekeeping protocol or policy, such as identifying remediation strategies that are congruent with the developmental needs of the student and arranging criteria such as the timeline, observable outcomes required, and other details that are required to fulfill the purpose of the meeting.
- *Documenter:* recording the events and decision of the meeting and overseeing the written communication following the meeting, such as distributing a summary of the meeting to all participants, constructing the formal remediation plan or letter, and sending notifications of decisions to all parties affected.

The roles outlined here are suggestions. Participating faculty (or supervisors) often assume multiple roles. Organizing and assigning functions helps organize and structure the process of the meeting. This process also serves to calm the anticipatory anxiety of those running the meeting (faculty and supervisors often find these meetings distressful) as well as that of the student, who senses the support offered by the structure of this approach when engaging in difficult interventions. In all gatekeeping activities, faculty support one another in filling their agreed-on roles and in modeling professionalism in the face of demanding events.

As students expand their self-understanding of intra- and interpersonal functions, such as encountering conflict, coping with emotions, and managing personal values, they build self-efficacy and increase their sense of personal control. This internal awareness in turn affects relational functioning in personal, professional, and therapeutic relationships. Pai (2015) found that self-reflection exercises that helped improve self-awareness were predictors of students' clinical competence. Self-reflection was also found to reduce trainee stress in this study. Exercises aimed at increasing awareness of internal functioning enhanced trainees' understanding of process issues in therapy and supported the development of competency in the expectations of professional standards and functioning (Schneider & Rees, 2012). These developmental shifts in self-understanding can also serve as a prevention measure in averting problematic behaviors. Alternatively, resistance to engaging in self-reflective processes may indicate to clinical educators and supervisors the potential for future challenges with those trainees.

Wellness and Self-Care Education

Counselor development is understood to be an iterative process that includes overlapping spheres, including academic development, social development, interpersonal relations, and intrapersonal professional identity development (Gibson, Dollarhide, & Moss, 2010). Training programs that emphasize the importance of clinicians' mental health as a component of clinical competence foster the value of healthy intra- and interpersonal qualities in their trainees. Witmer and Young (1996) acknowledged that the factors that lead to problematic clinicians or trainees are not clear; most likely, the paths are many and unique to the individual. These authors further suggested that adopting wellness strategies can contribute to the prevention of problematic or impaired clinicians. The opportunity to engage in environments that support holistic wellness practices should be available in both educational training programs as well as agency settings.

Witmer and Young (1996) suggested that faculty and supervisors embed into the training curriculum opportunities for students to develop their full potential of self-care strategies, including acquiring knowledge and skills for coping with stress and burnout. They also believed that faculty and supervisors should model the effect healthy personal functioning has on clinical and professional performance:

> The example set by the faculty and advanced students is integral to building a therapeutic community that cares and encourages its members to become whole. A dysfunctional faculty, like that of a dysfunctional family, creates conditions and experiences that result in unhealthy students. (p. 144)

Helping trainees recognize a range of self-care strategies for the variety of situations they may encounter in their clinical work is important. Distressed clinicians inadvertently permit external stressors to interfere with their clinical competency. Lawson (2007) reported that between 37% and 60% of psychologists admitted that their clinical work suffered because of high levels of distress. Ongoing and uncontrolled distress, vicarious traumatization, compassion fatigue, and burnout eventually lead to competency problems in clinical practice. Many students are engaged in juggling multiple responsibilities throughout their training experience—family, work, school, relationships, clinical caseloads—and will likely be able to identify with high levels of emotional exhaustion and reduced feelings of accomplishment; thus, training programs have the opportunity to promote knowledge of and support the development of wellness strategies that can be generalized to postdegree experiences and implemented as career-long habits.

Yager and Tovar-Blank (2007) introduced 10 strategies to address wellness in counselor (clinical) training:

1. Include wellness education as a specific content area in the graduate curriculum.
2. Emphasize self-growth and self-awareness learning experiences as proactive wellness strategies intended to circumvent the development of problematic behavior.

3. Model wellness as faculty and supervisors by setting examples for trainees.
4. Communicate that perfectionism is counterproductive to the goal of wellness.
5. Emphasize and encourage wellness as an important lifestyle choice for clinical practitioners that counters the effects of stress, compassion fatigue, or burnout.
6. Encourage personal counseling as a method of obtaining the psychological support needed to address self-care and personal growth efforts throughout one's career.
7. Review professional ethics codes and the literature to encourage the development and maintenance of wellness and self-care practices as a professional obligation for students and other clinicians.
8. Support the development of a wellness philosophy in course activities and supervisory settings.
9. Cultivate novel approaches to bolster students' and supervisees' attention to personal wellness.
10. Model a view of human nature for trainees that supports the quality of therapeutic relationships, values client strengths and resiliency, values prevention, and minimizes pathologizing clients.

Lawson (2007) reviewed similar career-sustaining behaviors as adaptive wellness strategies, such as "maintaining objectivity about clients, reflecting on positive experiences, participating in continuing education, and avoiding undue responsibility for clients' problems" (p. 22). Lawson found that the top career-sustaining behaviors were maintaining a sense of humor, spending time with family, achieving a balance between one's professional and personal lives, maintaining self-awareness, and retaining a sense of control over work responsibilities. Trainees can begin developing these protective factors as they create their own comprehensive wellness plans.

There are many wellness models for clinicians and clinicians-in-training (J. E. Myers & Sweeney, 2008; Wolf, Thompson, Thompson, & Smith-Adcock, 2014). Lenz, Sangganjanavanich, Balkin, Oliver, and Smith (2012) believed that supervisors can use the supervisory relationship to monitor and promote the development of a holistic wellness approach in supervisees. Their approach includes the creation of a personal wellness definition accompanied by supervisory interventions that support the application of holistic wellness approaches that extend trainees' perspectives of client functioning. Lenz et al. discovered that their supervisory approach improved the well-being of supervisees, despite challenges encountered during their practicum work. Their approach also may have enhanced the development of counseling skills in trainees.

As Lawson, Venart, Hazler, and Kottler (2007) discovered, a culture of wellness in the field of professional practice includes the use by clinicians of proactive self-care strategies to enhance their well-being and prevent "the devastation, fatigue, and distress" (p. 6) that can lead to impaired functioning, such as clinicians fulfilling their personal needs at the expense of clients. Young and Lambie (2007) suggested that clinicians need to advocate for healthy organizations with policies that promote wellness in their employees. This occurs when site agencies and graduate programs promote healthy lifestyles among students, supervisees, faculty, and supervisors. Mental health training programs and agencies can reduce job stress by improving interpersonal relationships, increasing teamwork, and clarifying roles and expectations to reduce ambiguity and incongruence (Young & Lambie, 2007). These efforts can also be extended to the culture of graduate training programs.

It is helpful for trainees to learn about wellness approaches and identify strategies that are effective while navigating challenges with the encouragement of faculty and supervisors. Being able to implement coping strategies during the challenging processes of receiving feedback or participating in a remediation plan is an example of applying the strategies of a personal wellness plan. The development of self-care strategies can mitigate the development of problematic behavior, such as emotional dysfunction, interpersonal conflict, or unprofessional conduct, that interfere with learning and effective clinical work.

Self-Reflection and Self-Supervision

The ultimate goal of clinical training is to facilitate a trainee's ability to successfully self-monitor his or her own practice as a clinician. This includes developing the capacity to reflect on personal experiences and interpersonal systems to accurately assess how they influence one's clinical work. Examples include ongoing assessment of emotional reactions and regulation, personal wellness, and ethical decision-making practices. The intention of self-monitoring is to continuously enhance one's ability to create effective therapeutic relationships with clients and cooperative interactions with colleagues. The commitment to self-assessment and self-supervision engages clinicians in the ongoing practice of propelling their professional growth to become better practitioners. Furthermore, self-reflective practice is considered essential for professional competence as part of the process inherent in integrating theory and practice (Mann, Gordon, & MacLeod, 2009).

According to Morrissette (1999), "Self-supervision has been defined as a systematic process in which professionals work independently to monitor and direct their own professional development" (p. 165). Ideally, ongoing self-supervision allows clinicians and clinicians-in-training to "identify blind spots, strengths, and needs which may go undetected without careful reflection" (pp. 165–166). The process facilitates the examination of one's rationale for choices and is an important strategy to help clinicians understand their own experiences as information on which to base future actions (Australian Institute of Professional Counsellors, 2009).

To engage in the self-reflective and self-assessment processes that lead to self-supervision, trainees need to learn how to accurately observe internal reactions, collect external data, and access other professional resources to make informed decisions about their own personal performance (Sargeant, 2008). Assessing one's strengths and areas of growth as a clinician is also a preventive measure to deter the occurrence of unethical, illegal, or unprofessional behavior. Instituting the ongoing practice of self-monitoring is essential in proactive professional functioning. Epstein, Siegel, and Silberman (2008) believed that "self-monitoring allows for the early recognition of cognitive biases, technical errors, and emotional reactions and may facilitate self-correction and development of therapeutic relationships" (p. 5), consequently improving future behavior and skills. Essentially, a routine self-monitoring approach will continue beyond the conclusion of formal training and the postdegree supervisory period.

Facilitating ongoing self-supervision skills, especially regarding intrapersonal, interpersonal, and professional behaviors, can assist trainees in reducing problematic behaviors. Thus, it is important that personal reflectivity and critical self-assessment are actively connected to knowledge of clinical practice guidelines, ethical and legal standards, and professional conduct expectations taught during the training process. Mann et al. (2009) found that the elements that are most effective in "enabling the development of reflection and reflective practice are a supportive environment, both intellectually and emotionally; an authentic context; accommodation for individual differences in learning style; mentoring; group discussion; support; and, free expression of opinions" (p. 608). Morrissette (1999) offered multiple methods for fostering advancement of this skill in the clinical curriculum and noted that

> self-supervision is a complex endeavor that moves beyond a general discernment and encompasses (a) introspection, (b) self-awareness, and (c) self-evaluation culminating in greater insight, skill, and functioning on the part of therapists. To achieve these goals, family therapists are required to assume an active self-regulating role to evaluate their professional development. Consequently, they become responsible for their clinical decisions, actions, and remain individually accountable.. . . Through the reflective process, the less obvious aspects of one's experience become more apparent and can be connected to his or her present and future activities. (pp. 168–169)

The Australian Institute of Professional Counsellors (2009) proposed a self-assessment process for clinicians that includes identifying an issue or event they experienced that requires reflection; describing the event and associated context; assessing and analyzing the event;

appraising their own behavior and reactions through self-assessment, which requires vulnerability and nondefensive analysis; and transforming their self-understanding, approach, and future practice based on their analyses. The authors of this model acknowledged that self-assessment and self-reflection are individual processes that require time, patience, and a supportive environment. The Australian Institute of Professional Counsellors also provided a series of guided journaling activities to support the process.

As discussed previously in this chapter, trainees learn appropriate professional functioning by observing role models as they develop their own identities as clinicians. When students and supervisees are subsequently able to develop the skills of self-reflection and assessment, particularly in relation to personal and professional conduct, they can make preemptive decisions that circumvent engagement in unethical or other problematic behaviors. If supervisees are incapable of self-assessment or self-reflection, they may also be unable to self-supervise, behave appropriately, or adapt their own interpersonal and intrapersonal functioning to professional expectations.

Ethical Conduct and Professionalism

One of the first and most critical steps a training program undertakes is educating students about professional ethics and standards, a process that continues under the guidance of supervisors at clinical sites and into professional practice via continuing education requirements and lived experiences. Facilitating professional conduct that includes a thorough understanding of legal regulations, ethical doctrines, and best practice standards assists trainees in avoiding violating these critical professional principles. Students new to the mental health field are typically not familiar with the standards of professional performance. It is incumbent on educators to set students up for success in becoming clinical professionals. This effort extends well beyond the acquisition of knowledge and skills and ties in closely to professional identity development. Preparing students to learn expectations for professional conduct entails a comprehensive effort of providing information (as discussed in Chapter 8), modeling appropriate professional behavior (as encouraged previously in this chapter and in Chapter 5), and supporting trainees in the developmental process of professional identity development (as presented in Chapter 4). Preparing trainees also extends to helping reshape problematic behavior with early and responsive interventions (as described in Chapter 3).

Fostering essential ethical and legal behavior in students is particularly critical early in the educational process. The correlation between ethical complaints and marginal education is the reason most jurisdictions require clinical licensees to complete a portion of their continuing education requirements on ethical practice (Grenyer & Lewis, 2012; M. E. Johnson, Brems, Warner, & Roberts, 2006). Preventing lapses in professional conduct is also the motive behind professional liability or malpractice insurance companies offering discounts on premiums in return for policyholders taking continuing education courses on ethics.

Education on and awareness of effective ethical and legal practices supports trainees in preventing problematic behavior that might otherwise occur without adequate knowledge of the law or ethics codes. Tjeltveit and Gottlieb (2010) suggested that problems of professional behavior were reduced when clinicians attended to building ethical resilience, bolstering protective factors, and confronting personal vulnerabilities that may lead to ethics violations by facilitating self-examination and awareness. Thus, the development of one's internal resource of critical thinking connected to ethical issues is particularly important. The development of internal cognitive and awareness abilities serves as a protective factor that can mitigate the development of problematic professional behavior:

> Not all trainees in professional preparation programs have the opportunity to acquire these skills at an optimal level. Too many professionals complete their training without the emotional education and awareness needed to avoid self-deception and to act in the prudent, considered manner that society expects and that represents professional ethical excellence. (p. 105)

It is the task of faculty and supervisors to go beyond simply teaching information about ethical and legal standards. Programs and agencies should offer opportunities for trainees to develop reflective and critical thinking strategies that aspire to a committed best practice of professional standards throughout their careers. Examples include experience applying ethical and legal codes to case studies, practice applying ethical decision-making models in classroom and clinical activities (Cottone & Claus, 2000; Pope & Vasquez, 2016), and assistance reconciling personal and professional values (Ametrano, 2014). Advanced development of ethical decision-making skills will occur only if the educational groundwork is first laid in the classroom in conjunction with attentive supervisors committed to supporting supervisees' person-as-professional development as they navigate the ambiguous challenges of actual practice (Francis & Dugger, 2014). As Tjeltveit and Gottlieb (2010) noted,

> Learning the ethics code and attending risk management workshops are necessary but not sufficient to avoid ethical problems, much less to practice at the highest levels. To do so, we must look more deeply within ourselves and come to a better understanding of our personal feelings and values. (p. 108)

Consider the real-life situation experienced in Orlando, Florida, after the Pulse nightclub tragedy to apply the knowledge and information discussed in this chapter and book. See What Would You Do? 12.1.

As discussed in Chapter 2, *professionalism* is a construct that has not been clearly defined as it applies to the clinical professions, but general agreement indicates that professionalism is composed of the

What Would You Do? 12.1

In the aftermath of a community tragedy—in this case the Pulse nightclub massacre in Orlando, Florida, on June 12, 2016—you are heartened to witness the amazing response by local members of the clinical professions as they appear within hours at community centers frequented by the most affected groups, staging sites, and other public gathering places to actively provide support to those affected by the tragedy. The turnout of professionals is overwhelming because everyone wants to do something to help using their clinical skills.

Yet you notice several concerning things, including the following:

1. Many clinicians who are not trained in immediate crisis counseling strategies are responding with traditional counseling approaches. They are asking questions and suggesting strategies for coping that can prove damaging to the individuals stunned by the incomprehensibility of the situation, and who are still actively in fear for their own safety because facts about the situation remain unknown.
2. In an effort to be helpful, newly graduated and inexperienced mental health professionals are volunteering for responsibilities that are beyond their scope of practice or level of experience.
3. In managing their own reactions of shock and grief, therapists are sharing stories in informal settings with others and on social media about the individuals they counseled or the stories they heard.

You notice that some of the individuals engaging in these actions are recent graduates of your program in their postdegree supervisory period required prior to licensure.

What would you do to inform the clinical community at large regarding your concerns about appropriate interventions and maintaining confidentiality?

How might you specifically address the emerging ethical issues?

What can you do to specifically address the recent graduates of your program in their developmental understanding of scope of practice in crisis situations, realizing that they along with everyone else are pulled by a strong need to do whatever they can to help those victimized by the tragedy?

How might you support the community of helpers by fostering the development of their professional conduct in the following categories:

Self-awareness of their actions and behaviors?

Wellness and self-care during a time of crisis for the community and themselves?

Self-reflection and self-supervision about the activities or practices in which they are engaging?

qualities and behaviors that characterize or mark a given profession as generally expected by those within and outside of the profession. For clinical practitioners, this includes a commitment to abide by the ethics code and the collective values and norms of the profession (Francis & Dugger, 2014). Professionalism is also a pattern of performance of expected behaviors in the categories of interpersonal, intrapersonal, and professional functioning, which are the foundational concerns of gatekeeping activities.

Entering students may or may not be acquainted with the qualities of professionalism in clinical practice, or they may be unfamiliar with professional behavior in general, depending on their previous employment experience or exposure to professional work. Consistent with the goal of fostering adaptive development in clinical trainees as a prevention effort, educators and supervisors have the opportunity and responsibility to help trainees grow as professionals in terms of both their identity development and conduct. The value of developing trainee professionalism should be integrated into the foundational expectations of graduate programs and clinical training sites. Professionalism can be reflected as an aspect of the mission or a goal of the program, emphasized in the program's published standards and expectations of students, and included as a topic for discussion throughout the curriculum or as a focus of training site discussions. Program faculty can unite to develop a professionalism statement that appears in every course syllabus or a set of general competencies that are part of the student evaluation process. Ideally, the foundational tenets of professionalism as an underlying program value should also be successively reinforced at all appropriate transitional points, such as during new student orientation, before launching into practicum or other field experiences, and in preparation for graduation and job seeking—whenever the expectations for professional conduct are expanded to accommodate progressive levels of advancement in the training process. Appendix I provides ideas for incorporating expectations for professionalism across the curriculum.

Supervisors at field sites can also promote the development of professionalism by serving as role models when engaged with trainees in cotherapy or case consultation and when cultivating trainees' professional identity development during supervision or mentoring activities. The establishment of agency or program-wide norms for professionalism and prosocial behaviors should be accompanied by multiple opportunities to adopt and reinforce trainees' professional identity development and professional conduct. Clear expectations, evaluation opportunities, and ongoing thoughtful feedback on trainees' professional conduct can proactively shape their behavior and prevent problematic unprofessional behaviors from developing.

Admissions Processes That Screen for Problematic Trainees

An additional preventive measure that has been discussed across the professional literature is advanced screening of individuals seeking to enter the profession or receive supervisory oversight. Advanced assessment prior to accepting trainees as supervisees or students is one of the first steps of the gatekeeping process (Kerl & Eichler, 2005). At the point of admission, clinical educators can control entry to the profession when considering prospective students who show behaviors that would result in the inability to meet professional competencies (Brown-Rice & Furr, 2016). Once a trainee has been accepted into a program, that program has a dual responsibility to both the student and the standards of the profession; thus, the admissions process is a checkpoint for preventing trainees who are likely unsuited for the profession from entering the profession.

Unfortunately, implementing admissions screening processes cannot guarantee the elimination of problematic trainees; however, it may deter individuals who are not appropriate for the clinical professions from beginning a program. McCaughan and Hill (2015) suggested that programs clearly articulate the characteristics expected of a clinician to prospective applicants, including "desired personality characteristics such as empathy, warmth, genuineness, emotional stability, and sensitivity" (p. 37). Crawford and Gilroy (2012) found that clinical graduate programs considered the following personal characteristics important to consider in admissions: "interpersonal skills, interpersonal maturity, self-awareness, the ability to perceive one's areas for growth, the ability to perceive one's strengths, openness to feedback, and potential for growth" (p. 31) along with the additional qualities of humility, career goals, and the ability to work with others. Many of these qualities align with the proposed standards discussed in detail in Chapter 8. Openly conveying the qualities expected of trainees may encourage self-assessment for goodness of fit between one's personal qualities and the clinical profession. This may result in deterring applicants from pursuing a profession that is not a good match. The same holds true for supervisees who might be considered a high liability risk because of problematic professional behavior, especially if expectations and candidate qualities are made very clear prior to the application and acceptance processes. This attempt to encourage self-assessment may not be fully successful, and clinical programs are reminded that "it is the ethical duty of the faculty and supervisors in the training program, not of the individual entering the training program, to gatekeep for the profession" (McCaughan & Hill, 2015, p. 37).

Some ethics codes and program accreditation standards offer guidance in the admissions process. For example, the Council for Accreditation of Counseling and Related Educational Programs (2015) recommends an admissions screening process for identifying applicants' appropriateness as the first opportunity to formally evaluate person–profession suitability:

> Entry-level admission decision recommendations are made by the academic unit's selection committee and include consideration of each applicant's (1) relevance of career goals, (2) aptitude for graduate-level study, (3) potential success in forming effective counseling relationships, and (4) respect for cultural differences. (p. 5)

Despite these guidelines and others like them, there is not agreement across the clinical professions about which personal characteristics should be assessed during the selection process, nor is there empirical evidence that supports any particular admissions strategy as a predictor of students' desired personal characteristics (Hatchett, Lawrence, & Coaston, 2017; McCaughan & Hill, 2015). The lack of empirically validated methods for screening character and fitness is a shortcoming of the profession (W. B. Johnson & Campbell, 2002) and makes the process of admissions selections very challenging for clinical faculty and supervisors. Most instruments that assess the personal and professional qualities of trainees are designed for use during the training program after admissions. "Counselor educators articulated a strong and overarching concern about how to evaluate students in a fair and reliable manner, identify professional dispositions, and screen for psychological impairment" (Swank & Smith-Adcock, 2014, p. 58). Admissions procedures rely heavily on academic aptitude criteria, such as Graduate Record Exam scores and undergraduate grade point averages. Predictors of academic achievement are relevant but not solely adequate when determining the functional interpersonal success of future mental health clinicians (Leverett-Main, 2004; McCaughan & Hill, 2015).

Despite the lack of supportive evidence for useful admissions procedures, scholars have offered suggestions that support some methods of screening. Most common among these are admissions requirements that provide insight into applicants' personal functioning, including a personal statement, particularly one that requests responses to very specific questions; previous clinical experience or exposure; and applicant interviews, held individually or in group settings. Swank and Smith-Adcock (2014) reported that 82% of master's programs and 85% of doctoral programs in their study identified interviews as part of the admissions process. These authors proposed a structured group interview approach to observe the interactional styles of applicants. Other examples offered in the literature include role-play vignettes; specific or structured questions during interviews; and informal discussions conducted during, before, and after formal interviews as useful in evaluating applicants' interpersonal skills, cultural sensitivity, and professional potential (Ziomek-Daigle & Christensen, 2010).

McCaughan and Hill (2015) proposed that programs construct admissions criteria and processes that align with the program-designated instruments used to assess trainees' personal and professional qualities. They suggested developing admissions rubrics that correlate with clearly defined preferred characteristics informed by research and the lived experience of program faculty. The rubrics should clearly connect the assessment domain to the methods for assessing such qualities. Doing so provides "a framework for applicants, counselor trainees, and counselor educators and supervisors to understand the purpose and focus of the admission process in identifying these characteristics" (p. 37).

For example, multicultural competence as a disposition is challenging in evaluating in the admissions process. To address this issue, one training program added a question in its admissions packet that inquired about applicants' understanding of the profession's commitment to diversity and included an opportunity for self-reflection in essay form in response to the following statement and query:

> The [name of university and graduate program] and the American Counseling Association (ACA) are known for valuing diversity and social justice for oppressed groups. [Quotation of specific ethical standards, i.e., Standard A.4.b. (Personal Values) and Standard C.5. (Nondiscrimination) of the *ACA Code of Ethics* (American Counseling Association, 2014a).] With these ethical expectations in mind, how will you begin the process of reflecting on and addressing any personal attitudes, beliefs, assumptions, or feelings that may prevent you from working with a client or a colleague holding an identity or a social status different than your own? (Rollins College, 2017a, p. 1)

As this example illustrates, the need for thoughtful construction of questions to elicit applicant reflection during admission protocols is important and can both steer applicant self-selection and contribute to the screening of applicants by admissions committees.

Lack of empirically validated approaches limits the level of gatekeeping effectiveness during the admissions process but does not eliminate gatekeeper responsibility. Clinical training programs can utilize a range of screening strategies that reflect the value of interpersonal, intrapersonal, and professional expectations of their programs. They can design creative assessment measures and activities to evaluate applicant goodness of fit. As McCaughan and Hill (2015) suggested,

> An intentional commitment within counseling and counselor education to screen for personal characteristics prior to enrollment upholds a best practice approach, through encouraging counselor training programs to embrace their gatekeeping functions by not introducing individuals into the field who possess the potential for dismissal or uncertain advancement later due to personal and professional conflict. (p. 39)

All clinical training programs can minimize the enrollment of students or supervisees with potentially problematic behavior if careful attention is paid to applicant qualities during admissions processes.

Conclusion

The purpose of this chapter was to focus on preventing problematic behavior by supporting the professional development of clinical trainees and supervisees. Modeling appropriate behavior, clarifying appropriate professionalism, and providing opportunities for learning about self-care and wellness are strategies that not only support the prevention of problematic behaviors in trainees but will also become career-sustaining protective practices. Incorporating into the admissions process education and reflection on the personal and professional characteristics of mental health clinicians offers the opportunity to start gatekeeping at the entry point to the profession.

Key Points and Best Practices

- The ultimate goal of clinical training is to facilitate a trainee's ability to successfully self-monitor his or her own practice as a clinician.
- As a form of prevention, design and implement admissions screening procedures based on gatekeeping strategies and competencies that will be evaluated in the program.
- Students and trainees learn behaviors through observing faculty and supervisors' behaviors, which are later transferred into their future professional actions.
- Students entering a training program may not know the expectations of or operational definitions for professional conduct, confidentiality, self-reflection, and other expected intra- and interpersonal abilities; faculty and supervisors must explain these definitions, preferably in written form.
- The benefits of identifying and implementing intentional prevention steps throughout a training program to support trainees will not only serve students/trainees in a positive manner but also alleviate faculty involvement in gatekeeping tasks and build the reputation of the program and institution.

Appendix A

Ethical Mandates for Gatekeeping Practices in Clinical Training and Supervision

Throughout this book, specific ethics codes guiding the gatekeeping process are cited from the four major professional associations:

- American Counseling Association. (2014). *ACA code of ethics.* Retrieved from https://www.counseling.org/Resources/aca-code-of-ethics.pdf
- American Psychological Association. (2017). *Ethical principles of psychologists and code of conduct.* Retrieved from www.apa.org/ethics/code/ethics-code-2017.pdf
- National Association of Social Workers. (2017). *Code of ethics of the National Association of Social Workers.* Retrieved from https://www.socialworkers.org/About/Ethics/Code-of-Ethics/Code-of-Ethics-English
- American Association for Marriage and Family Therapy. (2015). *Code of ethics.* Retrieved from www.aamft.org/iMIS15/AAMFT/Content/Legal_Ethics/Code_of_Ethics.aspx

The following clinical professional associations also maintain ethical standards that include guidelines for the processes inherent in gatekeeping. Although these are written for the association membership within the specific clinical field of practice, the codes can be used by those in other clinical professions as suggestions for best practice guidelines.

American School Counselor Association. (2016). *ASCA ethical standards for school counselors*. Retrieved from https://www.schoolcounselor.org/asca/media/asca/Ethics/EthicalStandards2016.pdf

D. School Counseling Intern Site Supervisors
Field/intern site supervisors:

c. Use a collaborative model of supervision that is on-going and includes, but is not limited to, the following activities: promoting professional growth, supporting best practices and ethical practice, assessing supervisee performance and developing plans for improvement, consulting on specific cases and assisting in the development of a course of action.

i. Ensure supervisees are aware of policies and procedures related to supervision and evaluation and provide due-process procedures if supervisees request or appeal their evaluations.

j. Ensure performance evaluations are completed in a timely, fair and considerate manner, using data when available and based on clearly stated criteria.

k. Use evaluation tools measuring the competence of school counseling interns. These tools should be grounded in state and national school counseling standards. In the event no such tool is available in the school district, the supervisor seeks out relevant evaluation tools and advocates for their use.

l. Are aware of supervisee limitations and communicate concerns to the university/college supervisor in a timely manner.

m. Assist supervisees in obtaining remediation and professional development as necessary.

n. Contact university/college supervisors to recommend dismissal when supervisees are unable to demonstrate competence as a school counselor as defined by the ASCA School Counselor Competencies and state and national standards. Supervisors consult with school administrators and document recommendations to dismiss or refer a supervisee for assistance. Supervisors ensure supervisees are aware of such decisions and the resources available to them. Supervisors document all steps taken.

American Mental Health Counselors Association. (2015, October). *AMHCA code of ethics.* Retrieved from http://connections.amhca.org/HigherLogic/System/DownloadDocumentFile.ashx?DocumentFileKey=d4e10fcb-2f3c-c701-aa1d-5d0f53b8bc14

II. Commitment to Other Professionals

A. Relationship with Colleagues

6. When mental health counselors have knowledge of the impairment, incompetence, or unethical conduct of a

mental health professional, they are obliged to attempt to rectify the situation. Failing an informal solution, mental health counselors should bring such unethical activities to the attention of the appropriate state licensure board and/or the ethics committee of the professional association.

III. Commitment to Students, Supervisees and Employee Relationships

A. Relationship with Students, Interns and Employees

Mental health counselors have an ethical concern for the integrity and welfare of supervisees, students, and employees. These relationships typically include an evaluative component and therefore need to be maintained on a professional and confidential basis.

8. Supervisors provide written informed consent prior to beginning a supervision relationship that documents . . . evaluation procedures in the supervisory relationship; the limits and scope of confidentiality and privileged communication within the supervisory relationship; . . . and procedures for supervisee endorsement for certification and/or licensure, or employment to those whom are competent, ethical, and qualified.

B. Commitment for Clinical Supervision

Clinical supervision . . . is also a gatekeeping process to ensure safety to the client, the profession and to the supervisee.

2. Clinical Supervision Contract

A clinical supervision contract signed by both supervisor and supervisee, . . . [shall include information about the following components:]

b) Compliance with the AMHCA Code of Ethics: The supervisor should provide a copy of the AMHCA Code of Ethics to the supervisee, or ensure that the supervisee has obtained a copy. The supervisee must agree to comply AMHCA Code of Ethics with the AMHCA Code of Ethics in all treatment provided. As needed, the supervisor and supervisee will discuss the principles contained in the AMHCA Code of Ethics. The supervisor needs to be aware of other codes of ethics which may apply to the supervisee.

c) State Licensing Board Rules: The supervisee needs to obtain a copy of the appropriate State Licensing Board Rules, and agree to comply with them. As needed, the supervisor and supervisee will discuss the provisions of board rules. The supervisor will be aware of all credentials and membership organizations regulating the supervisee.

d) Compliance with State Laws: The supervisor should inform the supervisee of state laws contained in the

Practice Act for counselors, and other legal provisions which apply to treatment, requirements for licensure, billing, and the discipline of counselors.

e) Duty of the Clinical Supervisor: The contract should specify that the duty of the clinical supervisor will be to direct the treatment process, and to assist the supervisee in complying with all legal and ethical standards for treatment.

Commission on Rehabilitation Counselor Certification. (2017). *Code of professional ethics for rehabilitation counselors.* Retrieved from https://www.crccertification.com/filebin/pdf/ethics/CodeOfEthics_01-01-2017.pdf
(*Note:* As a division of the American Counseling Association [ACA], the American Rehabilitation Counseling Association relies on the *ACA Code of Ethics.*)

SECTION H: Supervision, Training, and Teaching

H.1. CLINICAL SUPERVISOR RESPONSIBILITIES

a. CLIENT WELFARE. A primary obligation of rehabilitation counselor supervisors is to monitor client welfare by overseeing supervisee performance and professional development. To fulfill these obligations, rehabilitation counselor supervisors meet or communicate regularly with supervisees to review the supervisees' work and help them become prepared to serve a diverse client population.

d. SUPERVISEE RIGHTS AND INFORMED CONSENT FOR SUPERVISION. Rehabilitation counselor supervisors have an obligation to review, in writing and verbally, the rights and responsibilities of both the supervisor and supervisee. Rehabilitation counselor supervisors disclose to supervisees organizational policies and procedures to which supervisors are to adhere and the mechanisms for due process appeal of individual supervisor actions. Issues unique to the use of distance supervision are included.

H.4. SUPERVISION EVALUATION, REMEDIATION, AND ENDORSEMENT

a. EVALUATION OF SUPERVISEES. Rehabilitation counselor supervisors document and provide supervisees with ongoing feedback regarding their performance and schedule periodic formal evaluative sessions throughout the supervisory relationship.

b. GATEKEEPING AND REMEDIATION FOR SUPERVISEES. Through initial and ongoing evaluation, rehabilitation counselor supervisors are aware of and address supervisee limitations that might impede performance. If remedial assistance does not resolve concerns regarding supervisee performance and supervisees are unable to demonstrate they can provide competent professional services to a range of diverse clients, rehabilitation counselor supervisors may recommend dismissal from training programs or supervision settings. Rehabilitation counselor supervisors seek consultation and document their decisions to recommend dismissal. They make reasonable efforts to ensure that supervisees are aware of options available to them to address such decisions.

c. REFERRING SUPERVISEES FOR COUNSELING. If supervisees request counseling or if counseling services are suggested as part of a remediation process, rehabilitation counselor supervisors assist supervisees in identifying appropriate services. Rehabilitation counseling supervisors do not provide counseling services to supervisees but may address interpersonal competencies in terms of the impact of these issues on the supervisory relationship, professional functioning, and/or clients.

d. ENDORSEMENT. Rehabilitation counselor supervisors endorse supervisees for certification, licensure, employment, or completion of academic or training programs based on satisfactory progress and observations while under supervision or training. Regardless of qualifications, rehabilitation counselor supervisors do not endorse supervisees whom they believe to be impaired in any way that would interfere with the performance of the duties associated with the endorsement.

H.5. REHABILITATION COUNSELOR EDUCATOR RESPONSIBILITIES

a. PROGRAM INFORMATION AND ORIENTATION. Rehabilitation counselor educators recognize that orientation is a developmental process that continues throughout the educational and clinical training of students. Rehabilitation counselor educators have an ethical responsibility to provide enough information to prospective or current students about program expectations for them to make informed decisions about entering into and continuing in a program.

H.6. REHABILITATION COUNSELOR EDUCATOR COMPETENCE

a. EDUCATOR KNOWLEDGE AND SKILL. Rehabilitation counselor educators who are responsible for developing, implementing, and supervising educational programs are knowledgeable regarding the ethical, legal, and regulatory aspects of the profession, are skilled in applying that knowledge, and make students aware of their responsibilities. Rehabilitation counselor educators conduct counselor education and training programs in an ethical manner.

H.8. EDUCATION EVALUATION, REMEDIATION, AND ENDORSEMENT

a. EVALUATION OF STUDENTS. Rehabilitation counselor educators clearly state to students, prior to and throughout the training program, the levels of competency expected, appraisal methods, and timing of evaluations for both didactic and clinical competencies. Rehabilitation counselor educators provide students with ongoing feedback regarding their performance throughout the training program.

b. GATEKEEPING AND REMEDIATION FOR STUDENTS. Rehabilitation counselor educators, through ongoing evaluation, are aware of and address the inability of some students to achieve required competencies, which may be due to academic performance or personal concerns. Rehabilitation counselor educators do the following: (1) assist students in securing remedial assistance, including counseling, when needed; (2) seek professional consultation and document the decision to recommend dismissal or refer students for assistance; and (3) make reasonable efforts to ensure that students have recourse in a timely manner to address decisions requiring them to seek assistance, or to dismiss them and provide students with due process, according to institutional policies and procedures.

c. REFERRING STUDENTS FOR COUNSELING. If students request counseling or if counseling services are suggested as part of a remediation process, rehabilitation counselor educators assist students in identifying appropriate services. Rehabilitation counselor educators do not provide counseling services to currently enrolled students but may address interpersonal competencies in terms of the impact of these issues on academic performance, professional functioning, and/or clients.

d. ENDORSEMENT. Rehabilitation counselor educators endorse students for certification, licensure, employment, or completion of academic or training programs based on satisfactory progress and observations while under supervision or training. Regardless of qualifications, rehabilitation counselor educators do not endorse students whom they believe to be impaired in any way that would interfere with the performance of the duties associated with the endorsement.

Appendix B

Sample Appeals Process From a Published Student Handbook

Faculty Procedures for Assisting Students in Becoming Effective and Competent Counselors

Faculty members identify and address student concerns as they emerge throughout the program. The students' knowledge, interpersonal skills, and counseling skills are routinely evaluated to determine if the student is competent, if remedial work is necessary, or if a student should be withdrawn from the program.

If a student is not demonstrating personal qualities and skills related to becoming a competent and effective counselor, the instructor completes a Student Competency Summary and Requirements Form and Report of Concern. The instructor meets with the student, reviews the concerns and remediation requirements, and provides the student with a copy of the Student Competency Summary and Requirements form. The instructor also informs the student of their right to appeal. If the student believes the review is unjustified or does not want to adhere to the requirements, the student needs to follow these procedures.

Student Procedures for Appealing Remediation Requirements or Withdrawal

Student

1. The student must submit a written appeal documenting the rationale for the appeal. The appeal must be given to the department chair

within three weekdays or the right to appeal is forfeited and the student is required to follow the instructor's requirements.

Instructor

2. The instructor provides a copy of the Student Competency Summary and Requirements form to the department chair. During the next faculty meeting, the instructor provides an informational report regarding the student concern and outcome of the meeting.

Student

3. If the student chooses to adhere to the instructor's recommendations regarding (a) remedial procedures or (b) exit from the program, the following procedures will not be implemented.
4. When a student submits an appeal, the department chair meets with the student and instructor and seeks a resolution. (If the department chair is also the instructor who has completed the Competency Review and Requirements form, another tenured program faculty member reviews the appeal.)

Department Chair

5. If no resolution is reached, the department chair appoints an ad hoc hearing committee of three (3) faculty members normally within three (3) weekdays of receipt of the student's appeal.

Student, Instructor, and Committee

6. The student and instructor must submit a written statement to the committee. The committee meets, reviews each written statement and holds an oral hearing where the views of the instructor and the student are heard.

Committee

7. The committee determines whether the student continues in the program without restriction, continues in the program with remedial work, or is withdrawn from the program. The committee makes specific written recommendations within ten (10) days of its appointment. The decision is conveyed to the instructor, the student, and the department chair in writing.

Student

8. The student has ten (10) days to appeal in writing said ruling to the dean of the college of arts and science. The dean confers with the department chair. All decisions made by the dean and the chair are final.

Department Procedure

9. All records are filed in the student's departmental file.

Future Formal Evaluation of the Student

10. Once a Student Competency Summary and Requirements form is completed for a student, all of the student's future instructors complete a Student Competency Progress Report form during mid-semester.

Adapted from *Stetson University Department of Counselor Education Student Handbook*, by Department of Counselor Education, Stetson University, 2016, retrieved from www.stetson.edu/artsci/counselor/media/SH%202015-2016.pdf.

Appendix C

Sample Correspondence Following Up a Remediation Planning Meeting

[Date]
[Address]

Dear [student],

The faculty are concerned and recently met to discuss (a) your poor academic performance in COUN 506 Human Growth and Development and (b) a pattern of problematic academic behavior (i.e., failure to turn in several assignments or participate appropriately in course-required group assignments) and professional behavior (i.e., your self-report of DUI and use of behavior- or mind-altering substances) while enrolled in the program. This letter serves as a summary of the outcome of that meeting. First, we would like to commend you for your openness to feedback and willingness to take responsibility for your actions this semester in Dr. Wyatt's class.

As per the program guidelines specified in the *Counselor Education Graduate Student Handbook* (page 15), the Counselor Education faculty "... identify and address student concerns as they emerge throughout the program. The students' knowledge, interpersonal skills, and counseling skills are routinely evaluated to determine if the student is competent, if remedial work is necessary or if a student should be withdrawn from the program." As with all students, faculty members contribute input based on the student's academic performance, personal and professional behaviors in class, ability to get along with peers, openness to feedback and constructive criticism, as well as other aspects of his or her functioning as a future counselor.

At the most recent meeting of the Counselor Education program faculty on March 29, concerns were raised about your performance in the program and a plan was put into place in an attempt to remediate the faculty's concerns. A remediation plan is a structured process of defined interventions through which a struggling student has the opportunity to demonstrate competence. This letter, a copy of which will be placed in your student file, serves as notice of the current findings of the Counselor Education faculty.

As per the Due Process Policy (also found in the *Counselor Education Graduate Student Handbook*, pages 18–21) students may be remediated and later dismissed if found to be personally unsuitable for the profession. Given the unique nature of the field of counseling (requiring mastery of cognitive skills and demonstration of relevant and appropriate clinical and interpersonal skills), the faculty retains the right to remediate and/or "counsel out" of the program and/or not recommend for practicum or internship placement any student whose level of professional, interpersonal, and/or intrapersonal competence is considered incompatible with that required for effective functioning as a counselor.

For remediation of your personal and professional behaviors, it is required that you:

1. Receive the grade of "Incomplete" for COUN 506 Human Growth and Development for this spring semester. Any currently outstanding projects or assignments will not be accepted for credit at this juncture.
2. Refrain from taking classes until spring semester of next year, at which time you will be required to retake COUN 506 Human Growth and Development with Dr. Wyatt and COUN 503 Human Relations, Methods, and Skills with Dr. Jones. You will not be required to pay for these courses, but you will be required to adhere to strict assignment and attendance guidelines as set forth by your advisor and your professors (i.e., no missing classes, no late assignments, and passing with a B or better).
3. Attend a minimum of two weekly 12-step meetings (i.e., Alcoholics Anonymous and/or Narcotics Anonymous) during your time off from classes (from now until January 1). You must also submit proof of attendance with documentation that will be provided to you by your advisor.
4. Attend a minimum of 12 personal counseling sessions with a counselor experienced in working in addictions. You will need to submit proof of your completion of 12 sessions prior to December 1.
5. By December 1, you will need to submit and present to the faculty a written wellness action plan.

Adherence to these requirements will be assessed by the faculty at the end of next year's spring semester (by April 29) and by your faculty advisor during individual advising sessions until that time. If satisfactory progress has not occurred, as determined by 1) the faculty advisor in consultation with the Counselor Education faculty and 2) documented evidence that demonstrates satisfactory progress in the identified areas of remediation by the assigned deadline of April 29 next year, you will be dismissed from the Counselor Education program.

The Counselor Education program's goal is to educate and prepare competent counseling professionals, and thus our desire is to work *with* you as you work toward your stated goal of becoming a professional counselor. We are confident that if you thoughtfully and fully follow the requirements outlined in this letter, you will be able to continue the steps required to attain that goal.

By signing below, you acknowledge that you have received this letter, that you have had the opportunity to ask questions about and understand the content of this letter, and that you will engage in and follow up with this remediation plan to demonstrate a change in your personal and professional conduct as it affects your role as a counselor.

Student's Name *(printed)*	Signature	Date
Advisor/Instructor's Name *(printed)*	Signature	Date
Department Chair *(printed)*	Signature	Date

cc: Department chair/copy to be placed in student's file

Sample Student Action Plan Follow-Up Letter

[Date]
[Address]

Dear [student]:

On behalf of the Department of Social Work, we appreciate your openness and earnest self-reflections during our meeting on [date]. It was evident to us that you had given serious consideration to the matter of being dismissed from your position as a graduate assistant. You expressed increased self-awareness from your own reflections and consultations with others and conveyed an understanding of the issues that concerned the faculty and your graduate assistant supervisor.

Our goal as faculty members is to support you in changing the problematic behaviors we have noticed by providing concrete feedback for you to consider and use to improve your conduct as you continue in the graduate program. On behalf of the faculty, I would like to define in writing the discussion we had with you, because we realize that listening to our concerns regarding your professional behavior may have been difficult in the moment. To summarize, our primary concerns are that in the future you:

- Understand the impact your decisions and actions had on the problems you encountered in the graduate assistant situation and take responsibility for your part in the problems that arose.

- Exhibit awareness of others in making decisions about how to behave.
- Consider and incorporate the feedback provided by faculty.
- Respond to requests for information or decisions by faculty and supervisors.
- Follow through with commitments and responsibilities expected by the graduate program, your courses, and your other obligations.
- Maintain consistent performance in your academic and clinical work.
- Work respectfully with those having more knowledge and/or experience than you.
- Understand the gravity of this profession with regard to the importance of responsiveness, consistency, and responsibility.

[Student name], as we mentioned in the meeting, you clearly have many strengths, including leadership abilities, that will serve you and the profession of social work well. At the same time, these abilities can get in your way when you do not consider others or remain open to guidance from those who are in advanced positions of responsibility or knowledge.

To support you in your continued professional development, we would like for you to enroll in Dr. [professor name]'s section of Internship next year. This way, the core faculty can continue providing feedback about your progress.

Please let us know if you have any questions or need clarification of any of the statements above. Also let us know how we can support your progress.

Sincerely,

Professor and Department Chair

Note. In this example, the student's direct action to acknowledge receipt of this letter will be demonstrated through registration in the course section noted. That professor will also meet with the student in advance of the semester to discuss the student's strategy for success and remind the student that the points in the letter are areas of ongoing evaluation that the professor will be monitoring. Depending on the situation and student, the professor may find it helpful to also schedule advance supervision sessions as standing weekly or bimonthly meetings to provide active and regular feedback that will aid the student in his efforts to apply and integrate the behavioral changes that are expected.

Appendix D

Sample Professional Pledge for Entering Students

[Institution logo or letterhead]
[Department/program name]

The [Program/Department Name] Student Pledge

As I embark on the important professional and personal journey as a [university name] clinical mental health counselor-in-training, I understand that the [university and department or program name] program is rigorous and meets the highest standards of training as prescribed by the counselor education accrediting agency, CACREP. I understand that professional counselors must possess the awareness, knowledge, and skills to competently provide the highest quality services to our clients and to engage in advocacy and social change as prescribed by our American Counseling Association's ethical standards. Furthermore, as a counselor-in-training, I am called on to exhibit professional conduct that inspires confidence in the counseling profession.

Therefore, while enrolled in the [university name] Graduate Counseling program, I pledge to:

- Participate in an inclusive community of learners who value personal and intellectual growth through collaborative relationships among students, faculty, and staff;
- Conduct myself professionally in all public, social media, training, and classroom settings;
- Cultivate deep compassion and empathy for others; and

- Actively and responsibly complete each course, practicum, and internship with the goal of becoming an effective and ethical clinical mental health counselor who engages with clients in cultivating and increasing freedom in their lives.

By my signature, I affirm my commitment to this pledge.

______________________	______________________	______________________
Student's Name *(printed)*	Signature	Date

Appendix E

Sample Verification of Understanding Agreement (Informed Consent)

[Institution logo or letterhead]
[Department/program name]

Verification of Understanding Agreement

The [name] graduate program at [university] is charged with the task of preparing individuals to become [name of clinical specialty] in a variety of settings and to assume positions of leadership in the profession. In order to fulfill these responsibilities, faculty and supervisors continuously evaluate students based on their academic abilities, clinical skills, interpersonal behavior, and professional conduct. Successful completion of the graduate program as well as faculty endorsement for licensure and other professional pursuits depend on these factors.

In order to ensure proper training and client care, a counselor-in-training must be able to demonstrate professional character; the ability to communicate well and convey warmth, genuineness, and respect; and empathy in interactions with others, including clients, classmates, staff, and faculty. Counseling students are expected to be able to demonstrate the ability to accept and integrate feedback, be aware of their impact on others, accept personal responsibility for their actions, express emotions appropriately, resolve conflicts, and demonstrate professional judgment in decision making. Faculty and supervisors will evaluate students' level of clinical understanding and counseling skills and provide students with ongoing feedback as they progress through the program. This is consistent with the expectations of faculty and supervisors as gatekeepers of the profession as explained in the *ACA Code of Ethics* (American Counseling Association, 2014a).

It is the aim of the [name] program at [university] to foster ethical and professional behavior in our students in preparation for a career as clinical mental health counselors and to provide an environment conducive to positive learning and teaching. Students are expected to be familiar and comply with the [university] *Code of Community Standards*, the *Academic Honor Code*, the policies published in the most recent editions of the [university] *Graduate Studies Catalog* and the [name] program *Graduate Student Handbook*, and the *ACA Code of Ethics* and practice recommendations of the American Counseling Association. Student progress in the program may be interrupted for failure to comply with professional ethical standards or when intrapersonal, interpersonal, or professional behavior interferes with education and training requirements for self or others. Therefore, it is crucial to become familiar with the policies and procedures of [university] and [name] program in order to create an environment that is conducive to student learning and growth.

Civility in the Classroom and All Learning Settings

Civility is expected in all interactions and learning settings connected to the [name] graduate program. Civility in the classroom, during off-campus assignments, during small-group work, and in field site settings reflects a student's ability to maintain the professional behavior expected of a practicing counseling professional. Student incivility interferes with student learning and the teaching environment. Therefore, all students are expected to assist in providing a positive learning environment for other students as well as themselves. Disruptive behaviors such as arriving late, leaving early, arriving under the influence of substances, side discussions during class time, talking over or interrupting other students, and actions that inhibit or disparage the contributions of others are not acceptable. Inappropriate use of technology in the classroom will not be tolerated. Aggressive/volatile behaviors that lead to a negative working environment will be addressed with the individual, and if prosocial changes do not occur, faculty are permitted to and will be supported in asking students to leave the class and/or withdraw from the course. The student's final course grade will reflect the unarranged absence penalty described in the course attendance policy. The faculty will address inappropriate, unprofessional, and uncivil behaviors directly with the student in the weekly faculty meeting and during student review periods.

Acknowledgment of [Name] Graduate Program and Course Policies and Procedures

Students are asked to affirm the following statement with their signature:

I have received a copy of the checked off documents:

- ❑ [University and program name] *Student Handbook*
- ❑ [University] *Graduate Studies Catalog*
- ❑ *ACA Code of Ethics*
- ❑ [University] *Code of Community Standards*
- ❑ [University] *Academic Honor Code*

I verify that I have read each of the documents named above, including the referenced documents, and understand and agree to abide by the expectations, policies, and procedures of the [name] graduate program, [university], and the ethical standards of the profession.

- **I agree to participate in the ongoing self-evaluation process as described therein.**
- **I understand that I am responsible for following my planned program of study in sequence and if I do not, there will likely be a delay in completing the program.**
- **I confirm that I have taken responsibility for asking the faculty any questions I may have in order to fully clarify my understanding of these expectations.**

I further understand that my failure to fulfill the expectations of any course, of the ethics of the profession, of the graduate program, and/or of [university] may necessitate a review by the faculty and may result in the implementation of a remediation plan, suspension, or dismissal from the [name] graduate program.

______________________	______________________	______________
Student's Name *(printed)*	Signature	Date

Appendix F

Sample Supervision Contracts

[Institutional logo or letterhead]
[Department/program name]

Supervision Contract for [Course Number and Name]

Supervision is an important part of each student's professional development and is a place of learning with respect to your varied roles as developing counselors. The functions of supervision are to provide safety for the student and client alike, to enable the student to function with optimum effectiveness in the practicum/internship experience, and to provide the student with an opportunity for professional development.

Supervisor Information: [Supervisor name, credentials]

I have a master's and a doctoral degree in counselor education and am a licensed mental health counselor [license number] and registered play therapist–supervisor [number] in the state of [name of state]. In addition, I am a national certified counselor [certificate number] and a qualified supervisor for mental health counseling. I have significant additional training in both infant mental health and play therapy, and much of my past clinical experience involved working with families of very young children recovering from the experience of high levels of trauma and neglect. My clinical experience includes providing individual, family, and/or group counseling in the outpatient, partial-program, inpatient, home, and school settings. I consider my primary theoretical orientation to be Adlerian, although I will also provide child-centered play therapy and filial therapy when I find either to be appropriate. The tenets of

Adlerian therapy that I most closely identify with are the collaborative nature of the relationship with clients and supervisees, the importance of insight with regard to change, the belief that human beings need to feel a sense of belonging, the belief that all behavior has a purpose, and the importance of past experiences in understanding current functioning. I tend to employ expressive arts techniques (clay, drawing, painting, sand tray, etc.) in both my counseling and supervision because I find that they typically enhance insight and facilitate exploration and expression of inner feelings and beliefs.

Supervision

Supervision is one of the processes used to ensure students are accountable and encouraged to develop their skills and abilities. In this context, accountability means to clients, to oneself, to the community, and to the university.

Benefits of supervision:

- Ensure the student is clear about roles and responsibilities
- Encourage the student to meet the profession's objectives
- Encourage quality of service to clients
- Encourage professional development
- Assist in identifying and managing stress in the student
- Consider the resources available to the student in the practicum/internship and discuss issues arising where resources are inadequate
- Provide a positive environment and personal support for the student

1. ***Organizational***
   Group supervision will take place every Monday for one and half hours in compliance with CACREP standards. Meetings will occur in Room 315 from 5:30 p.m. to 7:00 p.m. I ask that students please be on time to supervision so as not to interrupt the group process once it has begun. Students are allowed to miss two group supervision sessions without significant impact to their final grade, but attendance at all sessions is expected and highly encouraged. If a student must miss a group supervision session, he or she is expected to let me know as soon as possible, and there may be additional tasks or assignments required depending on the topics covered during the missed session.
2. ***Confidentiality***
   Confidentiality is a crucial element within the profession of counseling. In group supervision, students will often discuss clients' personal information as well as students' own vulnerable thoughts and feelings as they relate to their own counselor development. It is imperative that students respect and uphold the confidentiality of their peers. Disclosure of things shared in group supervision by peers to others outside of the group supervision class is considered an egregious violation of professional ethics and is therefore possible grounds for dismissal from the program, and at the least an indication that serious remediation is needed. In

addition, when students discuss client situations, they must make every effort to disguise the identity of their clients. Students may use a pseudonym or simply call the person "the client" but must refrain from using the person's given first and/or last names and avoid giving specific personal information (e.g., rather than saying, "The client attends the University of Central Florida," a student could say, "The client is getting her bachelor's degree in psychology"; or rather than saying, "The client is a nurse at Arnold Palmer," he or she could say, "The client is a nurse and typically works with children" if the population is pertinent). Information shared in group supervision may be disclosed by me to others outside of the group who are in faculty or administrative positions as it relates to students' counselor development. Information from group and/or individual supervision may be indicated when there is need for remediation and/or termination from the program.

3. ***Content***
   This supervision group will be a combination of psychoeducation and process oriented. The content of the supervision sessions will often depend on the group members and could include, among other topics:

   - **Professional** issues of
   - Ethics
   - Values
   - Theoretical orientation
   - Time management
   - **Personal** issues of
   - Parallel process
   - Transference and countertransference
   - Nurturing and burnout
   - **Education** in relation to
   - Skills enhancement
   - Topics of special populations
   - Advanced counseling techniques
   - Diagnosis, treatment planning, and goal setting
   - **Group process** among members
   - **Organizational** issues with regard to program completion
   - Capstone project
   - Portfolio (physical and presentation)

4. ***Accountability***
   At the midpoint and end of each semester, all students' progress in the course (skill development, use of supervision, observance of ethical and professional practices) will be evaluated in writing by the site supervisors (see Student Handbook for evaluation forms). I will contact site supervisors biweekly throughout each semester to discuss students' strengths and areas for continued growth. Throughout the semester, I may personally obtain information on students' performance by verbal report (case presentation), observation (being physically present), role play, and/or review of written case records. When observing and assessing

students' counseling related skills, I will utilize the Counseling Competencies Scale (CCS; Lambie, Mullen, Swank, & Blount, 2018), which facilitates evaluation of primary counseling skills, professional dispositions, and professional behaviors. I will then provide formative feedback to the student and suggest methods for increasing his or her skill level clinically, personally, professionally, and ethically.

During the semester, if the site supervisor and/or I have significant concerns about any of the following issues (or others as outlined in the syllabus and Student Handbook):

- Client safety
- The student's well-being
- The student's ability to carry out his or her role in an appropriate way
- The student's professional competence

and the issue or issues cannot be resolved within the supervision sessions, then it is my responsibility as a professional gatekeeper and counselor educator to discuss these with the student and begin a remediation process. In this event, I will put my concerns in writing and we will both sign the Student of Concern form, which will also outline a plan for remediation of the identified area(s).

5. ***Support***
   If at any time students need my support outside of our scheduled supervision meetings, they may contact me via cell phone at (222) 222-2222 or e-mail at email@universityname.edu. If I am unavailable, I will return messages within 24 hours. If unable to reach me, students may also call Dr. [department chair name], the department chair, at (555) 555-5555.

   In the case of an emergency involving a client, the student should first contact the site supervisor for immediate direction about how to handle the situation in compliance with the site's protocol and policies. The student will next contact me via phone call, text, or e-mail to report the emergency and update progress about the situation until the emergent aspect has been resolved. In compliance with Florida law for mandated reporters, the student may be responsible for directly reporting the suspected or reported abuse of a child or vulnerable adult by calling the state abuse hotline at 1-800-###-####. In addition, if it is suspected that a client is in danger of harming self or others, the student is obligated to call 911 and report the danger.
6. ***Responsibilities of the Student***
   - Clinical mental health counseling students must read and abide by the ethics codes of the American Counseling Association (ACA), and marriage, couple, and family counseling students will read and abide by the ethics codes of the American Association for Marriage and Family Therapy (AAMFT), regardless of membership status within these organizations.

- Students must provide proof of professional liability insurance that is to remain active throughout the time in which the student is in practicum and internship.
- Students are expected to maintain all professional documentation in a timely manner as determined by the site.
- Students must complete all requirements as outlined in the course syllabus and bring to supervision issues that arise in practicum/internship. Examples of such issues are:
  –Difficulties that arise in client work
  –Personal issues affecting working or client relationships (transference, countertransference, parallel process)
  –An awareness of their own personal process and a commitment to personal growth
  –Areas of work where they would like to develop skills
  –Reflections on work that has gone well

I voluntarily enter into this contract and have had the opportunity to read and ask any questions to clarify my understanding of this agreement.

______________________________	____________________	____________
Student's Name *(printed)*	Signature	Date
______________________________	____________________	____________
Practicum/Intership Supervisor's Name *(printed)*	Signature	Date

Sample Postdegree Supervision Contract

[Supervisor's name]
[Address]
[E-mail]
[Phone number]

Agreement for Postdegree Supervision

This agreement is made between ________________________, MHC Registered Intern #_________ and MFT Registered Intern # _________ (hereinafter referred to as the "supervisee") and [supervisor name], [license number], NCC [certificate number] and state qualified supervisor for MFT and MHC (hereinafter referred to as the "supervisor"). The supervisor agrees to provide supervision in compliance with the requirements for the Registered Internship as designated by the State of [state] and in accordance with the terms below. The supervisor and supervisee agree to the following:

1. DEFINITION OF SUPERVISION
   Supervision is the relationship between the qualified supervisor and intern that promotes the development of responsibility; skills; knowledge; attitudes; and adherence to ethical, legal and regulatory standards in the practice of clinical social work, marriage and family therapy, and mental health counseling. Supervision

is contact between an intern and a supervisor during which the intern apprises the supervisor of the diagnosis and treatment of each client; client cases are discussed; the supervisor provides the intern with oversight and guidance in diagnosing, treating, and dealing with clients; and the supervisor evaluates the intern's performance (F.A.C.64B4-2002; rev. 2/2016).

2. SUPERVISORY ROLE
As a supervisor, I believe my role is to develop supervision strategies that will prepare and inspire future counselors to be effective and responsible helping professionals who will serve their clients, the local community, and beyond by assisting a diverse clientele in an ethical manner with a multilevel perspective of interacting systems. This is accomplished by providing and overseeing a range of experiences that will assist in the development of competent intervention skills, therapeutic abilities, ethical practice, and a solid professional identity. As a supervisor, I believe that I have four major responsibilities:

   - Monitoring client welfare
   - Monitoring supervisee welfare
   - Enhancing the supervisee's clinical development and identity as a professional therapist
   - Facilitating the supervisee's ability to self-supervise

   Overall, supervision is a critical aspect of counselor development and to be effective must include a balance between supportive encouragement and challenging growth. Assisting supervisees with their own professional development in such areas as interpersonal assessment, therapeutic orientation, evaluation of the therapeutic process, and monitoring client care is inherent in the clinical supervision experience. For optimal learning to occur from actual field experience, it must be guided by professional supervision that expands on the learning opportunities that emerge from the actual counseling encounters. The ultimate goal in supervision is to help supervisees become self-supervising counselors with well-developed intervention skills, conceptual skills, and personalization skills that are used consciously, ethically, and effectively.

3. PHILOSOPHY OF SUPERVISION
In approaching supervision, I draw primarily on solution-oriented principles and apply this approach to a solution-oriented model of supervision, including (a) striving for supervisor/supervisee cooperation, (b) focusing on supervisee strengths rather than deficits, and (c) impressing on supervisees that they have the resources to overcome their therapeutic impasses with clients (Rudes, Shilts, & Berg, 1997). In addition, consistent with the solution-focused model, I believe that supervision should (d) emphasize collaboration between supervisor and supervisee, (e) focus on positive changes in the supervisee's behavior, (f) foster supervisee curiosity about his or her own counseling potential, and (g) assume that small changes make possible larger changes in the supervisee's counseling behaviors (Thomas, 1996). Ultimately,

it is my goal that a solution-focused approach to supervision enhances supervisees' competence, strengths, and potential as clinical practitioners and helps supervisees become aware of their inner resources and contribution of life experiences to the role of counselor. I endeavor to assist supervisees in constructing a vision for their success as counselors throughout their training experience and after licensure in independent practice.

4. FREQUENCY AND DURATION
   The supervisee agrees to follow the requirements defined by State Administrative Code 64B4-2.002 Definition of "Supervision" for Clinical Social Work, Marriage and Family Therapy and Mental Health Counseling—Revised 2/2016 (as quoted below) throughout the registered internship period.

   (1) An intern shall be credited for the time of supervision required by State Statute 491.005, if the intern:
       (a) received at least 100 hours of supervision in no less than 100 weeks; and,
       (b) provided at least 1500 hours of face-to-face psychotherapy with clients; and
       (c) received at least 1 hour of supervision every 2 weeks;
   (2) The supervision shall focus on the raw data from the intern's face-to-face psychotherapy with clients. The intern shall make the raw data directly available to the supervisor through such means as written clinical materials, direct observation and video and audio recordings.

Sessions will be one clock hour in length.

The supervisor agrees to the following:

5. The primary emphasis of supervision will be on the concerns and welfare of the clients. The secondary emphasis will be on concerns and needs of the supervisee. The supervisor will decide the following nature/style/manner of providing supervision to the supervisee (examples might include allowing supervisor to observe supervisee providing services; reviewing supervisee's work products, such as progress notes, reports, and other documentation; reviewing recordings of therapy sessions; discussing supervisee work concerns; structuring the supervisory sessions around selected topics, such as ethics or record keeping or other professional matters; communicating with supervisee's site employers/supervisors).
6. The supervisor will be available when the supervisee needs assistance in making decisions about the direction of a case in a timely, but not necessarily immediate, manner. Outside of scheduled supervision sessions, the supervisor will respond to text messages, e-mail messages, or voicemail message requests for contact within 24 hours unless she is out of the range of technological communication. In the event of an emergency that involves a client, the supervisee will first contact the direct employer or

clinical site's administrative chain of command for immediate direction about handling the situation based on site protocol and policy. The supervisee will next contact this supervisor via each and every means possible (text, e-mail, phone message) to report the emergency and update progress about the situation until the emergent aspect has subsided.

Emergency situations are defined to include the following (although these situations are not intended to be comprehensive): when a client reveals immediate threat of harm to self or to others, when abuse of a minor or vulnerable adult is discovered and an abuse report is necessary based on the laws of [state] for mandated reporters, when the supervisee becomes aware of legal issues or ethical conflicts that need to be addressed immediately, when the supervisee is experiencing excessive anxiety or distress about a case and needs immediate consultation. In the case of these events, the supervisor agrees to be available for emergency supervision and/or to require that the supervisee schedule an emergency supervision session.

7. The supervisor will continually evaluate the appropriateness of the services rendered and the professional development of the supervisee. Formal evaluation of the supervisee will occur every 4 months. The supervisor will evaluate the supervisee using the Counseling Competencies Scale (CCS) in the following areas: primary counseling skills, professional dispositions, and professional behaviors (copy attached to this contract). The supervisor will provide formative feedback to the supervisee and suggest methods for the supervisee to increase his or her skill level clinically, personally, professionally, and ethically.
8. In the event the supervisor does not believe the supervisee is progressing at a level appropriate for the stage of training clinically, personally, professionally, or ethically, the supervisor will apprise the supervisee in writing. The supervisor also has an obligation to the profession and will fulfill the role of gatekeeper, monitoring the supervisee's readiness or appropriateness for the licensees for which he or she is applying and, if necessary, reporting conduct that violates legal or ethical boundaries required of clinicians-in-training.
9. The supervisor will only endorse a supervisee for licensure if the supervisor believes the supervisee has met more than the minimum standards of performance in professional activities when measured against generally prevailing peer performance, pursuant to Section 491.009(1)(r) of the State Statutes.
10. The supervisor will maintain professional licensure as a licensed psychologist and a licensed marriage and family therapist. She will also maintain qualified supervisor status for mental health counseling and marriage and family therapy in good standing with the respective state licensure boards (and will provide documentation on request of the supervisee).
11. The supervisor will maintain professional liability insurance (and will provide documentation on request of the supervisee). The

supervisor will inform the supervisee of all facts about any alleged complaint or claim subject to the terms of the professional liability insurance policies and will cooperate with the supervisee in the defense of any such claim made against the supervisee.

12. The supervisor will follow the ethics codes of the American Counseling Association and the American Association for Marriage and Family Therapy as well as the legal requirements for the professions under which she is licensed.
13. The supervisor will avoid any dual or multiple relationships with the supervisee that could reasonably be expected to lead to exploitation or loss of objectivity. (Dual relationship means a situation wherein the supervisor and supervisee have both a professional relationship and a nonprofessional relationship, such as a personal friendship, business or financial ties, mutual club or social group activities, family or marital ties, or sexual relationship.) If a dual relationship does exist, the supervisor will be responsible for ensuring that the relationship does not hamper objectivity or exploit the supervisee and the means developed to prevent/resolve any problems that may arise from the supervisory relationship.

The supervisee agrees to the following:

14. The supervisee will disclose a correct accounting of all face-to-face services to clients at each supervision meeting.
15. The supervisee will document all clinical activities that occur between supervision meetings using a written log listing all activities and communications that have occurred with clients using client initials, dates, and clock times of direct client contact verifying any and all services to clients.
16. The supervisee will apprise the supervisor of the progress, or lack thereof, of each client at each supervisory session.
17. In the event of an emergency that involves a client, the supervisee will first contact the direct employer or clinical site's administrative chain of command for immediate direction about handling the situation based on site protocol and policy. The supervisee will next contact the supervisor via each and every means possible (text, e-mail, phone message) to report the emergency and update progress about the situation until the emergent aspect has subsided.

    Emergency situations are defined to include the following (although these situations are not intended to be comprehensive): when a client reveals immediate threat of harm to self or to others, when abuse of a minor or vulnerable adult is discovered and an abuse report is necessary based on the laws of [state] for mandated reporters, when the supervisee becomes aware of legal issues or ethical conflicts that need to be addressed immediately, when the supervisee is experiencing excessive anxiety or distress about a case and needs immediate consultation. In the case of these events, the supervisor agrees to be available for emergency supervision and/or to require that the supervisee schedule an emergency supervision session.

18. The supervisee is responsible for scheduling and obtaining the requisite supervision hours per amount of client services provided as defined by State Licensure Code 64B4-2.002 (above).
19. If the supervisee chooses to supplement his or her supervision with services from another supervisor for individual supervision, the supervisor named in this contract must be first notified in writing and must agree to the source of and plan for the additional supervision. The supervisor and supervisee will construct an addendum to this contract defining the roles and responsibilities of each supervisor. This does not apply to supplemental group supervision.
20. The supervisee understands that according to State Licensure Code 64B4-3.008 he or she must remain under supervision and use the title "Registered Intern" until he or she is in receipt of a license to practice the profession for which he or she has applied or receives a letter from the licensure board stating he or she is licensed, even if the two (2) year post-master's supervision requirement has been satisfied, 1,500 client hours have been obtained, and 100 hours of supervision have been fulfilled.
21. The supervisee will inform all employers and clients about his or her status as a registered intern receiving supervision, as mandated by state law; will provide clients and employers with the name and contact information of the supervisor; and will obtain written acknowledgment of the supervisory relationship from each client prior to the commencement of professional services.
22. Pursuant to State Statute 491.0149, the supervisee will include the words "Registered Marriage and Family Therapist Intern" or "Registered Mental Health Counselor Intern" on all promotional materials, including business cards, brochures, stationery, advertisements, websites, and signs, naming the registered intern/supervisee.
23. The supervisee agrees to strictly follow all laws and rules identified by the State Board of Clinical Social Work, Marriage and Family Therapy, and Mental Health Counseling. The supervisee will also read and abide by the ethics codes of the American Counseling Association (ACA) if a registered mental health counselor intern and, if a marriage and family therapy intern, will abide by the ethics code of the American Association for Marriage and Family Therapy (AAMFT) whether or not he or she is a member of the professional association.
24. The supervisee will attend supervision on the agreed-on basis and will:

    a. Consider the registered internship period as a learning opportunity and seek the benefit of the supervisor's instruction and oversight as well as respect the supervisor's obligations and liability in the provision of supervision.
    b. Apprise the supervisor of the diagnoses, case conceptualization, and treatment of each client.
    c. Make available appropriate and current raw data and clinical materials that are representative of the supervisee's practice and for cases in which more guidance and direction are needed.

d. Participate in supervision with the goal of increasing competency and skill in ethical clinical practice.
e. Arrive at supervision sessions prepared to discuss cases and problems and take an active role in his or her clinical and professional growth.

25. The supervisee will attend supervision as scheduled, arriving on time and notifying the supervisor at least 24 hours in advance of absences or the need to reschedule. If 24-hour notice is not given, the supervisee is responsible for paying the session fee.
26. The supervisee will maintain registered internship status in good standing with the state licensure boards (and will provide documentation on request of the supervisor).
27. The supervisee will maintain professional liability insurance (and will provide documentation on request of the supervisor). Also, the supervisee will inform the supervisor of all facts about any alleged complaint or claim subject to the terms of the professional liability insurance policies and will cooperate with the supervisor in the defense of any such claim made against the supervisor as a result of the supervisee's actions.
28. In exchange for supervisor's time, expertise and licensure, the supervisor shall be compensated $65 per hour of supervision. If the session is dyadic supervision, each supervisee will pay $40. Payment will be in cash or by check and will be made at the beginning of each supervisory session.
29. Either party, on 14 days' notice in writing, may terminate this agreement. *The agreement may be terminated immediately if either party does not maintain necessary qualifications or fails to follow the identified code of ethics or state licensure board laws and rules.*
30. DURATION AND TERMINATION: The period of this agreement between the supervisor and supervisee shall be from ______________________________ [start date] until such time as the supervisee meets the hour and supervision requirements for licensure, or the agreement is otherwise terminated.

I have read the above, had an opportunity to discuss related questions, and agree to the provisions set forth.

____________________________	____________________	______________
Supervisor's Name *(printed)*	Signature	Date
____________________________	____________________	______________
Supervisee's Name *(printed)*	Signature	Date

[Address of License]
[Phone Number(s)]
[E-mail Address(es)]

Appendix G

Sample Documentation of Student Behavior and Faculty Action

Sample Concern Shared by a Student With a Faculty Member

[Date and time of interaction]

- Conversation initiated by student Jennifer W. in meeting with department chair
- Conversation approximately 45 minutes long
- Topic: student concerns about another student's problematic interpersonal behavior in [course name] and university honor code violations

Sample Student's Description of Situation

Jennifer requested meeting and asked for privacy with office door closed. She became emotional and tearful shortly after meeting began, stating that she hadn't slept for two nights because of being so upset about an interaction with another student in class earlier in the week.

Jennifer reported that on Monday night when the professor stepped out of class after distributing a take-home, open-book final exam, another student, Annie K., pulled out her calendar and said, "Okay everybody, when does everyone want to meet? We are going to have a discussion group about the take-home final exam for this class."

Jennifer asked, "Is that in compliance with the honor code?" and pointed to the poster in the classroom that displayed the honor code. Annie responded, "No, it's not!" (Jennifer noted the tone of Annie's voice was significantly admonishing.) "We are just going to have a 'discussion group' [air quotes], we aren't going to do anything wrong, we are just going to write down the page numbers for the questions and discuss those." Jennifer observed that other students in the class also indicated that they thought it was wrong but didn't speak up much.

Jennifer said she was still shook up that night and didn't want to stay after class to ask the professor directly, but from home she e-mailed the professor and asked, "Do you allow students to discuss the take-home final in study group? Just curious." The professor responded, "No." Jennifer forwarded the e-mail to five other students who had expressed doubts or didn't think the proposed study group was right.

Jennifer found out that there had been a similar study group for the midterm exam also. She learned that there were other students in the class, in addition to her, who were not included in the study group for the midterm.

Jennifer reported that Annie had left Jennifer several voice messages, which she has not returned because she was quite distressed and feared Annie's aggressive manner and potential confrontation if Annie learned of Jennifer "ratting her out."

The documentation of this conversation will be shared with the core faculty and affected professor. There has been a pattern of concern about Annie's professional and interpersonal behavior over several semesters as well as possible evidence of another violation of the university's honor code.

Sample Documentation of Student Behaviors of Concern

Notes prepared by [professor's name; course name] on [date].

During class on [date] (Week 2 of the semester), students were asked to engage in a class exercise that would assist with continued group cohesion development for the class. Given that all students have taken at least two prior courses together, this exercise was not expected to be a challenge, as rapport between students was established. All students participated in the exercises and appeared to be engaged in a positive and dynamic manner.

Following the closure of the exercise, students were asked to bring their chairs back into a circle to engage in a whole-class discussion and debrief about the exercise. During the group discussion, Samantha J. had positioned her chair just outside of the circle. None of the other students commented on the positioning of her chair, yet a space remained in the circle for her chair to be moved up and included with the rest of the class. As the group discussion began, Samantha pulled out her cell phone and seemed focused on the phone and using it, attempting to hide her behaviors by repositioning how she was seated in her chair. She would verbally participate randomly, often agreeing automatically no matter what was said. After a few students shared their thoughts, one student, Heather S., challenged Samantha by asking her why she was on her phone during our class time and why she had chosen not to be a part of the circle. Heather seemed concerned more than upset or irritated by Samantha's behaviors. Samantha appeared embarrassed by Heather's comment and responded by saying, "Fine, I didn't realize it was a big deal," in what seemed to be a defensive tone. She moved her chair forward to join the circle, sat back down, and crossed her arms and legs in her chair. Samantha did not use her phone for the rest of class but did look down at it occasionally. The group reluctantly resumed the discussion and appeared to be disturbed by these events. When time ended for class, Samantha hurried out of the room. Heather seemed confused by the reaction, and other students appeared to have concerned reactions or appeared indifferent. The remainder of the group discussions stayed on task.

The following day, I left a phone message with Samantha to touch base with her and better understand her actions and reactions. I will e-mail as a second follow-up before class meets next week, letting her know I wish to speak with her before class meets next week.

Sample E-Mail Recounting Student Meeting[1]

Thanks to all of you for your participation in the meeting that took place on [date] to support Jason S., who is enrolled in the [university] Marriage and Family Therapy program. The meeting was requested by Jason's academic advisor, Dr. [name], based on concerns about Jason's declining academic performance. Two of Jason's instructors had contacted his advisor about their concerns, and an individual meeting between Jason and his advisor occurred earlier this semester. Jason attributed his declining performance to changes in his family situation and the extraordinary amount of distress it has caused him. He also reported working two part-time jobs.

Now that we are at the midterm point of this semester, Jason's status in all courses indicates that he may not meet the minimum overall final course grade of a B or better as defined by the university grading policy found in the graduate catalog. If his grades do not improve, Jason is in jeopardy of being placed on academic probation and will be ineligible to continue on to his first semester of field experience. The meeting we had today was to discuss what has worked well this semester and plan adjustments Jason can make moving forward to support his success.

Dr. [name of advisor] shared in our meeting her recommendation that Jason seek services from the Accessibility and Resource Office on campus for an evaluation and initiate counseling at the university's Counseling and Psychological Services Office. Jason will schedule these meetings for early next week and keep his advisor informed of his actions. It is possible that the Accessibility and Resource Office may request information to document a decline in course performance. Only if that request is officially made should Jason's course grades be shared. He will be included on all communications if this information is required.

Jason, thank you for your willingness to share your current personal challenges in our meeting today and to self-reflect on some of the processes you have been experiencing that have contributed to your current level of stress. In addition to following through with the university resources listed above, you are encouraged to meet with Dr. [name

[1]*Note.* It is recommended that this document be e-mailed within 24 hours to all participants present at the meeting, including the student.

of advisor] as regularly as you will find helpful. We also suggest that you take responsibility for speaking directly to your course instructors to inform them that you are navigating personal challenges that have impacted your academic performance and that you are working toward remedying the problems. Although this does not mean you will automatically receive opportunities to revise or redo work that has already been completed in your courses, it will be a productive and adaptive way to engage in open communication with your course instructors, who are there to help support your learning and training as a marriage and family therapist.

Ultimately, the responsibility for managing your personal situations and your academic performance is yours. Dr. [name of advisor] can assist you in preparing for these conversations if you'd find that helpful. As therapists, it is important to know how to engage in difficult conversations. We invite you to consider this opportunity not only one that will support your self-advocacy as a student and a learner but also one that can assist you in practicing skills required for the professional field for which you are training.

Please let us know if you have any questions or need clarification. We can reevaluate your progress next month to help guide course registration for next semester.

Sincerely,

Professor and Director of Training

Appendix H

Sample Student Progress Evaluation Rating Form and Accompanying Rubric for Evaluating Multiple Students

Appendix H

Sample Student Progress Evaluation Rating Form

This evaluation system can be utilized annually or each semester.

Year Admitted: ____________________ GPA: __________
Student Name: ____
Faculty Advisor: ____

Rating Scale: 0 = *unsatisfactory*; 1 = *marginal*; 2 = *competent*; 3 = *exemplary*

Academic Performance: ❑ 0 ❑ 1 ❑ 2 ❑ 3
Clinical Skills Performance: ❑ 0 ❑ 1 ❑ 2 ❑ 3
Professional Conduct/Disposition: ❑ 0 ❑ 1 ❑ 2 ❑ 3

Comments/Source: ____
____
____

Actions to take: ____
____
____

Rubric for Evaluating Student Progress

Academic Performance (33% of overall rating):

_____ *Unsatisfactory* (0 points): Student does not demonstrate satisfactory academic performance or progress across multiple academic areas.

_____ *Marginal* (1 point): Student demonstrates marginal academic knowledge and performance across multiple academic areas.

_____ *Competent* (2 points): Student demonstrates competent knowledge and performs well across multiple academic areas.

_____ *Exemplary* (3 points): Student demonstrates exemplary academic knowledge and/or performs extremely well across multiple academic areas.

Clinical Skills Performance (33% of overall rating):

_____ *Unsatisfatory* (0 points): Student does not demonstrate satisfactory performance or progress in clinical skill development.

_____ *Marginal* (1 point): Student demonstrates marginal therapeutic awareness and/or skill performance in clinical skill development.

_____ *Competent* (2 points): Student demonstrates competent and progressively appropriate clinical skill development.

_____ *Exemplary* (3 points): Student demonstrates exemplary therapeutic abilities and clinical skill development.

Professional Conduct and Disposition (33% of overall rating):

_____ *Unsatisfatory* (0 points): Student engages in unprofessional conduct and does not demonstrate appropriate intra- or interpersonal dispositions or behavioral change when provided the opportunity.

_____ *Marginal* (1 point): Student demonstrates marginal professional conduct and intra- or interpersonal dispositions expected of a counselor trainee.

_____ *Competent* (2 points): Student demonstrates professional conduct and intra- or interpersonal dispositions that are developmentally appropriate for a counselor trainee.

_____ *Exemplary* (3 points): Student demonstrates exemplary professional conduct and intra- or interpersonal dispositions.

Comment Examples

Academic Performance:

Student engages in academic performance that is consistent with expectations published in the [university] *Graduate Studies Catalog* and the *Graduate Studies Student Handbook*, including the following: maintains a 3.0 grade point average; engages in the learning process and educational opportunities and supports the learning process of others; completes non-course-related program requirements in timely manner in compliance with requirements of the graduate counseling program and university policies and procedures; and participates in remediation processes, if recommended.

Clinical Skills Performance:

Student demonstrates levels of counseling skills, knowledge, and awareness developmentally appropriate for the given point in the training program; establishes effective counseling relationships and progresses in his or her ability to work with clients; assesses and conceptualizes cases accurately; implements and evaluates counseling interventions; responds appropriately to and integrates feedback and engages effectively in supervision; maintains appropriate boundaries and establishes professional interactions with colleagues and supervisors; integrates multicultural awareness, knowledge, and skills into professional interactions; integrates theory and research into clinical practice; and maintains professional ethics.

Professional Conduct and Disposition:

Student engages in conduct that is consistent with expectations of professional counselors as published in the [university] *Graduate Studies Catalog* and the *Graduate Studies Student Handbook*, including the following: understands and maintains ethical guidelines of the profession; abides by the academic honesty policy of the university; respects the privacy and confidentiality needs of others; engages in learning and experiential opportunities for personal and professional development; prioritizes interests of clients over self when providing professional services; remains open to ideas, learning, and change; fulfills obligations promptly, consistently, reliably, and according to expectations stated by the professor or supervisor; cooperates with remediation plans and endeavors to adjust or improve behavior; maintains sensitivity to role differences and power dynamics that may exist in relationships and settings and manages them appropriately; seeks professional consultation with regard to recognized personal areas of growth; maintains a professional appearance appropriate for the setting; and supports the learning process of others. Student also engages in intra- and interpersonal growth and behaviors that are consistent with expectations of professional counselors, including the following: exhibits awareness of personal beliefs, values, needs, strengths, and limitations; respects the autonomy and beliefs of others and refrains from imposing his or her personal beliefs on others; demonstrates genuineness, empathy, and interest in the welfare of others; establishes and maintains effective and functional relationships personally, professionally, and therapeutically; exhibits sensitivity to the individual and cultural identities of others and displays cultural competence; communicates respectfully and professionally; exhibits appropriate interpersonal boundaries; resolves interpersonal conflicts with colleagues and others in a timely and professional manner; interacts with appropriate assertiveness and emotional control; accepts responsibility for actions and problems; manages personal mental health, emotional problems, stress, and/or interpersonal issues effectively; demonstrates personal and professional integrity in stated thoughts and actions; participates in self-reflection and self-exploration; exhibits emotional self-control; manages personal wellness; and participates in personal growth and self-development activities.

Appendix I

Sample Strategies for Reinforcing Professionalism at Transition Points in a Graduate Program

1. Standardized statement printed in all program syllabi:

   Professionalism and Classroom Civility: Graduate students are expected to observe a level of professional conduct in the classroom reflective of practicing mental health professionals and in keeping with the professional ethics code adopted by this program and the policies of the university. *Students failing to act professionally will be asked to leave the class. Your final grade will reflect an unarranged absence penalty described in the Attendance and Participation Policy section of this syllabus.*

2. Rubric categories designated to measure professionalism and participation in the course grading system:

   Professionalism [Consider constructing a rubric to describe specific expectations for each item]

   - Attendance and Promptness
   - Level of Engagement in Class Discussions
   - Level of Engagement While Working in Small Groups
   - Listening Skills
   - Professional Behavior
   - Preparation

3. Components of the agreement for practicum and internship field site placement that reference professional expectations of the student. This agreement includes the agency/field site supervisor, university faculty supervisor, and student, all of whom sign to affirm agreement.

The student counselor agrees to:

1. Behave in a professional and ethical manner at all times in accordance with the ethical guidelines of the [name of professional association], the laws of the State of [name], and the policies of [name of academic institution] and the [name] program.
2. Abide by the administrative policies, standards, regulations, schedules, and practices of the agency site.
3. Behave in accordance with the role expectations of a trainee.
4. Consistently and punctually attend all scheduled training activities and meetings onsite and on campus as agreed on by the faculty supervisor, site supervisor and/or onsite mentor, and counseling student.
5. Attend all scheduled individual supervision sessions and group supervision sessions consistently and on time.
6. Arrive prepared for all scheduled individual and group supervision sessions (i.e., completed case presentation, readings, and other assigned activities).
7. Notify the site supervisor and the faculty supervisor of illness, accident, or any other situation that prevents the counseling student from meeting the prearranged schedule at the agency site as soon as possible.
8. Complete all required paperwork and documentation by the scheduled due dates.
9. Continuously strive to improve counseling performance and accept feedback from supervisors in a professional manner.
10. Ensure a valuable clinical learning experience by communicating with the faculty supervisor and/or site supervisor if there are difficulties.

References

Alexander, P. A. (2004). A model of domain learning: Reinterpreting expertise as a multidimensional, multistage process. In D. Y. Dai & R. J. Sternberg (Eds.), *Motivation, emotion and cognition: Integrative perspectives on intellectual functioning and development* (pp. 273–298). Mahwah, NJ: Erlbaum.

Althouse, L. A., Stritter, F. T., & Steiner, B. D. (1999). Attitudes and approaches of influential role models in clinical education. *Advances in Health Sciences Education*, *4*, 111–122.

American Association for Marriage and Family Therapy. (2014). *Approved supervision designation: Standards handbook.* Retrieved from https://dx5br1z4f6n0k.cloudfront.net/imis15/Documents/Approved_Supervisor_Handbook_2014.pdf

American Association for Marriage and Family Therapy. (2015). *Code of ethics.* Retrieved from https://www.aamft.org/Documents/Approved_supervisor_handbook_2014.pdf

American Counseling Association. (2005). *ACA code of ethics.* Alexandria, VA: Author.

American Counseling Association. (2009). *The ACA encyclopedia of counseling.* Alexandria, VA: Author.

American Counseling Association. (2014a). *ACA code of ethics.* Alexandria, VA: Author.

American Counseling Association. (2014b). *States that have adopted the* ACA Code of Ethics. Retrieved from https://www.counseling.org/docs/default-source/licensure/state-licensure-boards-that-have-adopted-the-aca-code-of-ethics-(pdf).pdf?sfvrsn=9331cb46_2

American Mental Health Counselors Association. (2015, October). *AMHCA code of ethics*. Retrieved from http://connections.amhca.org/HigherLogic/System/DownloadDocumentFile.ashx?DocumentFileKey=d4e10fcb-2f3c-c701-aa1d-5d0f53b8bc14

American Psychological Association. (2006). *Final report of the APA Task Force on the Assessment of Competence in Professional Psychology*. Retrieved from www.apa.org/ed/resources/competence-report.aspx

American Psychological Association. (2011). Model act for state licensure of psychologists. *American Psychologist, 66*, 214–226.

American Psychological Association. (2012). *A practical guidebook for the competency benchmarks*. Retrieved from www.apa.org/ed/graduate/benchmarks-guide.aspx

American Psychological Association. (2014). *Guidelines for clinical supervision in health service psychology*. Retrieved from https://www.apa.org/about/policy/guidelines-supervision.pdf

American Psychological Association. (2015a). Professional practice guidelines: Guidance for developers and users. *American Psychologist, 70*, 823–831.

American Psychological Association. (2015b). *Serving a diverse public*. Retrieved from www.apa.org/ed/graduate/diversity-preparation.aspx?tab=2

American Psychological Association. (2017a). *About accreditation: What is the purpose of accreditation?* Retrieved from www.apa.org/ed/accreditation/about/about-accreditation.aspx_

American Psychological Association. (2017b). *Competency initiatives in professional psychology*. Retrieved from www.apa.org/ed/graduate/competency.aspx

American Psychological Association. (2017c). *Ethical principles of psychologists and code of conduct: Including 2010 and 2016 amendments*. Retrieved from www.apa.org/ethics/code/

American Psychological Association Commission on Accreditation. (2015). *Standards of accreditation for health service psychology*. Retrieved from www.apa.org/ed/accreditation/about/policies/standards-of-accreditation.pdf

American Psychological Association Working Group on Restrictions Affecting Diversity Training in Graduate Education. (2013). *Serving a diverse public*. Retrieved from www.apa.org/ed/graduate/diversity-preparation.aspx

American School Counselor Association. (2016). *ASCA ethical standards for school counselors*. Retrieved from https://www.schoolcounselor.org/asca/media/asca/Ethics/EthicalStandards2016.pdf

Americans with Disabilities Act Amendments Act of 2008, Pub. L. No. 110-325, 122 Stat. 3553 (2008).

Americans with Disabilities Act of 1990, Pub. L. No. 101-336, 104 Stat. 328 (1990).

Ametrano, I. M. (2014). Teaching ethical decision making: Helping students reconcile personal and professional values. *Journal of Counseling & Development*, *92*, 154–161.

Andrews, E. E., Kuemmel, A., Williams, J. L., Pilarski, C. R., Dunn, M., & Lund, E. M. (2013). Providing culturally competent supervision to trainees with disabilities in rehabilitation settings. *Rehabilitation Psychology*, *58*(3), 233–244.

Arredondo, P., Shealy, C., Neale, M., & Winfrey, L. L. (2004). Consultation and interprofessional collaboration: Modeling for the future. *Journal of Clinical Psychology*, *60*, 787–800.

Artman, L. K., & Daniels, J. A. (2010). Disability and psychotherapy practice: Cultural competence and practical tips. *Professional Psychology: Research and Practice*, *41*, 442–448.

Association for Counselor Education and Supervision. (2011, April). *Best practices in clinical supervision*. Retrieved from www.acesonline.net/sites/default/files/ACES-Best-Practices-in-clinical-supervision-document-FINAL_0.pdf

Association of State and Provincial Psychology Boards. (2015, August). *Supervision guidelines for education and training leading to licensure as a health service provider*. Retrieved from https://c.ymcdn.com/sites/asppb.site-ym.com/resource/resmgr/Guidelines/Final_Supervision_Guidelines.pdf

Australian Institute of Professional Counsellors. (2009). *Reflective practice, supervision, and self-care* (Counsellor Skills Series Report No. 4). Retrieved from www.counsellingconnection.com/wp-content/uploads/2009/10/report-4-reflective-practice-supervision-self-care.pdf

Baldo, T. D., Softas-Nall, B. C., & Shaw, S. F. (1997). Student review and retention in counselor education: An alternative to Frame and Stevens-Smith. *Counselor Education and Supervision*, *36*, 245–254.

Baldwin, J. R., Faulkner, S. L., Hecht, M. L., & Lindsley, S. L. (2008). *Redefining culture: Perspectives across disciplines*. Mahwah, NJ: Erlbaum.

Bandura, A. (1986). *Social foundations of thought and action*. Englewood Cliffs, NJ: Prentice Hall.

Barber, J. P., Sharpless, B. A., Klostermann, S., & McCarthy, K. S. (2007). Assessing intervention competence and its relation to therapy outcome: A selected review derived from the outcome literature. *Professional Psychology: Research and Practice*, *38*, 493–500.

Barlow, C., & Coleman, H. (2003). Suitability for practice guidelines for students: A survey of Canadian social work programmes. *Social Work Education*, *22*(2), 151–163.

Behnke, S. (2005). The supervisor as gatekeeper: Reflections on Ethical Standards 7.02, 7.04, 7.05, 7.06, and 10.01. *Monitor on Psychology*, *36*(5), 90–91.

Behnke, S. H. (2008). Discussion: Toward elaborating and implementing a conceptualization of healthy, safe training environments. *Training and Education in Professional Psychology*, *2*(4), 215–218. doi:10.1037/a0014008

Belar, C. D., Brown, R. A., Hersch, L. E., Hornyak, L. M., Rozensky, R. H., Sheridan, E. P., . . . Reed, G. W. (2001). Self-assessment in clinical health psychology: A model for ethical expansion of practice. *Professional Psychology: Research and Practice*, *32*(2), 135–141. doi:10.1037/0735-7028.32.2.135

Belar, C. D., & Perry, N. W. (1992). National conference on scientist–practitioner education and training for the professional practice of psychology. *American Psychologist*, *47*, 71–75.

Bemak, F., Epp, L. R., & Keys, S. G. (1999). Impaired graduate students: A process model of graduate program monitoring and intervention. *International Journal for the Advancement of Counseling*, *21*, 19–30.

Bernard, J. M., & Goodyear, R. K. (2014). *Fundamentals of clinical supervision* (5th ed.). Upper Saddle River, NJ: Pearson.

Bhat, C. S. (2005). Enhancing counseling gatekeeping with performance appraisal protocols. *International Journal for the Advancement of Counseling*, *27*, 399–411.

Biaggio, M. K., Gasparikova-Krasnec, M., & Bauer, L. (1983). Evaluation of clinical psychology graduate students: The problem of the unsuitable student. *Professional Practice of Psychology*, *4*(1), 9–20.

Bigelow, J. R., & Johnson, W. B. (2001). Promoting mentor-protégé relationship formation in graduate school. *The Clinical Supervisor*, *20*, 1–23.

Birk, J. M., & Mahalik, J. R. (1996). The influence of trainee conceptual level, trainee anxiety, and supervision evaluation on counselor developmental level. *The Clinical Supervisor*, *14*, 123–137.

Black, P. N., Jeffreys, D., & Hartley, E. (1993). Personal history of psychosocial trauma in the early life of social work and business students. *Journal of Social Work Education*, *29*, 171–180.

Board of Curators of the University of Missouri v. Horowitz, 435 U.S. 78, 98 S.Ct. 948, 55 L.Ed.2n 124 (1978).

Bodner, K. E. (2012). Ethical principles and standards that inform educational gatekeeping practices in psychology. *Ethics & Behavior*, *22*(1), 60–74.

Borders, L. D. (1989). Developmental cognitions of first practicum supervisees. *Journal of Counseling Psychology*, *36*, 163–169.

Borders, L. D., Fong, M. L., & Neimeyer, G. J. (1986). Counseling students' level of ego development and perceptions of clients. *Counselor Education and Supervision*, *26*, 36–49.

Bradey, J., & Post, P. (1991). Impaired students: Do we eliminate them from counselor education programs? *Counselor Education and Supervision*, *31*, 100–108.

Brear, P., & Dorrian, J. (2010). Gatekeeping or gate slippage? A national survey of counseling educators in Australian undergraduate and postgraduate academic training programs. *Training and Education in Professional Psychology*, *4*, 264–273.

Brear, P., Dorrian, J., & Luscri, G. (2008). Preparing our future counseling professionals: Gatekeeping and the implications for research. *Counseling and Psychotherapy Research*, 8, 93–101.

Brew, L., Cervantes, J. M., & Shepard, D. (2013). Millennial counselors and the ethical use of Facebook. *The Professional Counselor*, *3*(2), 93–104.

Briggs, K., Fournier, D. G., & Hendrix, C. C. (1999). Evaluating trainees' skill development: The Family Therapy Skills Checklist. *Contemporary Family Therapy*, *21*(3), 353–371.

Bronfenbrenner, U. (1979). *The ecology of human development: Experiments by nature and design.* Cambridge, MA: Harvard University Press.

Brown, M. (2013). A content analysis of problematic behavior in counselor education programs. *Counselor Education and Supervision*, *52*, 179–192.

Brown-Rice, K. A., & Furr, S. (2013). Preservice counselors' knowledge of classmates' problems of professional competency. *Journal of Counseling & Development*, *91*, 224–233.

Brown-Rice, K., & Furr, S. (2016). Counselor educators and students with problems of professional competence: A survey and discussion. *The Professional Counselor*, *6*, 134–146.

Bruff v. North Mississippi Health Services, Inc., 244 F.3d 495 (5th Cir. 2001).

Burkholder, D., & Hall, S. F. (2014). *Ward v. Wilbanks:* Students respond. *Journal of Counseling & Development*, *92*, 232–240.

Burkholder, D., Hall, S. F., & Burkholder, J. (2014). *Ward v. Wilbanks:* Counselor educators respond. *Counselor Education and Supervision*, *53*, 267–283.

Busseri, M. A., Tyler, J. D., & King, A. R. (2005). An exploratory examination of student dismissals and prompted resignations from clinical psychology PhD training programs: Does clinical competency matter? *Professional Psychology: Research and Practice*, *36*, 441–445. doi:10.1037/0735-7028.36.4.441

Carkhuff, R. R. (1969). Critical variables in effective counselor training. *Journal of Counseling Psychology*, *16*(3), 238–245.

Cass, V. C. (1979). Homosexual identity formation: A theoretical model. *Journal of Homosexuality*, *4*(3), 219–235.

Center for Credentialing and Education. (2016). *Code of ethics.* Retrieved from www.cce-global.org/Assets/Ethics/ACScodeofethics.pdf

Chang, V. Y. (2017). *A grounded theory approach to faculty experiences and perspectives on gatekeeping in counselor education programs* (Unpublished doctoral dissertation). Oregon State University, Corvallis.

Christensen, J. K. (2015). *Building a consensus on the professional dispositions of counseling students: A content analysis on counseling student retention policies* (Unpublished doctoral dissertation). The College of William and Mary, Williamsburg, VA.

Christensen, J. (2016). *FIASCO rubric.* Unpublished scale, Lewis & Clark, Psychology Department.

Cobb, N. H. (1994). Court-recommended guidelines for managing unethical students and working with university lawyers. *Journal of Social Work Education, 30*(1), 18–31.

Cobb, N. H., & Jordan, C. (1989). Students with questionable values of threatening behavior: Precedent and policy from discipline to dismissal. *Journal of Social Work Education, 25*, 87–97.

Cobia, D. C., & Boes, S. R. (2000). Professional disclosure statements and formal plans for supervision: Two strategies for minimizing the risk of ethical conflicts in post-master's supervision. *Journal of Counseling & Development, 78*, 293–296.

Cohn, L. D., & Westenberg, P. M. (2004). Intelligence and maturity: Meta-analytic evidence for the incremental and discriminant validity of Loevinger's measures of ego development. *Journal of Personality and Social Psychology, 86*, 760–772.

Cole, B. S. (1991). Legal issues related to social work program admissions. *Journal of Social Work Education, 27*(1), 18–24.

Cole, B. S., & Lewis, R. G. (1993). Gatekeeping through termination of unsuitable social work students: Legal issues and guidelines. *Journal of Social Work Education, 29*(2), 150–159.

Commission on Accreditation for Marriage and Family Therapy Education. (2017, August). *Accreditation standards: Graduate and post-graduate marriage and family therapy training programs.* Retrieved from http://dx5br1z4f6n0k.cloudfront.net/imis15/Documents/COAMFTE/Accreditation%20Resources/2018%20COAMFTE%20Accreditation%20Standards%20Version%2012.pdf

Commission on Rehabilitation Counselor Certification. (2017). *Code of professional ethics for rehabilitation counselors.* Retrieved from https://www.crccertification.com/filebin/pdf/ethics/CodeOfEthics_01-01-2017.pdf

Constangy, Brooks, Smith, & Prophete, LLP. (2008, October 2). *Client bulletins: ADA Amendments Act to take effect January 1* [Web log post]. Retrieved from www.constangy.com/communications-185.html

Corey, G., Corey, M. S., Corey, C., & Callanan, P. (2015). *Issues and ethics in the helping professions* (9th ed.). Boston, MA: Brooks/Cole.

Cornell Law School Legal Information Institute. (2017). *Respondeat superior.* Retrieved from https://www.law.cornell.edu/wex/respondeat_superior

Cottone, R. R., & Claus, R. E. (2000). Ethical decision-making models: A review of the literature. *Journal of Counseling & Development, 78*, 275–283.

Council for Accreditation of Counseling and Related Educational Programs. (2015). *2016 CACREP standards.* Alexandria, VA: Author.

Council on Social Work Education Commission on Accreditation. (2015). *Educational policy and accreditation standards.* Retrieved from https://www.cswe.org/getattachment/Accreditation/Accreditation-Process/2015-EPAS/2015EPAS_Web_FINAL.pdf.aspx

Crawford, M., & Gilroy, P. (2012). Professional impairment and gatekeeping: A survey of master's level training programs. *Journal of Counselor Preparation and Supervision, 2*, 28–37.

Crewe, N. M. (1994). Implications of the Americans with Disabilities Act for the training of psychologists. *Rehabilitation Education, 8*, 9–16.

Cruise, T. K., & Swerdlik, M. E. (2010). Problematic behaviors: Mediating differences and negotiating change. In J. Kaufman, T. L. Hughes, & C. A. Riccio (Eds.), *Handbook of education, training, and supervision of school psychologists in school and community: Vol. 2. Bridging the training and practice gap: Building collaborative university/field practices* (pp. 129–152). New York, NY: Routledge.

Cunningham, M. (2003). Impact of trauma work on social work clinicians: Empirical findings. *Social Work, 48*, 451–459.

Cunningham, M. (2004). Teaching social workers about trauma: Reducing the risks of vicarious traumatization in the classroom. *Journal of Social Work Education, 40*(2), 305–317.

Custer, G. (1994). Can universities be liable for incompetent grads? *APA Monitor, 25*(11), pp. 6–7.

D'Augelli, A. R. (1994). Identity development and sexual orientation: Toward a model of lesbian, gay, and bisexual development. In E. J. Trickett, R. J. Watts, & D. Birman (Eds.), *Human diversity: Perspectives on people in context* (pp. 312–333). San Francisco, CA: Jossey-Bass.

Darr, J., Moore, H., & Snyder, C. (2003). Gatekeeping: Preparing quality counselors. *Journal of the Pennsylvania Counseling Association, 5*, 51–55.

Delunas, L. R., & Rouse, S. (2014). Nursing and medical student attitudes about communication and collaboration before and after an interprofessional education experience. *Nursing Education Perspectives, 35*(2), 100–105. doi:10.548Q/11-716.1

Department of Counselor Education, Stetson University. (2016). *Stetson University Department of Counselor Education student handbook.* Retrieved from www.stetson.edu/artsci/counselor/media/SH%20 2015-2016.pdf

Disney, M. J., & Stephens, A. M. (1994). *Legal issues in clinical supervision* (Vol. 10). Alexandria, VA: American Counseling Association.

Donaldson, S. I. (2003). Theory-driven program evaluation in the new millennium. In S. I. Donaldson & M. Scriven (Eds.), *Evaluating social programs and problems: Visions for the new millennium* (pp. 109–141). Mahwah, NJ: Erlbaum.

Dreyfus, H. L., & Dreyfus, S. E. (1986). *Mind over machine: The power of human intuition and expertise in the era of the computer.* New York, NY: Free Press.

Duba, J. D., Paez, S. B., & Kindsvatter, A. (2010). Criteria of nonacademic characteristics used to evaluate and retain community counseling students. *Journal of Counseling & Development, 88*, 154–162.

Dufrene, R. L., & Henderson, K. L. (2009). A framework for remediation plans for counseling trainees. In G. Walz, J. Bleuer, & R. Yep (Eds.), *Compelling counseling images: The best of VISTAS 2009* (pp. 149–159). Alexandria, VA: American Counseling Association.

Dugger, S. M., & Francis, P. C. (2014). Surviving a lawsuit against a counseling program: Lessons learned from *Ward v. Wilbanks*. *Journal of Counseling & Development, 92*, 135–141.

Duys, D. K., & Hedstrom, S. M. (2000). Basic counselor skill training and counselor cognitive complexity. *Counselor Education and Supervision, 40*, 8–18.

Ellis, A. (1972). Psychotherapy without tears. In A. Burton (Ed.), *Twelve therapists* (pp. 103–126). San Francisco, CA: Jossey-Bass.

Elman, N. S., & Forrest, L. (2004). Psychotherapy in the remediation of psychology trainees: Exploratory interviews with training directors. *Professional Psychology: Research and Practice, 35*(2), 123–130.

Elman, N. S., & Forrest, L. (2007). From trainee impairment to professional competence problems: Seeking new terminology that facilitates effective action. *Professional Psychology: Research and Practice, 38*, 501–509.

Elman, N. S., Forrest, L., Vacha-Haase, T., & Gizara, S. (1999). Rejoinder: A systems perspective on trainee impairment: Continuing the dialogue. *The Counseling Psychologist, 27*, 712–721. doi:10.1177/0011000099275005

Enochs, W. K., & Etzbach, C. A. (2004). Impaired student counselors: Ethical and legal considerations for the family. *The Family Journal, 12*, 396–400.

Epstein, R. M., & Hundert, E. M. (2002). Defining and assessing professional competence. *Journal of the American Medical Association, 9*, 226–235.

Epstein, R. M., Siegel, D. J., & Silberman, J. (2008). Self-monitoring in clinical practice: A challenge for medical educators. *Journal of Continuing Education in the Health Professions, 2*, 5–13.

Falender, C. A., Collins, C. J., & Shafranske, E. P. (2009). "Impairment" and performance issues in clinical supervision: After the 2008 ADA Amendments Act. *Training and Education in Professional Psychology, 3*(4), 240–249.

Falender, C. A., Ellis, M. V., & Burnes, T. R. (2013). Response to reactions to major contribution: Multicultural clinical supervision and benchmarks. *The Counseling Psychologist, 41*(1), 140–151.

Family Educational Rights and Privacy; final rule. (2008, December 9). Retrieved from https://www2.ed.gov/legislation/FedRegister/finrule/2008-4/120908a.pdf

Flanders, J. M. (2008). Academic student dismissals at public institutions of higher education: When is academic difference not an issue? *Journal of College and University Law, 34*, 19–73.

Florida Board of Clinical Social Work, Marriage & Family Therapy and Mental Health Counseling. (2016). *Rule: 64B4-5.001*. Retrieved from https://www.flrules.org/gateway/RuleNo.asp?title=DISCIPLINE&ID=64B4-5.001

Fly, B. J., van Bark, W. P., Weinman, L., Kitchener, K. S., & Lang, P. R. (1997). Ethical transgressions of psychology graduate students: Critical incidents with implications for training. *Professional Psychology: Research and Practice, 28*, 492–495. doi:10.1037/0735-7028.28.5.492

Fong, M. L., Borders, L. D., Ethington, C. A., & Pitts, J. H. (1997). Becoming a counselor: A longitudinal study of student cognitive development. *Counselor Education and Supervision, 37*, 100–114.

Forrest, L., Elman, N. S., Gizara, S., & Vacha-Haase, T. (1999). Trainee impairment: A review of identification, remediation, dismissal and legal issues. *The Counseling Psychologist, 27*, 627–686. doi:10.1177/0011000099275001

Forrest, L., Shen-Miller, D. S., & Elman, N. S. (2008). Psychology trainees with competence problems: From individual to ecological conceptualizations. *Training and Education in Professional Psychology, 2*(2), 183–192. doi:10.1037/1931-3918.2.4.183

Foster, J. M., Leppma, M., & Hutchinson, T. S. (2014). Students' perspectives on gatekeeping in counselor education: A case study. *Counselor Education and Supervision, 53*, 190–203.

Foster, V. A., & McAdams, C. R., III. (2009). A framework for creating a climate of transparency for professional performance assessment: Fostering student investment in gatekeeping. *Counselor Education and Supervision, 48*, 271–284.

Fouad, N. A., Grus, C. L., Hatcher, R. L., Kaslow, N. J., Smith Hutchings, P., Madson, M. B., . . . Crossman, R. E. (2009). Competency benchmarks: A model for understanding and measuring competence in professional psychology across training levels. *Training and Education in Professional Psychology, 3*, S5–S26. doi:10.1037/a0015832

Foundation for Individual Rights in Education. (2016). *FIRE's guide to due process and campus justice*. (2016). Retrieved from https://www.thefire.org/fire-guides/fires-guide-to-due-process-and-campus-justice/fires-guide-to-due-process-and-fair-procedure-on-campus-full-text/

Frame, M. W., & Stevens-Smith, P. (1995). Out of harm's way: Enhancing monitoring and dismissal processes in counselor education programs. *Counselor Education and Supervision, 35*, 118–129.

Francis, P. C., & Dugger, S. M. (2014). Professionalism, ethics, and value-based conflicts in counseling. *Journal of Counseling & Development, 92*, 131–134.

Fraser, S. W., & Greenhalgh, T. (2001). Coping with complexity: Educating for capability. *British Medical Journal, 323*, 799–803.

Freeman, B., Coll, K., Juhnke, J., & Martinez, M. (2017, October). *Teaching gatekeeping to doctoral students: A ten step approach*. Session presented at the meeting of the Association for Counselor Education and Supervision, Chicago, IL.

Gaubatz, M. D., & Vera, E. M. (2002). Do formalized gatekeeping procedures increase programs' follow-up with deficient trainees? *Counselor Education and Supervision*, *41*, 294–305.

Gaubatz, M. D., & Vera, E. M. (2006). Trainee competence in master's-level counseling programs: A comparison of counselor educators' and students' views. *Counselor Education and Supervision*, *46*, 32–43.

Gibson, D. M., Dollarhide, C. T., & Moss, J. M. (2010). Professional identity development: A grounded theory of transformational tasks of new counselors. *Counselor Education and Supervision*, *50*, 21–38.

Gilfoyle, N. (2008). The legal exosystem: Risk management in addressing student competence problems in professional psychology training. *Training and Education in Professional Psychology*, *2*(4), 202–209.

Gill, C. J. (1995). A psychological view of disability culture. *Disability Studies Quarterly*, *15*, 15–19.

Gill, C. J. (1997). Four types of integration in disability identity development. *Journal of Vocational Rehabilitation*, *9*, 39–46.

Gill, C. J. (2001). Divided understanding: The social experience of disability. In G. L. Albrecht, K. D. Seelman, & M. Bury (Eds.), *Handbook of disability studies* (pp. 351–372). Thousand Oaks, CA: Sage.

Gillis, H., & Lewis, J. S. (2004). Addressing the issue of psychiatric disability in social work interns: The need for a problem-solving framework. *Journal of Social Work Education*, *40*, 391–402.

Gizara, S. S., & Forrest, L. (2004). Supervisors' experiences of trainee impairment and incompetence at APA-accredited internship sites. *Professional Psychology: Research and Practice*, *35*(2), 131–140. doi:10.1037/0735-7028.35.2.131

Glance, D., Fanning, G., Schoepke, A., Soto, W., & Williams, M. A., Sr. (2012). *Gatekeeping in counselor education*. Retrieved from https://www.counseling.org/resources/library/VISTAS/vistas12/Article_11.pdf

Gonsalvez, C. J., & Freestone, J. (2007). Field supervisors' assessments of trainee performance: Are they reliable and valid? *Australian Psychologist*, *42*(1), 23–32. doi:10.1080/00050060600827615

Goodrich, K. M., & Luke, M. (2012). Problematic student in the experiential group: Professional and ethical challenges for counselor educators. *Journal for Specialists in Group Work*, *37*, 326–346.

Goodrich, K. M., & Shin, R. Q. (2012). A culturally responsive intervention for addressing problematic behaviors in counseling students. *Counselor Education and Supervision*, *52*, 43–55.

Gordon, R. M. (2010). The *Psychodynamic Diagnostic Manual* (PMD). In I. Weiner & E. Craighead (Eds.), *Corsini's encyclopedia of psychology* (4th ed., Vol. 3, pp. 1312–1315). Hoboken, NJ: Wiley.

Granello, D. H. (2002). Assessing the cognitive development of counseling students: Changes in epistemological assumptions. *Counselor Education and Supervision, 41*, 279–293.

Granello, D. H. (2006). Promoting student cognitive development in counselor preparation: A proposed expanded role for faculty advisers. *Counselor Education and Supervision, 46*, 116–130.

Grenyer, K. L., & Lewis, B. F. S. (2012). Prevalence, prediction, and prevention of psychologist misconduct. *Australian Psychologist, 47*, 68–76.

Guest, C. L., Jackson, R., & Dooley, K. (1999). Supervisor malpractice: Liability to the supervisee in clinical supervision. *Counselor Education and Supervision, 38*, 269–279.

Handelsman, M. M., Gottlieb, M. C., & Knapp, S. (2005). Training ethical psychologists: An acculturation model. *Professional Psychology: Research and Practice, 36*, 59–65.

Harris v. Blake and the Board of Trustees of the University of Northern Colorado, 798 F.2d 419 (CO10 1986).

Hatcher, R. L., Fouad, N. A., Grus, C. L., Campbell, L. F., McCutcheon, S. R., & Leahy, K. L. (2013). Competency benchmarks: Practical steps toward a culture of competence. *Training and Education in Professional Psychology*, 7(2), 84–91.

Hatcher, R. L., & Lassiter, K. D. (2007). Initial training in professional psychology: The practicum competencies outline. *Training and Education in Professional Psychology, 1*(1), 49–63.

Hatchett, G. T., Lawrence, C., & Coaston, S. C. (2017). Re-examination of traditional admissions criteria in predicating academic success in a counselor education program. *International Journal for the Advancement of Counselling, 39*, 70–81.

Hauser, P. C., Maxwell-McCaw, D. L., Leigh, I. W., & Gutman, V. A. (2000). Internship accessibility issues for deaf and hard-of-hearing applications: No cause for complacency. *Professional Psychology: Research and Practice, 31*, 569–574.

Haynes, R., Corey, G., & Moulton, P. (2003). *Clinical supervision in the helping professions: A practical guide*. Pacific Grove, CA: Books/Cole.

Henderson, K. L. (2010). *The remediation of students in counseling graduate programs: Behavioral indicators, terminology, and interventions* (Doctoral dissertation). Available from the University of New Orleans Theses and Dissertations database (No. 1135).

Henderson, K. L., & Dufrene, R. L. (2011). *Student remediation: Practical considerations for counselor educators and supervisors*. Retrieved from https://www.counseling.org/knowledge-center/vistas/by-subject2/vistas-education-and-supervision/docs/default-source/vistas/vistas_2011_article_45

Henderson, K. L., & Dufrene, R. L. (2012). Student behaviors associated with remediation: A content analysis. *Counseling Outcome Research and Evaluation, 3*, 48–60. doi:10.1177/2150137812437364

Henderson, K. L., & Dufrene, R. L. (2013). Student behaviors and remediation: An empirical study. *Journal of Professional Counseling: Practice, Theory, and Research*, *40*(2), 2–14.
Henderson, K. L., & Dufrene, R. L. (2015). A contributor's perspective: Boundary issues with supervisee incompetence. In B. Herlihy & G. Corey (Eds.), *Boundary issues in counseling: Multiple roles and responsibilities* (3rd ed., pp. 147–151). Alexandria, VA: American Counseling Association.
Hensley, L. G., Smith, S. L., & Thompson, R. W. (2003). Assessing competencies of counselors-in-training: Complexities in evaluating personal and professional development. *Counselor Education and Supervision*, *42*, 219–229.
Herlihy, B. J., Hermann, M. A., & Greden, L. R. (2014). Legal and ethical implications of using religious beliefs as he basis for refusing to counsel certain clients. *Journal of Counseling & Development*, *92*, 148–153.
Hermann, M. A., & Herlihy, B. R. (2006). Legal and ethical implications of refusing to counsel homosexual clients. *Journal of Counseling & Development*, *84*, 414–418.
Hermann, M., Spurgeon, S., & Watts, R. (2014, October). *The new 2014 ACA Code of Ethics.* Paper presented at the annual conference of the Southern Association for Counselor Education and Supervision, Birmingham, AL.
Holloway, E. L., & Wampold, B. E. (1983). Patterns of verbal behavior and judgments of satisfaction in the supervision interview. *Journal of Counseling Psychology*, *28*, 373–376.
Holloway, E. L., & Wampold, B. E. (1986). Relation between conceptual level and counseling-related tasks: A meta-analysis. *Journal of Counseling Psychology*, *33*, 310–319.
Holloway, E. L., & Wolleat, P. (1980). Relationship of counselor conceptual level to clinical hypothesis information. *Journal of Counseling Psychology*, *27*, 539–545.
Homrich, A. M. (2009). Gatekeeping for personal and professional competence in graduate counseling programs. *Counseling and Human Development*, *41*(7), 1–24.
Homrich, A. M., DeLorenzi, L. D., Bloom, Z. D., & Godbee, B. (2014). Making the case for standards of conduct in clinical training. *Counselor Education and Supervision*, *53*, 126–144.
Huprich, S. K., & Rudd, M. D. (2004). A national survey of trainee impairment in clinical, counseling, and school psychology doctoral programs and internships. *Journal of Clinical Psychology*, *60*, 43–52. doi:10.1002/jclp.10233
Hutchens, N., Block, J., & Young, M. (2013). Counselor educators' gatekeeping responsibilities and students' first amendment rights. *Counselor Education and Supervision*, *52*, 82–95.
Ivey, A. E., Ivey, M. B., & Zalaquett, C. P. (2014). *Intentional interviewing and counseling: Facilitating client development in a multicultural society* (8th ed.). Belmont, CA: Brooks/Cole.

Jackson-Cherry, L. R. (2006). *Protecting our gatekeepers? Hard lessons learned from the dismissal of a graduate counseling student.* Retrieved from https://www.counseling.org/docs/default-source/vistas/protecting-our-gatekeepers-hard-lessons-learned-from-the-dismissal-of-a-graduate-counseling-student.pdf?sfvrsn=14

Jacobs, S. C., Huprich, S. K., Grus, C. L., Cage, E. A., Elman, N. S., Forrest, L., . . . Kaslow, N. J. (2011). Trainees with professional competency problems: Preparing trainers for difficult but necessary conversations. *Training and Education in Professional Psychology, 5*, 175–184.

Jasonson, W. B., Elman, N. S., Forrest, L., Robiner, W. N., Rodolfa, E., & Schaffer, J. B. (2008). Addressing professional competence problems in trainees: Some ethical considerations. *Professional Psychology: Research and Practice, 39*, 589–599.

Jochemsen-van der Leeuw, H. G. A., van Dijk, N., van Etten-Jamaludin, F. S., & Wieringa-de Waard, M. (2013). The attributes of the clinical trainer as a role model: A systematic review. *Academic Medicine, 88*, 26–34.

Johnson, M. E., Brems, C., Warner, T. D., & Roberts, L. W. (2006). The need for continuing education in ethics as reported by rural and urban mental health care providers. *Professional Psychology: Research and Practice, 37*, 183–189.

Johnson, W. B. (2002). The intentional mentor: Strategies and guidelines for the practice of mentoring. *Professional Psychology: Research and Practice, 33*, 88–96.

Johnson, W. B. (2007). Transformational supervision: When supervisors mentor. *Professional Psychology: Research and Practice, 38*, 259–267.

Johnson, W. B., & Campbell, C. D. (2002). Character and fitness requirements for professional psychologists: Are there any? *Professional Psychology: Research and Practice, 33*(1), 46–53.

Johnson, W. B., & Campbell, C. D. (2004). Character and fitness requirements for professional psychologists: Training directors' perspectives. *Professional Psychology: Research and Practice, 35*, 405–411.

Johnson, W. B., Elman, N. S., Forrest, L., Robiner, W. N., Rodolfa, E., & Schaffer, J. B. (2008). Addressing professional competence problems in trainees: Some ethical considerations. *Professional Psychology: Research and Practice, 39*, 589–599. doi:10.1037/a0014264

Johnson, W. B., Porter, K., Campbell, C. D., & Kupko, E. N. (2005). Character and fitness requirements for professional psychologists: An examination of state licensing application forms. *Professional Psychology: Research and Practice, 36*, 654–662.

Kaplan, D. M. (2014). Ethical implications of a critical legal case for the counseling profession: *Ward v. Wilbanks. Journal of Counseling & Development, 92*, 142–146.

Kaplan, D. M., & Gladding, S. T. (2011). A vision for the future of counseling: The 20/20 principles for unifying and strengthening the profession. *Journal of Counseling & Development, 89*, 367–372.

Kaplan, D., & Martz, E. (2014, August). *Preamble scramble.* Retrieved from https://www.counseling.org/docs/default-source/ethics/ethics_august_2014.pdf?sfvrsn=2

Karau, S. J., & Williams, K. D. (1993). Social loafing: A meta-analytic review and theoretical integration. *Journal of Personality and Social Psychology, 65*, 681–706. doi:10.1037/0022-3514.65.4.681

Kaslow, N. J. (2004). Competencies in professional psychology. *American Psychologist, 59*, 774–781. doi:10.1037/0003-066X.59.8.774

Kaslow, N. J., Borden, K. A., Collins, F. L., Jr., Forrest, L., Illfelder-Kaye, J., Nelson, P. D., . . . Willmuth, M. E. (2004). Competencies conference: Future directions in education and credentialing in professional psychology. *Journal of Clinical Psychology, 60*, 699–712.

Kaslow, N. J., Grus, C. L., Campbell, L. F., Fouad, N. A., Hatcher, R. L., & Rodolfa, E. R. (2009). Competency assessment toolkit for professional psychology. *Training and Education in Professional Psychology, 3*(4S), S27–S45.

Kaslow, N. J., Rubin, N. J., Forrest, L., Elman, N. S., Van Horne, B. A., Jacobs, S. C., . . . Thorn, B. E. (2007). Recognizing, assessing and intervening with problems of professional competence. *Professional Psychology: Research and Practice, 38*, 479–492.

Kaslow, N., Rubin, N., Leigh, I., Portnoy, S., Lichtenberg, J., & Smith, L. (2006). *APA Task Force on the Assessment of Competence in Professional Psychology: Final report.* Retrieved from https://www.scribd.com/document/147279537/APA-Task-Force-Competencies

Keeton v. Anderson-Wiley, 733 F. Supp. 2d 1368 (Dist. Ct., S.D. Ga. 2010).

Keeton v. Anderson-Wiley, 664 F.3d 865 (U.S. Ct. App., 11th Cir. 2011).

Kegan, R. (1982). *The evolving self: Problems and process in human development.* Cambridge, MA: Harvard University Press.

Kelly, V. A. (2011). Assessing individual student progress: Meeting multiple accreditation standards and professional gatekeeping responsibilities. *Journal of Counselor Preparation and Supervision, 3*(2), 111–123.

Kerl, S., & Eichler, M. (2005). The loss of innocence: Emotional costs to serving as gatekeepers to the profession. *Journal of Creativity in Mental Health, 1*, 71–88.

Kerl, S. B., Garcia, J. L., McCullough, S., & Maxwell, M. E. (2002). Systematic evaluation of professional performance: Legally supported procedure and process. *Counselor Education and Supervision, 41*, 321–332.

Khan, M. (1974). *The privacy of the self.* New York, NY: International Universities Press.

Kindsvatter, A., Haag Granello, D., & Duba, J. (2008). Cognitive techniques as a means for facilitating supervisee development. *Counselor Education and Supervision, 47*, 179–192.

Klimoski, R., & Palmer, S. (1994). The ADA and the hiring process in organizations. In S. Bruyere & J. O'Keefe (Eds.), *Implications of the Americans with Disabilities Act for psychology* (pp. 37–84). Washington, DC: American Psychological Association.

Knapp, S., Younggren, J. N., VandeCreek, L., Harris, E., & Martin, J. N. (2013). *Assessing and managing risk in psychological practice: An individualized approach* (2nd ed.). Rockville, MD: The Trust.

Knoff, H. M., & Prout, H. T. (1985). Terminating students from professional psychology programs: Criteria, procedures, and legal issues. *Professional Psychology: Research and Practice, 16*, 789–797. doi:10.1037/0735-7028.16.6.789

Kocet, M. M., & Herlihy, B. J. (2014). Addressing value-based conflicts within the counseling relationship: A decision-making model. *Journal of Counseling & Development, 92*, 180–186.

Koerin, B., & Miller, J. (1995). Gatekeeping policies: Terminating students for nonacademic reasons. *Journal of Social Work Education, 31*(2), 247–260.

Koppel Mitnick, M. (2001). Internships and the law. *Association of Psychology Postdoctoral and Internship Centers Newsletter, 26*(2), p. 25.

Kress, V. E., & Protivnak, J. J. (2009). Professional development plans to remedy problematic counseling student behaviors. *Counselor Education and Supervision, 48*, 154–166.

Kutz, S. L. (1986). Defining "impaired psychologist." *American Psychologist, 41*, 220.

L'Abate, L. (2008). *Toward a science of clinical psychology: Laboratory evaluations and interventions.* Hauppauge, NY: Nova Science.

Lafrance, J., Gray, E., & Herbert, M. (2004). Gatekeeping for professional social work practice. *Social Work Education, 23*, 325–340.

Laliotis, D. A., & Grayson, J. H. (1985). Psychologist heal thyself: What is available for the impaired psychologist? *American Psychologist, 40*(1), 84–96.

Lamb, D. H. (1999). Addressing impairment and its relationship to professional boundary issues: A response to Forrest, Elman, Gizara, and Vacha-Haase. *The Counseling Psychologist*, 27, 702–711. doi:10.1177/0011000099275004

Lamb, D. H., Cochran, D. J., & Jackson, V. R. (1991). Training and organizational issues associated with identifying and responding to intern impairment. *Professional Psychology: Research and Practice, 22*(4), 291–296. doi:10.1037/0735-7028.22.4.291

Lamb, D. H., Presser, N. R., Pfost, K. S., Baum, M. C., Jackson, V. R., & Jarvis, P. A. (1987). Confronting professional impairment during the internship: Identification, due process, and remediation. *Professional Psychology: Research and Practice, 18*, 597–603. doi:10.1037/0735-7028.18.6.597

Lamb, D. H., & Swerdlik, M. E. (2003). Identifying and responding to problematic school psychology supervisees: The evaluation process and issues of impairment. *The Clinical Supervisor, 22*(1), 87–110. doi:10.1300/J001v22n01_07

Lambert, M. J., & Barley, D. E. (2001). Research summary on the therapeutic relationship and psychotherapy outcome. *Psychotherapy, 28*(4), 357–361.

Lambie, G. W., Mullen, P. R., Swank, J. M., & Blount, A. (2018). The Counseling Competencies Scale: Validation and refinement. *Measurement and Evaluation in Counseling and Development, 51*, 1–15.

Larson, L. M., Suzuki, L. A., Gillespie, K. N., Potenza, M. T., Bechtel, M. A., & Toulouse, A. L. (1992). Development and validation of the Counseling Self-Estimate Inventory. *Journal of Counseling Psychology, 39*(1), 105–120.

Lawson, G. (2007). Counselor wellness and impairment: A national survey. *Journal of Humanistic Counseling, Education & Development, 46*, 20–34.

Lawson, G., Venart, E., Hazler, R. J., & Kottler, J. A. (2007). Toward a culture of counselor wellness. *Journal of Humanistic Counseling, Education & Development, 46*, 5–19.

Le Maistre, C., Boudreau, S., & Pare, A. (2006). Mentor or evaluator? Assisting and assessing newcomers to the professions. *Journal of Workplace Learning, 18*, 344–354.

Lent, R. L., Hackett, G., & Brown, S. D. (1998). Extending social cognitive theory to counselor education: Problems and prospects. *The Counseling Psychologist, 26*(2), 295–306.

Lenz, A. S., Sangganjanavanich, V. F., Balkin, R. S., Oliver, M., & Smith, R. L. (2012). Wellness model of supervision: A comparative analysis. *Counselor Education and Supervision, 57*, 207–221.

Leverett-Main, S. (2004). Program directors' perceptions of admission screening measures and indicators of student success. *Counselor Education and Supervision, 43*, 207–219.

Levinson, F., & Parritt, S. (2006). Against stereotypes: Experiences of disabled psychologists. In D. Goodley & R. Lawthorn (Eds.), *Disability and psychology: Critical introductions and reflections* (pp. 111–122). Basingstoke, UK: Palgrave-Macmillan.

Lewis & Clark, Psychology Department. (2016). *Professional qualities evaluation.* Unpublished scale adapted from the Professional Counseling Performance Evaluation.

Li, C., Lampe, R., Trusty, J. G., & Lin, Y. (2009). Cluster analysis of impaired counseling students: A survey of master's level CACREP-accredited programs. *Journal of Professional Counseling: Practice, Theory, and Research, 27*(1), 38–50.

Li, C., Trusty, J., Lampe, R., & Lin, Y. (2008). *Remediation and termination of impaired students in CACREP-accredited counseling programs.* Retrieved from http://cnx.org/contents/X0YerrJq@2/Remediation-and-Termination-of

Lichtenberg, J. W., Portnoy, S. M., Bebeau, M. J., Leigh, I. W., Nelson, P. D., Rubin, N. J., . . . Kaslow, N. J. (2007). Challenges to the assessment of competence and competencies. *Professional Psychology: Research and Practice, 38*, 474–478.

Limberg, D., Bell, H., Super, J. T., Jacobson, L., Fox, J., DePue, M. K., . . . Lambie, G. W. (2013). Professional identity development of counselor education doctoral students: A qualitative investigation. *The Professional Counselor, 3*(1), 40–53.

Lockyer, J. (2003). Multisource feedback in the assessment of physician competencies. *Journal of Continuing Education in the Health Professions, 23*(1), 4–12.

Loevinger, J. (1998). *Technical foundations for measuring ego development: The Washington University Sentence Completion Test.* Mahwah, NJ: Erlbaum.

Lovell, C. W. (1999). Empathetic-cognitive development in students of counseling. *Journal of Adult Development, 6*, 195–203.

Lumadue, C. A., & Duffey, T. H. (1999). The role of graduate programs as gatekeepers: A model for evaluating student counselor competence. *Counselor Education and Supervision, 39*, 101–109.

Lund, E. M., Andrews, E. E., & Holt, J. M. (2014). How we treat our own: The experiences and characteristics of psychology trainees with disabilities. *Rehabilitation Psychology, 59*(4), 367–375.

Lyons, C., & Hazier, R. (2002). The influence of student development level on improving counselor student empathy. *Counselor Education and Supervision, 42*, 119–130.

Lysaght, R. M., & Altschuld, J. W. (2000). Beyond initial certification: The assessment and maintenance of competency of professionals. *Evaluation and Program Planning, 23*, 95–104.

Main, M., Kaplan, N., & Cassidy, J. (1985). Security in infancy, childhood and adulthood: A move to the level of representation. *Monographs for the Society for Research in Child Development, 50*, 66–106.

Mann, K., Gordon, J., & MacLeod, A. (2009). Reflection and reflective practice in health professions education: A systematic review. *Advances in Health Sciences Education: Theory and Practice, 14*, 595–621.

Marsh, S. R. (1988). Antecedents to choice of a helping career: Social work vs. business majors. *Smith College Studies in Social Work, 58*, 85–100.

Martin, D. J., Garske, J. P., & Davis, M. K. (2000). Relation of the therapeutic alliance with outcome and other variables: A meta-analytic review. *Journal of Consulting and Clinical Psychology, 68*, 438–450.

Martin, J., Slemon, A. G., Hiebert, B., Hallberg, E. T., & Cummings, A. L. (1989). Conceptualization of novice and experienced counselors. *Journal of Counseling Psychology, 36*, 359–400.

Martz, E., & Kaplan, D. (2014, October). *New responsibilities when making referrals.* Retrieved from https://www.counseling.org/docs/default-source/ethics/ethics_ocober-2014.pdf?sfvrsn=2

McAdams, C. R., III., & Foster, V. A. (2007). A guide to just and fair remediation of counseling students with professional performance deficiencies. *Counselor Education and Supervision, 47*, 2–13.

McAdams, C. R., III, Foster, V. A., & Ward, T. J. (2007). Remediation and dismissal policies in counselor education: Lessons learned from a challenge in federal court. *Counselor Education and Supervision, 46*, 212–229.

McCarn, S. R., & Fassinger, R. (1996). Revisioning sexual minority identity formation: A new model of lesbian identity and its implications for counseling and research. *The Counseling Psychologist, 24*, 508–534.

McCarthy, J. (2008). Helping counselor trainees overcome barriers to seeking help. *Journal of Humanistic of Counseling and Development, 47*, 71–81.

McCaughan, A. M., & Hill, N. R. (2015). The gatekeeping imperative in counselor education admission protocols: The criticality of personal qualities. *International Journal for the Advancement of Counselling, 37*, 28–40.

McKnight, D. (2004). An inquiry of NCATE's move into virtue ethics by way of dispositions (Is this what Aristotle meant?). *Educational Studies, 35*, 214–230.

Mearns, J., & Allen, G. J. (1991). Graduate students' experiences in dealing with impaired peers, compared with faculty predictions: An exploratory study. *Ethics & Behavior, 1*(3), 191–202.

Meyers, F. J., Hales, R. E., Young, H. M., Nesbitt, T. S., & Pomeroy, C. (2013). Restructuring academic health centers to advance interdisciplinary collaborations: Opportunities for psychiatry departments. *Academic Psychiatry, 37*(2), 72–75. doi:10.1176/appi.ap.11120209

Miller, C. M. (2010). *Endorsement for licensure: Practices and challenges reported by counselor supervisors* (Doctoral dissertation). Retrieved from http://libra.virginia.edu/catalog/libra-oa:5256

Miller, J., & Koerin, B. B. (2002). Gatekeeping in the practicum. *The Clinical Supervisor, 20*(2), 1–18. doi:10.1300/J001v20n02_01

Miller, R. K., & Van Rybroek, G. J. (1988). Internship letters of recommendation: Where are the other 90%? *Professional Psychology: Research and Practice, 19*, 115–117.

Mintrom, M. (2014). Creating cultures of excellence: Strategies and outcomes. *Cogent Education, 1*, 1–13.

Mintz, L. B., & Bieschke, K. J. (2009). Counseling psychology model training values statement addressing diversity. *The Counseling Psychologist, 37*, 634–640.

Mintz, L. B., Jackson, A. P., Neville, H. A., Illfelder-Kaye, J., Winterowd, C. L., & Loewy, M. I. (2009). The need for a counseling psychology model training values statement addressing diversity. *The Counseling Psychologist, 37*, 644–675.

Morrissette, P. J. (1999). Family therapist self-supervision. *The Clinical Supervisor, 18*, 165–184.

Myers, J. E., & Sweeney, T. J. (2008). Wellness counseling: The evidence base for practice. *Journal of Counseling & Development, 86*, 482–493.

Myers, S. B., Endres, M. A., Ruddy, M. E., & Zelikovsky, N. (2012). Psychology graduate training in the era of online social networking. *Training and Education in Professional Psychology*, *6*, 28–36.

National Association of School Psychologists. (2010). *Professional ethics*. Retrieved from https://www.nasponline.org/standards-and-certification/professional-ethics

National Association of Social Workers. (2015). *National Committee on Lesbian, Gay, Bisexual, and Transgender Issues position statement: Sexual orientation change efforts (SOCE) and conversion therapy with lesbians, gay men, bisexuals, and transgender persons*. Retrieved from https://www.socialworkers.org/LinkClick.aspx?fileticket=yH3UsGQQmYI%3d&portalid=0

National Association of Social Workers. (2017). *Code of ethics of the National Association of Social Workers*. Retrieved from https://www.socialworkers.org/LinkClick.aspx?fileticket=ms_ArtLqzeI%3d&portalid=0

National Association of Social Workers & Association of Social Work Boards. (2013). *Best practice standards in social work supervision*. Retrieved from www.socialworkers.org/LinkClick.aspx?fileticket=GBrLbl4BuwI%3D&portalid=0

National Board for Certified Counselors. (2016). *National Board for Certified Counselors (NBCC) code of ethics*. Retrieved from www.nbcc.org/Assets/Ethics/NBCCCodeofEthics.pdf

Nelson, K. W., Oliver, M., Reeve, J., & McNichols, C. (2010). *Gatekeeping and supervisory intervention: Complex ethical processes*. Retrieved from https://www.counseling.org/Resources/Library/VISTAS/2010-V-Online/Article_42.pdf

Nelson, P. D. (2007). Striving for competence in the assessment of competence: Psychology's professional education and credentialing journey of public accountability. *Training and Education in Professional Psychology*, *1*(1), 3–12.

Nelson, T. S., & Johnson, L. N. (1999). The basic skills evaluation device. *Journal of Marital and Family Therapy*, *25*(1), 15–30.

Neukrug, E. S., Lovell, C., & Parker, R. J. (1996). Employing ethical codes and decision-making models: A developmental process. *Counseling and Values*, *40*, 98–106.

Norcross, J. C., Strausser-Kirtland, D. J., & Faltus, F. J. (1988). The therapist's therapist. *American Journal of Psychotherapy*, *42*, 53–66.

Nugent, F. A., & Jones, K. D. (2009). *Introduction to the profession of counseling* (5th ed.). Boston, MA: Pearson.

Okech, J. E. A., & Geroski, A. M. (2015). Interdisciplinary training: Preparing counselors for collaborative practice. *The Professional Counselor*, *5*, 458–472. doi:10.15241/jeo.5.4.458

Oliver, M. N., Bernstein, J. H., Anderson, K. G., Blashfield, R. K., & Roberts, M. C. (2004). An exploratory examination of student attitudes toward "impaired" peers in clinical psychology training programs. *Professional Psychology: Research and Practice*, *35*(2), 141–147.

Olkin, R., & Gaughen, S. (1991). Evaluation and dismissal of students in master's level clinical programs: Legal parameters and survey results. *Counselor Education and Supervision, 30*, 276–288.

Osborn, C. J., & Davis, T. E. (1996). The supervision contract: Making it perfectly clear. *The Clinical Supervisor, 14*(2), 121–134.

Osborn, C. J., Paez, S. B., & Carrabine, C. L. (2007). Reflections on shared practices in a supervisory lineage. *The Clinical Supervisor, 26*(1/2), 119–139.

Pai, H.-C. (2015). The effect of a self-reflection and insight program on the nursing competence of nursing students: A longitudinal study. *Journal of Professional Nursing, 31*, 424–431.

Paice, E., Heard, S., & Moss, F. (2002). How important are role models in making good doctors? *British Medical Journal, 325*, 707–710.

Papadakis, M. A., Hodgson, C. S., Teherani, A., & Kohatsu, N. D. (2004). Unprofessional behavior in medical school is associated with subsequent disciplinary action by a state medical board. *Academic Medicine, 79*(3), 244–249.

Parker, L. K., Change, C. Y., Corthell, K. K., Walsh, M. E., Brack, G., & Grubbs, N. K. (2014). A grounded theory of counseling students who report problematic peers. *Counselor Education and Supervision, 53*, 111–125.

Pearlman, L. A., & Saakvitne, K. W. (1996). *Transforming the pain: A workbook on vicarious traumatization.* New York, NY: W. W. Norton.

Perosa, L. M. (2010). Assessing competencies in couples and family therapy/counseling: A call to the profession. *Journal of Marital and Family Therapy, 36*, 126–143.

Perry, W. G., Jr. (1970). *Forms of intellectual and ethical development in the college years.* New York, NY: Holt, Rinehart & Winston.

Pham, A. V. (2014). Navigating social networking and social media in school psychology: Ethical and professional considerations in training programs. *Psychology in the Schools, 51*, 767–778.

Phelps v. Washburn University of Topeka, 634 F. Supp. 556 (U.S.D. Ct., D. 1986).

Plaintiff v. Rector and Board of Visitors of The College of William and Mary, No. 03-2119 (4th Cir. February 8, 2005).

Pollock, C. S., & Poteet, C. W. (1983). Diminishing faculty liability. *Nurse Educator, 8*(1), 31–34.

Polychronis, P. D., & Brown, S. G. (2016). The strict liability standard and clinical supervision. *Professional Psychology: Research and Practice, 47*(2), 139–146.

Pope, K. S. (2005). Disability and accessibility in psychology: Three major barriers. *Ethics & Behavior, 15*, 103–106.

Pope, K. S., & Vasquez, M. J. T. (2016). *Ethics in psychotherapy and counseling: A practical guide* (5th ed.). New York, NY: Wiley.

Procidano, M. E., Busch-Rossnagel, N. A., Reznikoff, M., & Geisinger, K. F. (1995). Responding to graduate students' professional deficiencies: A national survey. *Journal of Clinical Psychology, 51*, 426–433.

Rapp, M., Moody, S., & Stewart, L. (2017, October). *Developing a gatekeeper identity in counselor education: Preparing doctoral students.* Session presented at the meeting of the Association for Counselor Education and Supervision, Chicago, IL.

Reber, A. S., Allen, R., & Reber, E. S. (2009). *The Penguin dictionary of psychology.* New York, NY: Penguin Books.

Regehr, C., Stalker, C. A., Jacobs, M., & Pelech, W. (2001). The gatekeeper and the wounded healer. *The Clinical Supervisor, 20*(1), 127–143.

Regulations to implement the Equal Employment Provisions of the Americans With Disabilities Act, as amended; final rule. (2011, March 25). Retrieved from https://www.gpo.gov/fdsys/pkg/FR-2011-03-25/pdf/2011-6056.pdf

Remley, T. P., & Herlihy, B. (2014). *Ethical, legal, and professional issues in counseling* (4th ed.). Upper Saddle River, NJ: Pearson Education.

Roberts, M. C., Borden, K. A., Christiansen, M. D., & Lopez, S. J. (2005). Fostering a culture shift: Assessment of competence in the education and careers of professional psychologists. *Professional Psychology: Research and Practice, 36*(4), 355–361.

Rollins College. (2017a). *Clinical Mental Health Counseling application instructions.* Retrieved from www.rollins.edu/evening/how-to-apply/master-of-arts-in-counseling-application-instructions.html

Rollins College. (2017b). *Graduate counseling program.* Retrieved from www.rollins.edu/counseling/current-students/index.html

Rompf, E. L., & Royce, D. (1994). Choice of social work as a career: Possible influences. *Journal of Social Work Education, 30*, 163–171.

Rosenberg, J. I., Getzelman, M. A., Arcinue, F., & Orin, C. Z. (2005). An exploratory look at students' experiences of problematic peers in academic professional psychology programs. *Professional Psychology: Research and Practice, 36*, 665–673.

Rudes, J., Shilts, L., & Berg, I. K. (1997). Focused supervision seen through a recursive frame analysis. *Journal of Marital and Family Therapy, 23*(2), 203–215.

Russell, C. S., & Peterson, C. M. (2003). Student impairment and remediation in accredited marriage and family therapy programs. *Journal of Marital & Family Therapy, 29*(3), 329–337. doi:10.1111/j.1752-0606.2003.tb01210.x

Russel, R., Gill, P., Coyne, A., & Woody, J. (1993). Dysfunction in the family of origin of MSW and other graduate students. *Journal of Social Work Education, 29*, 121–129.

Rust, J. P., Raskin, J. D., & Hill, M. S. (2013). Problems of professional competence among counselor trainees: Programmatic issues and guidelines. *Counselor Education and Supervision, 52*, 30–42. doi:10.1002/j.1556-6978.2013.00026

Saccuzzo, D. P. (1997). Liability for failure to supervise adequately mental health assistants, unlicensed practitioners and students. *California Wester Law Review, 34*(1), 115–152.

Sargeant, J. (2008). Toward a common understanding of self-assessment. *Journal of Continuing Education in the Health Professions, 28*, 1–4.

Savin-Williams, R. C. (1988). Theoretical perspectives accounting for adolescent homosexuality. *Journal of Adolescent Health, 9*(6), 95–104.

Schneider, K., & Rees, C. (2012). Evaluation of a combined cognitive behavioural therapy and interpersonal process group in the psychotherapy training of clinical psychologists. *Australian Psychologist, 47*, 137–146.

Schoener, G. R. (1999). Practicing what we preach. *Counseling Psychologist, 27*, 693–701. doi:10.1177/0011000099275003

Sehgal, R., Saules, K., Young, A., Grey, M. J., Gillem, A. R., Nabors, N. A., & Jefferson, S. (2011). Practicing what we know: Multicultural counseling competence among clinical psychology trainees and experienced multicultural psychologists. *Cultural Diversity and Ethnic Minority Psychology, 17*(1), 1–10.

Sekach, M. F., Perelygina, E. B., & Zotova, O. Y. (2013). Intensity of psychological health and personality psychological resistance. *Procedia—Social and Behavioral Sciences, 86*, 88–92.

Shen-Miller, D. S., Forrest, L., & Elman, N. S. (2009). Training directors' conceptualizations of the intersections of diversity and trainee competence problems: A preliminary analysis. *The Counseling Psychologist, 37*, 482–518.

Shen-Miller, D. S., Grus, C. L., Van Sickle, K., Schwartz-Mette, R., Cage, E. A., Elman, N. S., . . . Kaslow, N. J. (2011). Trainees' experiences with peers having competence problems: A national survey. *Training and Education in Professional Psychology, 5*(2), 112–121. doi:10.1037/a0023824

Shirk, S. R., & Karver, M. (2003). Prediction of treatment outcomes from relationship variables in child and adolescent therapy: A meta-analytic review. *Journal of Consulting and Clinical Psychology, 71*, 452–464.

Skovholt, T. M., & Ronnestad, M. H. (1992). Themes in therapist and counselor development. *Journal of Counseling & Development, 70*, 505–515.

Sowbel, L. R. (2012). Gatekeeping: Why shouldn't we be ambivalent? *Journal of Social Work Education, 48*, 27–44.

Springer, A. D. (2009, May). *The impact of FERPA/HIPAA regulations on addressing trainees with problems of professional competence: HIPAA and FERPA: Privacy alphabet soup.* Paper presented to the Accreditation Assembly APA Commission on Accreditation, San Diego, CA.

Spruill, J., Rozensky, R. H., Stigall, T. T., Vasquez, M., & Bingham, R. P. (2004). Becoming a competent clinician: Basic competencies in intervention. *Journal of Clinical Psychology, 60*, 741–754.

Stakeholder. (2014). *The glossary of education reform.* Retrieved from http://edglossary.org/stakeholder/

Stoltenberg, C. D. (2005). Enhancing professional competence through developmental approaches to supervision. *American Psychologist, 60*, 857–864.

Stoltenberg, C. D., & Delworth, U. (1987). *Supervising counselors and therapists: A developmental approach.* San Francisco, CA: Jossey-Bass.

Stoltenberg, C. D., & McNeill, B. W. (2010). *IDM supervision: An integrative developmental model for supervising counselors and therapists* (3rd ed.). New York, NY: Routledge.

Stoppard, J. M., & Miller, A. (1985). Conceptual level matching in therapy: A review. *Current Psychological Research and Reviews, 4*, 47–68.

Swank, J. M., Lambie, G. W., & Witta, E. L. (2012). An exploratory investigation of the Counseling Competencies Scale: A measure of counseling skills, dispositions, and behaviors. *Counselor Education and Supervision, 51*, 189–206.

Swank, J. M., & Smith-Adcock, S. (2014). Gatekeeping during admissions: A survey of counselor education programs. *Counselor Education and Supervision, 53*, 47–61.

Tabachnick, B. G., Keith-Spiegel, P., & Pope, K. S. (1991). Ethics of teaching. *American Psychologist, 46*, 506–515.

Tanenbaum, R. L., & Berman, M. A. (1990). Ethical and legal issues in psychotherapy supervision. *Psychotherapy in Private Practice, 8*(1), 65–77.

The Constitution: Amendments 11-27. (1886). Retrieved from https://www.archives.gov/founding-docs/amendments-11-27

Thomas, F. N. (1996). Solution-focused supervision: The coaxing of expertise. In S. D. Miller, M. A. Hubble, & B. L. Duncan (Eds.), *Handbook of solution-focused brief therapy* (pp. 128–151). San Francisco, CA: Jossey-Bass.

Thomas, J. T. (2007). Informed consent through contracting for supervision: Minimizing risks, enhancing benefits. *Professional Psychology: Research and Practice, 38*(3), 221–231.

Thomas, J. T. (2010). *The ethics of supervision and consultation: Practical guidance for mental health professionals.* Washington, DC: American Psychological Association.

Tjeltveit, A. C., & Gottlieb, M. C. (2010). Avoiding the road to ethical disaster: Overcoming vulnerabilities and developing resilience. *Psychotherapy: Theory, Research, Practice, Training, 47*, 98–110.

Torres-Rivera, E., Wilbur, M. P., Maddux, C. D., & Smaby, M. H. (2002). Factor structure and construct validity of the Counselor Skills Personal Development Rating Form. *Counselor Education and Supervision, 41*, 268–278.

Tracey, T. J., Ellickson, J. L., & Sherry, P. (1989). Reactance in relation to different supervisory environments and counselor development. *Journal of Counseling Psychology, 36*, 336–344.

Trimble, L. D., Stroebel, S. S., Krieg, F. J., & Rubenstein, R. L. (2012). Problematic students of NASP-approved programs: An exploratory study of graduate student views. *Psychology in the Schools, 49*, 589–605.

Troiden, R. R. (1979). Becoming homosexual: A model of gay identity acquisition. *Psychiatry, 42*, 362–373.

Troiden, R. R. (1988). Homosexual identity development. *Journal of Adolescent Health Care*, *9*, 105–113.

Turnbull, J., Gray, J., & MacFadyen, J. (1998). Improving in-training evaluation programs. *Journal of General Internal Medicine*, *13*(5), 317–323.

Tweed, A., Graber, R., & Wang, M. (2010). Assessing trainee clinical psychologists' clinical competence. *Psychology Learning & Teaching*, *9*, 50–60.

Urwin, C. A., Van Soest, D., & Kretzschmar, J. A. (2006). Key principles for developing gatekeeping standards for working with students with problems. *Journal of Teaching in Social Work*, *26*(1/2), 163–180.

U.S. Department of Education. (2015). *Family educational rights and privacy act (FERPA)*. Retrieved from https://www2.ed.gov/policy/gen/guid/fpco/ferpa/index.html?src=rn

U.S. Department of Health and Human Services. (2013). *Summary of the HIPAA privacy rule*. Retrieved from https://www.hhs.gov/hipaa/for-professionals/privacy/laws-regulations/index.html

Vacha-Haase, T., Davenport, D. S., & Kerewsky, S. D. (2004). Problematic students: Gatekeeping practices of academic professional psychology programs. *Professional Psychology: Research and Practice*, *35*(2), 115–122. doi:10.1037/0735-7028.35.2.115

van der Kolk, B., Hostetler, A., Herron, N., & Fisler, R. (1994). Trauma and the development of borderline personality disorder. *Psychiatric Clinics of North America*, *17*, 715–730.

Vande Kemp, H., Chen, J. S., Erickson, G. N., & Friesen, N. L. (2003). ADA accommodation of therapists with disabilities in clinical training. *Women & Therapy*, *26*, 155–168.

Vasquez, M. J. T. (1999). Trainee impairment: A response from a feminist/multicultural retired trainer. *Counseling Psychologist*, *27*, 687–692. doi:10.1177/0011000099275002

Vincent, J. (1996). Why ever do we do it? Unconscious motivation in choosing social work as a career. *Journal of Social Work Practice*, *10*, 63–69.

Ward v. Polite, 667 F.3d 727 (6th Cir. 2012).

Ward v. Wilbanks, Case No. 09-CV-11237 (E.D. Mich. July 26, 2010).

Wayne, R. H. (2004). Legal guidelines for dismissing students because of poor performance in the field. *Journal of Social Work Education*, *40*, 403–414.

Welch, B. (2003). Supervising with liability in mind. *Insight: Safeguarding Psychologists Against Liability Risks*, *1*, 1–6.

Welfel, E. R. (2006). *Ethics in counseling and psychotherapy: Standards, research, and emerging issues* (3rd ed.). Belmont, CA: Brooks/Cole.

West, J. D., Bubenzer, D. L., Osborn, C. J., Paez, S. B., & Desmond, K. J. (2006). Leadership and the profession of counseling: Beliefs and practices. *Counselor Education and Supervision*, *46*, 2–16. doi:10.1002/j.1556-6978.2006.tb00008.x

Wester, S. R., Christianson, H. F., Fouad, N. A., & Santiago-Rivera, A. L. (2008). Information processing as problem solving: A collaborative approach to dealing with students exhibiting insufficient competence. *Training and Education in Professional Psychology*, *2*(4), 193–201. doi:10.1037/1931-3918.2.4.193

Wester, S. R., Danforth, L., & Olle, C. (2013). Social networking site and the evaluation of applicants and students in applied training programs in psychology. *Training and Education in Professional Psychology*, 7(3), 145–154.

Wheeler, A. M., & Bertram, B. (2015). *The counselor and the law: A guide to legal and ethical practice* (7th ed.). Alexandria, VA: American Counseling Association.

Whitman, J. S., Glosoff, H. L., Kocet, M. M., & Tarvydas, V. (2013, January 16). *The latest news from ACA: Ethical issues related to conversion or reparative therapy*. Retrieved from https://www.counseling.org/news/updates/2013/01/16/ethical-issues-related-to-conversion-or-reparative-therapy

Wilkerson, K. (2006). Impaired students: Applying the therapeutic process model to graduate training programs. *Counselor Education and Supervision*, *45*, 207–217.

Witmer, J. M., & Young, M. E. (1996). Preventing counselor impairment: A wellness approach. *Journal of Humanistic Education and Development*, *34*, 141–155.

Wolf, C. P., Thompson, I. A., Thompson, E. S., & Smith-Adcock, S. (2014). Refresh your mind, rejuvenate your body, renew your spirit: A pilot wellness program for counselor education. *Journal of Individual Psychology*, *70*, 57–75.

Yager, G. G., & Tovar-Blank, Z. G. (2007). Wellness and counselor education. *Journal of Humanistic Counseling, Education & Development*, *46*, 142–153.

Yalom, I. D., & Leszcz, M. (2005). *Theory and practice of group psychotherapy*. New York, NY: Basic Books.

Young, M. (2017). *Learning the art of helping: Building blocks and techniques* (6th ed.). Boston, MA: Pearson.

Young, M. E., & Lambie, G. W. (2007). Wellness in school and mental health systems: Organizational influences. *Journal of Humanistic Counseling, Education and Development*, *46*, 98–113.

Ziomek-Daigle, J., & Christensen, T. M. (2010). An emergent theory of gatekeeping practices in counselor education. *Journal of Counseling & Development*, *88*, 407–415.

Index

Figures and tables are indicated by "f" and "t" following page numbers.

A

B

(continued)

D

(continued)

F

G

H

I

(continued)

R

(continued)

T

U

V

W